Research Methods in Health Promotion

Crosby

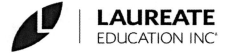

LAUREATE
EDUCATION INC°

Wiley Custom Learning Solutions

To order books or for customer service, please call
1(800)-CALL-WILEY (225-5945).

Printed in the United States of America.

ISBN 978-1-118-68877-9
Printed and bound by EPAC.

10 9 8 7 6 5 4 3

RESEARCH METHODS IN HEALTH PROMOTION

RESEARCH METHODS IN HEALTH PROMOTION

Richard A. Crosby
Ralph J. DiClemente
Laura F. Salazar

Editors

Foreword by Lawrence W. Green

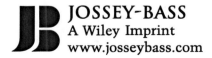

JOSSEY-BASS
A Wiley Imprint
www.josseybass.com

Published by Jossey-Bass
A Wiley Imprint
989 Market Street, San Francisco, CA 94103-1741   www.josseybass.com

Jossey-Bass books and products are available through most bookstores. To contact Jossey-Bass
directly, call our Customer Care Department within the U.S. at 800-956-7739 or outside the U.S.
at 317-572-3986, or fax to 317-572-4002.

Jossey-Bass also publishes its books in a variety of electronic formats. Some content that appears in print
may not be available in electronic books.

This publication is designed to provide accurate and authoritative information in regard to the subject
matter covered. It is sold with the understanding that the publisher is not engaged in rendering
professional services. If professional advice or other expert assistance is required, the services of a
competent professional person should be sought.

Library of Congress Cataloging-in-Publication Data

Research methods in health promotion / Richard A. Crosby, Ralph J.
    DiClemente, Laura Francisca Salazar, editors.
       p. ; cm.
    Includes bibliographical references and index.
    ISBN-13: 978-0-7879-7679-8 (alk. paper)
    ISBN-10: 0-7879-7679-2 (alk. paper)
    1. Health promotion—Research—Methodology. I. Crosby, Richard
A., 1959-   . II. DiClemente, Ralph J. III. Salazar, Laura Francisca,
1960-   .
    [DNLM: 1. Health Promotion. 2. Research—methods.   WA 590
R432 2006]
    RA427.8.R46 2006
    613'.072—dc22

                                                                    2005016228

Printed in the United States of America
FIRST EDITION
HB Printing   10 9 8 7 6 5 4 3 2 1

CONTENTS

PART ONE: FOUNDATIONS OF HEALTH PROMOTION RESEARCH   1

PART FOUR: CORE SKILLS RELATED TO HEALTH PROMOTION RESEARCH 369

FIGURES, TABLES, AND BOXES

Figures

Tables

Boxes

FOREWORD

Much that has been written on research methods misses the mark for students of the health professions because academic authors tend to emphasize research methods that will meet scientific needs rather than practitioner needs. They often start with theory or research questions from more basic disciplines and ask what opportunities or challenges clinical, school, or community health situations offer to test those theories. It seems too often that preprofessional students are being trained to turn their practices into community laboratories to serve the cause of science and theory testing, rather than using science and theory to solve their problems in practice. The editors of this volume have challenged their contributing authors (and themselves, with the many chapters they have written) to show how their research methods can answer the questions that practitioners are asking. They acknowledge the growing demand for evidence-based practice and theory-based practice, but they demonstrate that these will come most effectively when we have more practice-based evidence and practice-based theory.

Rather than starting with theories and asking what practice situations can offer to test them, practice-based research starts with problems in practice and asks what research and theory can offer to solve them. It is that twist that sets this book apart from the usual emphasis of textbooks often used in professional preparation programs.

Each chapter offers applied examples from health promotion that illustrate the key concepts or research methods presented in that chapter. The chapters present a series of pros and cons for the methods presented, and case studies that challenge readers to apply what they have learned. Another added value of this book as distinct from the numerous textbooks available on research methods for each of the cognate disciplines (for example, epidemiology, psychology, sociology, anthropology, political science, economics) underpinning health promotion practice, is that this book seeks the multidisciplinary blending of methods necessary to understand, predict, and address the several ecological levels at which causation happens and change must occur. Any of the excellent research methods books from other disciplines would deal only with a relatively narrow slice of the multilayered reality that health promotion must address. Research methods in health promotion must blend methods from psychology and sociology, for example, to encompass the ecological reality of reciprocal determinism between individual behavior and environment.

While integrating these several complexities of multiple methods and multiple levels of analysis, the editors have strived to give cohesiveness to varied research methods by maintaining a consistent theme that "research involves a predetermined series of well-defined steps." They revisit these steps throughout in a common sequential format. They seek to present a cohesive understanding of the role of science in public health and, more specifically, in health promotion. At the same time that they are ecumenical in their admission of the methods from various disciplines, they are critical in evaluating their use and their limitations in health promotion research, and the ethical issues surrounding some methods of experimental design, sampling, and randomization in the health promotion context.

The editors have drawn on their considerable academic experience in teaching students of health promotion, and their field experience in practice-based research in HIV/AIDS, school health, reducing health disparities, and numerous other areas of public health, to represent research methods specifically for students in health promotion.

November 2005   Lawrence W. Green
Adjunct Professor, Department of Epidemiology and Biostatistics
School of Medicine and Comprehensive Cancer Center
University of California at San Francisco

ACKNOWLEDGMENTS

We would not have been able to produce this volume without our contributors. Each contributor spent a great deal of time, effort, and careful thought in organizing and clearly presenting his or her subject.

Furthermore, we extend our thanks to Becky Flannagan for her superb editorial acumen as well as her stellar figures and tables; to Justin Wagner for his original artwork and conceptualization of Dincus and Mincus; and to Dr. Roger Bakeman, for his helpful review and insightful comments on the statistics chapters.

Also, we wish to acknowledge our Jossey-Bass editor, Andy Pasternack, who has been instrumental in producing this volume. He has been diligent in guiding its preparation, thoughtful in conceptualization of the format, understanding of our needs, and helpful in ways uncountable. He has become a dear friend and a valued resource. The editorial team at Jossey-Bass has been tremendous. Seth Schwartz, Catherine Craddock, Susan Geraghty, and David Horne have made the process enjoyable and have contributed greatly.

Finally, we wish to acknowledge all scholars who aspire to make the world a safer and healthier place to live and those students who will shape and guide the future of health promotion research and practice.

Thanks to my family for their continued inspiration, and especially
to my wife for her love, support, and perseverance in my years
of growth as a scholar.
—R.A.C.

To my lovely wife, Gina, and beautiful daughter, Sahara Rae,
for their love, support, patience, and encouragement.
They are always in my thoughts.
—R.J.D

I would like to thank my wonderful husband, Chuck,
whose support and love sustained me through the process,
and my amazing children, who inspire me every single day.
—L.F.S.

THE EDITORS

Richard A. Crosby is an associate professor in the Department of Health Behavior in the College of Public Health at the University of Kentucky. Crosby received his B.A. degree (1981) in school health education from the University of Kentucky and his M.A. degree (1984) in health education from Central Michigan University. His Ph.D. degree (1998) is in health behavior and is from Indiana University.

Crosby was formerly an assistant professor at the Rollins School of Public Health, and previous to that appointment he was a Fellow of the Association of Teachers of Preventive Medicine. He currently teaches graduate courses in public health and research methods. Crosby's research interests include development and application of behavioral theory to health promotion, particularly in adolescent and young adult populations. He is primarily involved in health promotion practice and research that contributes to reducing the incidence of sexually transmitted diseases, especially infection with the human immunodeficiency virus. Also affiliated with the Rural Center for AIDS and STD Prevention, Crosby has published numerous journal articles that report empirical findings relevant to the sexual risk behaviors of adolescents and adults.

Ralph J. DiClemente is Charles Howard Candler Professor of Public Health and associate director, Emory Center for AIDS Research. He holds concurrent appointments as professor in the School of Medicine, the Department of Pediatrics, in the Division of Infectious Diseases, Epidemiology, and Immunology;

the Department of Medicine, in the Division of Infectious Diseases; and the Department of Psychiatry. He was recently chair, the Department of Behavioral Sciences and Health Education at the Rollins School of Public Health, Emory University. DiClemente was trained as a health psychologist at the University of California, San Francisco, where he received his Ph.D. degree (1984) after completing an S.M. degree (1978) in behavioral sciences at the Harvard School of Public Health and his B.A. degree (1973) at the City University of New York.

DiClemente's research interests include developing decision-making models of adolescents' risk and protective behaviors. He has a particular interest in the development and evaluation of theory-driven HIV/STD-prevention programs for adolescents and young adult women. He has published numerous books and journal articles in the fields of adolescent health and HIV/STD prevention. He currently teaches a course on adolescent health and serves on numerous editorial boards and national prevention organizations.

Laura F. Salazar is currently an assistant research professor in behavioral sciences and health education at the Rollins School of Public Health at Emory University. Salazar completed her B.S. degree (1982) in business management from the State University of New York at Buffalo. After a brief career in business, and raising a family, she pursued an M.A. degree (1996) and a Ph.D. degree (2001) in community psychology at Georgia State University in Atlanta, Georgia.

Salazar's research interests focus on examining the societal, community, and institutional influences of certain health risk behaviors, such as sexual risk behavior and violence against women. She also holds a keen interest in examining the intersection of these two health risks and how they should be addressed simultaneously through the development of innovative programs. She currently teaches graduate courses in theory and applied research methods. She has published many scientific articles in peer-reviewed journals related to these health issues, and is also the author of numerous book chapters.

THE CONTRIBUTORS

Katherine A. Atwood, Sc.D., is an assistant professor in the Department of Health Behavior of the College of Public Health at the University of Kentucky in Lexington, Kentucky.

Richard R. Clayton, Ph.D., is the chairperson and a professor in the Department of Health Behavior of the College of Public Health at the University of Kentucky in Lexington, Kentucky.

Pamela K. Cupp, Ph.D., is project director for the Institute for HIV, Other STDs, and Pregnancy Prevention and research assistant professor in the Department of Communication at the University of Kentucky in Lexington, Kentucky.

David R. Holtgrave, Ph.D., is professor and vice-chair in the Department of Behavioral Sciences and Health Education at the Rollins School of Public Health at Emory University.

Michelle C. Kegler, Dr. P.H., M.P.H., is an associate professor in the Department of Behavioral Sciences and Health Education at the Rollins School of Public Health, and deputy director of the Emory Prevention Research Center at Emory University.

John F. Santelli, M.D., M.P.H., is professor and chairperson in the Heilbrunn Department of Population and Family Health at the Mailman School of Public Health, Columbia University in New York City.

Nancy Thompson, M.P.H., Ph.D., is an associate professor in the Department of Behavioral Sciences and Health Education at the Rollins School of Public Health at Emory University.

Rick S. Zimmerman, Ph.D., is a professor in the Department of Communication at the University of Kentucky in Lexington, Kentucky.

RESEARCH METHODS
IN HEALTH PROMOTION

PART ONE

FOUNDATIONS OF HEALTH PROMOTION RESEARCH

CHAPTER ONE

KEY STEPS IN THE RESEARCH PROCESS

Richard A. Crosby, Ralph J. DiClemente, and Laura F. Salazar

Health promotion has become a cornerstone of efforts designed to prevent morbidity and premature mortality (Smedley and Syme, 2000). Indeed, many nations have embraced health promotion as an approach to enriching and extending the lives of their people. Core tasks of health promotion include the primary and secondary prevention of disease and health-compromising conditions. These tasks are reflected in two overarching goals established by the United States Department of Health and Human Services: to "increase the quality and years of healthy life" and to "eliminate health disparities" (Department of Health and Human Services, 2000). Of course, the broad scope of these tasks presents an enormous challenge to the discipline of health promotion. This challenge demands that the efforts and resources of health promotion practitioners must be firmly grounded in the context of research findings.

To begin, then, it is important to state that health promotion research is the harbinger of effective health promotion practice. Thus, a great deal of time and attention should be devoted to research agendas before health promotion programs are designed and widely implemented. In turn, successful research endeavors must ensure rigor. Rigor may best be viewed as the hallmark of science.

Rigor is properly thought of as a quantity—it exists (or fails to exist) in varying degrees. Although no study can be "perfect" in rigor, studies can have a high degree of rigor. As rigor increases, confidence in the findings also increases. Therefore, rigorous studies have great potential to shape health promotion practice.

Although this book focuses on the application of research methods to health promotion, there are at least two frameworks that address a number of other issues relevant to the conceptualization, design, implementation, evaluation of programs. In particular, an emerging framework, RE-AIM (Glasgow, Vogt, and Boles, 1999) can be used as both a design and an evaluation tool for health promotion planning. Also, the PRECEDE-PROCEED Model (Green and Kreuter, 2005) is a comprehensive framework for organizing the health promotion planning process from its inception to its widespread implementation and ongoing evaluation.

Illustration of Key Concepts

As was ancient Rome, rigor is built "one brick at a time." Fortunately, clear blueprints exist for building rigorous studies. In fact, successful research can be characterized by a series of well-defined steps. Although some of these steps may appear tedious, they are all essential. Following the steps sequentially is equally important. In this chapter we provide an overview of the process and then illustrate each of the essential and sequential steps in detail.

Discovery

Without question, one of greatest rewards of health promotion research is the excitement generated by evidence-based conclusions. Health promotion research is a process that reveals insights into human behavior as it pertains to health and wellness. This exploration into people's lives should never be taken for granted; indeed, the opportunity provides health promotion practitioners a partial blueprint for the design, implementation, and justification of behavioral and structural interventions.

The process of discovery in health promotion research is iterative. Each time a research question is addressed successfully, several new questions emerge. The diversity of potential research questions in any one aspect of health promotion creates an unending challenge (see Chapter Four for more detail regarding potential research purposes and questions). Research questions can be appear quite humble, yet demand rather complex and intense investigation efforts. Consider, for example, a question as simple as determining why people consume large amounts of saturated fats despite widespread awareness that these fats cause heart disease. An investigator could pursue cognitive reasons (for example, "those foods taste really good" or "those foods are satisfying"), social reasons (such as "most party foods are not healthy, but having fun is more important"), cultural reasons (for instance, "those foods are a tradition in our house"), or economic reasons (for example, "fatty foods are usually more filling and less expensive than healthy foods"). An investigator could also approach the question based on perceived vulnerability of the study participants to the multiple forms of disease associated with a diet high in saturated fats (such as heart disease, stroke, obesity, and some forms of cancer). Obviously then, the seemingly humble research question is actually an entire research career. In fact, successful researchers typically devote themselves to only one or two areas of inquiry. This focus enables them to use the findings from one study as a platform to formulate subsequent research questions for the next study, and so on.

MINCUS "DISCOVERS" HIS RESEARCH IDEA.

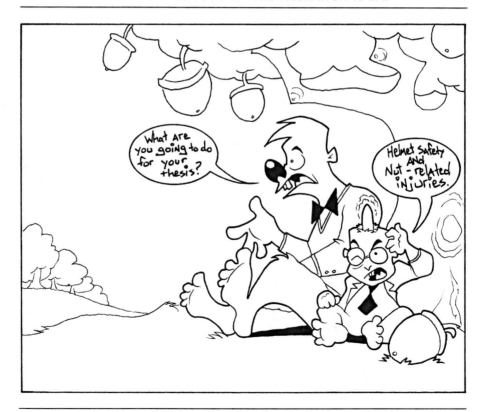

Copyright 2005 by Justin Wagner; reprinted with permission.

Because health promotion research is a discovery process it is also a public venture. Conclusions from health promotion research often have a direct impact on public health (for example, "evidence suggests that people who wear sunscreen are less likely to develop skin cancers") or an indirect impact on public health through changes in health promotion practice and policy (for example, the practice of providing same-day results for HIV testing is based on empirical findings that indicated low return rates for people testing positive). As a public venture, then, discovery through health promotion research is an indispensable contribution to maintaining the health and well-being of society. In the next section, we illustrate the discovery process using tobacco as the public health issue.

◆ ◆ ◆

In a Nutshell

As a public venture, then, discovery through health promotion research is an indispensable contribution to maintaining the health and well-being of society.

◆ ◆ ◆

Vignette: Preventing Tobacco Dependence

Globally, the use of tobacco is a behavior that leads to multiple forms of *morbidity* (incidence of disease in a given population) and premature *mortality* (incidence of death due to a particular disease in a given population). Thus, health promotion programs designed to prevent tobacco dependence among young people are strongly warranted. A substantial number of these programs seek to prevent youths from initial experimentation with tobacco. These approaches certainly have value; however, research suggests that among young people tobacco dependency may be an extended process, which may be amenable to intervention even after their initial use of the substance. Imagine, then, that you have been asked to determine the *efficacy* (that is, the ability to produce the desired effect) of providing behavioral interventions to youths who have recently begun to use tobacco, but have yet to develop a physical dependence.

A Nine-Step Model

The research process can easily become unwieldy. Even seemingly simple research questions may lead an investigator to wonder if he or she is "on the right track" with regard to the process. To streamline the thinking and actions involved in rigorous research, we have created a nine-step model that may be helpful.

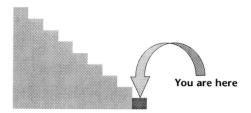

You are here

Step 1: Defining the Research Population. Given that the elimination of health disparities is a priority, health promotion research typically seeks solutions to problems that disproportionately exist among members of a defined population. Because *population* is a broad term and can be defined in many different ways, it is up to the researcher to specify the parameters that will describe the target population. For example, the researcher may define the population as "low-income youths, thirteen to nineteen years of age, residing in rural, tobacco-producing states."

Moreover, the process of defining the target population is far from arbitrary. Ideally, selecting the target population should be based on known *epidemiology* (the scientific discipline studying the distribution of disease in human populations) of the disease or health risk behavior under consideration. Generally speaking, health promotion programs should be delivered to epidemiologically defined populations on a prioritized basis (in other words, those with the greatest degree of burden—often expressed as the rate of disease per 100,000 people—are served first).

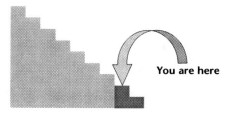

You are here

Step 2: Defining the Research Goal and Specifying the Exact Research Questions. This second step is a turning point for the remainder of the research process. As a rule, narrow and precisely defined goals and questions are far more amenable to rigorous research designs than broadly defined goals and questions. At times, new researchers propose goals and questions that are far too broad to be addressed with ample rigor. An effective strategy to avoid this pitfall is to thoroughly review the recent and relevant empirical literature. This can be a time-consuming process, but is nonetheless time well spent. Engaging in this process will inevitably yield a clear picture of gaps in the existing research. For new investigators, these gaps represent an opportunity to build on and extend the research literature, and should be a logical focus of their subsequent research.

In a Nutshell

As a rule, narrow and precisely defined goals and questions are far more amenable to rigorous research designs than broadly defined goals and questions.

Although conventional standards do not exist, from a practical standpoint many researchers restrict their review of the literature to the past five years. On-line search engines such as Medline® and PsychInfo® are invaluable assets to the review process. A thorough review should include articles directly related to the topic and those that are related tangentially. Articles directly related, for example, could include those that report findings from research designed to prevent tobacco dependence in new smokers. Indirectly related articles could include those involving different populations (for instance, middle-class urban high school students) and address broader issues such as use of other substances like alcohol or marijuana. When interpreting your review, it is important to assign a higher priority to directly related articles, whereas articles that are indirectly related should be applied judiciously.

Once the literature review is complete, a research goal can be formulated. The research goal is a general statement that conveys the purpose of the planned study. The following statement, "to determine the efficacy of providing behavioral interventions for youths who have recently begun to use tobacco" is the research goal as stated in the vignette. The goal provides an overview of purpose and scope, but it lacks precision and specificity. Rather, it is the research questions that provide the precision and specificity. Research questions are based on the research goal. In the given vignette, samples of a few appropriate research questions may be as follows.

- Will a twelve-hour small-group intervention promote tobacco cessation among a greater percentage of youths than a brief version (six hours) of the same program?
- Will a twelve-hour small-group intervention promote tobacco cessation among a greater percentage of youths as compared to youths who receive no program at all?
- Will a six-hour small-group intervention promote tobacco cessation among a greater percent of youths as compared to youths who receive no program at all?

Please notice that each question is a derivative of the overarching research goal. Thus, each research question should provide information that serves the research goal. This derivative approach to research questions ensures that research efforts are accurately directed. Research questions should be centered upon a common purpose: the research goal. This practice sets the stage for the next step.

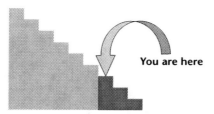

You are here

Step 3: Determining Whether the Research Should Be Observational or Experimental. Briefly stated, *observational research* refers to research in which variables are observed as they exist in nature—no manipulation of variables occurs. Observational research asks questions pertaining to "why people do what they do." This form of research *does not involve* treatment or intervention.

Experimental research, however, *does involve* manipulation of a variable (this could include education, policy changes, or changes in the environment). Thus, it builds upon observational research by asking, "How can we help people achieve positive change?" Experimental research is always concerned with the essential question of whether a given intervention program can produce outcomes of statistical significance and, more important, practical significance.

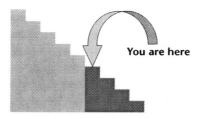

You are here

Step 4: Selecting a Research Design That Provides a Rigorous Test of the Research Questions. The choice of research designs ranges from simple observational studies (requiring relatively little time and generally manageable resources) to complex experimental studies (requiring several years to complete and the use of extensive resources).

The guiding principle in making the selection is parsimony. Parsimony implies that the need (that is, investigating the research questions) is met by a tool (that is, research design) that does the job well, without going beyond that which is necessary.

FIGURE 1.1.   A TRAJECTORY OF RESEARCH IN HEALTH PROMOTION.

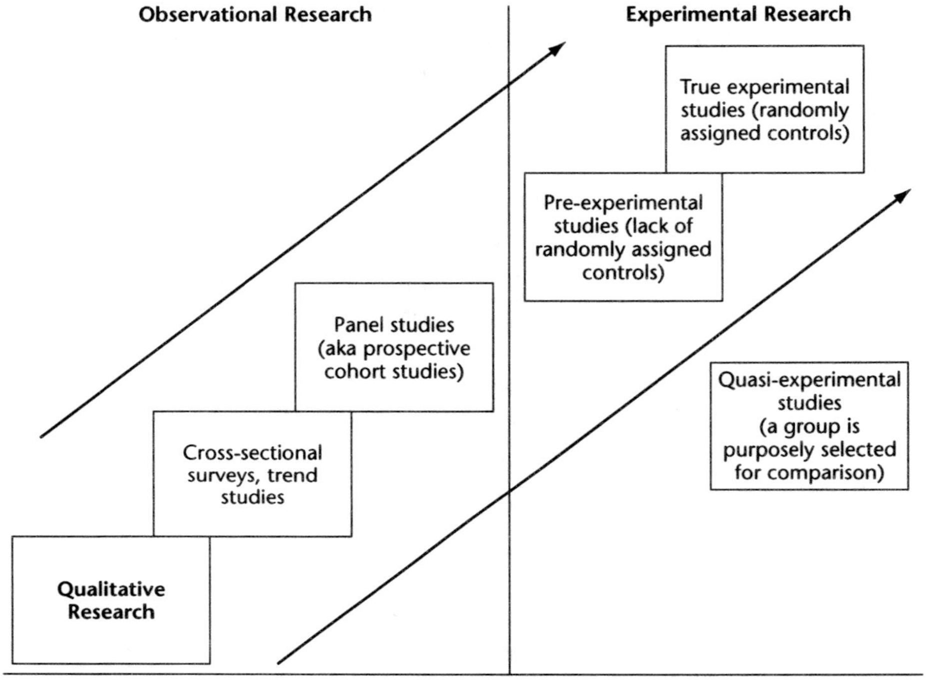

Figure 1.1 shows a trajectory of research designs that accommodate various forms of health promotion research. These designs are described in greater detail in Chapter Four. At the left and lower end of this trajectory, relatively simple research designs can be identified. Examples include qualitative studies and cross-sectional studies. As the level of complexity increases, the trajectory includes designs that necessitate the maintenance of a *cohort* (a cohort being a sample of research participants) over multiple assessment periods. A *cohort study* is synonymous with the terms *panel study, longitudinal study,* or *prospective study* and is located mid-level along the trajectory. Similarly, various levels of complexity exist among experimental designs, which are located toward the upper right end of the trajectory. The phrase "randomized, controlled, trial (RCT)" denotes a true experimental design located at the peak of the trajectory. Figure 1.1 also shows that quasi-experimental designs are located further along on the trajectory, but do not achieve the same "gold standard" status as the true experimental designs.

Quasi-experimental designs, however, are often necessary in health promotion, as certain intervention programs or structural-level interventions limit the ability to randomize (Murray, 1998).

As a rule, research should be constructed with designs that approximate the trajectory shown in Figure 1.1. That is, designs located to the left end of the trajectory serve as the building blocks for subsequent research questions that can then be addressed by progressively more complex designs.

◆ ◆ ◆

In a Nutshell

Designs located to the left end of the trajectory serve as the building blocks for subsequent research questions that can then be addressed by progressively more complex designs.

◆ ◆ ◆

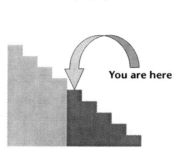

Step 5: Determining the Variables That Must Be Measured. First and foremost, the immediate goal is to be absolutely sure that every *variable* required for a rigorous study is identified. A variable is anything that changes, meaning it must assume a range of values. The research question and the literature review will inform variable selection. For example, suppose that the literature review indicated that efficacy of other tobacco-dependence programs was a function of participants' family environment (in other words, programs may work better for youths with a supportive family). Given even a remote chance that this same dynamic may operate in our hypothetical planned study of low-income youths residing in rural areas, it is incumbent upon the researchers to measure participants' perceived level of family support in addition to other critical variables.

The way in which the variables are measured is equally important. Indeed, rigor is dependent upon the selection of reliable and valid measurement instruments. Like research, measurement is a process. It involves identifying appropriate measures, or adapting existing measures to your unique research question, or creating new measures. Chapter Nine provides details about measurement issues in health promotion research.

Some variables may be measured directly using a physical instrument (for example, a sphygmomanometer for blood pressure, or a scale for weight), whereas other variables such as level of skill applying a condom to a penile model can be measured directly through observation. In health promotion research most variables are measured indirectly using participants' self-reports (See Chapter Ten for more detail regarding the use of self-report measures). In this case, a mode of administration (for example, paper and pencil, face-to-face interview, or computer-assisted self-interview) must be selected based upon previous knowledge of the research population and the nature of the previously identified research questions.

The process concludes with pilot testing designed to ensure that measures are appropriate for the planned study population. The pilot test also allows researchers to evaluate the psychometric properties of the self-report measures that purport to represent a *construct*. Constructs are defined concepts that would otherwise be considered abstractions. Examples of constructs used in health promotion research include self-esteem, depression, and self-efficacy.

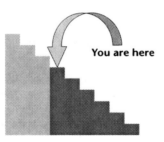

You are here

Step 6: Selecting the Sampling Procedure. As in other aspects of the research enterprise, there are numerous sampling procedures that can be used in health promotion research. Sampling exists across a continuum of complexity and rigor. The sampling procedure employed is one of the most critical determinants of *external validity. External validity* refers to the ability to generalize study findings to the population of individuals with similar characteristics represented in the study sample. It should be noted, however, that not all research studies need to use a sampling procedure that yields high external validity.

Sampling should also include specifying the number of study participants. This number is selected based on a *power analysis*. Stated simply, a power analysis is the estimated ability of a statistical test to find true differences between variables or between groups of study participants. Although a study's power is determined by multiple factors, sample size is one of the most important determinants. Planned sample sizes that provide inadequate power are crippling to the overall study. In the vignette, for example, a power analysis may suggest that each of the three study conditions should have one hundred participants. Having fewer participants in each condition could severely jeopardize the power of the study. More detailed descriptions of sampling procedures are presented in Chapter Eleven.

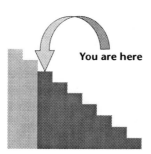

You are here

Step 7: Implementing the Research Plan. A basic requirement of *internal validity* is consistency in the implementation of all study protocols. *Internal validity* implies that the study is not confounded by design, measurement, or poor implementation of study procedures. Protocols spell out key procedures such as the sampling procedure to be used, how participants will be assigned to intervention conditions, when and where assessments will occur, who will provide the assessments, what participants will be told or not told about the research study, and how reticent participants will be enticed to return for follow-up programs or assessments. Because protocols are generally quite detailed, subtle departures from these detailed plans can be a common problem. Over time, however, this "drift" can amount to substantial changes in the way late-entry participants are treated as compared with those enrolling earlier in the study.

As an example of drift, consider the study of preventing tobacco dependence outlined in this chapter. The protocol specifies that teens will be "randomly assigned to either (1) the twelve-hour condition, (2) the six-hour condition, or (3) the no-treatment condition. Furthermore, assume that the protocol states that, "random assignment will be achieved by drawing colored marbles from an opaque container. Blue marbles signify assignment to the twelve-hour group, green marbles signify assignment to the six-hour group, and yellow marbles signify assignment to the no-treatment group. One hundred blue, one hundred green, and one hundred yellow marbles are placed in the container as the study begins. A dedicated research assistant has been charged with the implementation of this procedure.

In the first three months of the study, the research assistant performs flawlessly. Subsequently, however, the assistant learns that teens are benefiting from the twelve-hour and six-hour conditions. This perception leads the assistant to invite some teens (those who blindly pulled a yellow marble) to return the marble and "draw again." Repeated over time, this drift can create a systematic bias with respect to the composition of teens assigned to the three conditions.

Other common forms of drift include departure from the planned intervention (perhaps the health educator for the six-hour program develops an "improved" method), deviations in how assessments are administered (perhaps research assistants change the way they perform interviews), and departure from sampling protocols. Fortunately, drift can be averted by vigilant attention to an established set of quality-assurance procedures. Ultimately, then, the principle investigator is the one person who must be accountable for implementing these procedures, thereby ensuring that drift does not occur.

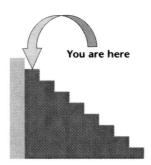

You are here

Step 8: Analyzing the Data. Once all the assessments have been conducted, a data set can be established. The data set consists of the variables measured for each participant. The data set is, of course, quite valuable, as it can subsequently be used to answer the research questions that were formulated in step 2. After the data are checked for logical inconsistencies (called "cleaning"), the research process becomes dependent on the statistical skills of the research team. Again, parsimony is important at this step—the goal is *not* to perform a sophisticated analysis; instead, the goal is to perform an analysis that provides a rigorous and fair test of the research questions while avoiding the introduction of artificially imposed procedures.

In the tobacco-dependence vignette, a parsimonious analysis would be to simply compare the mean number of cigarettes smoked in the past week in each group, assessed at a designated point in time after the interventions have been completed. Suppose the means are (1) 8.3 for the twelve-hour condition, (2) 12.1 for the six-hour condition, and (3) 17.2 for the no-treatment condition. The means can be compared using a very simple test (a one-way analysis of variance), which answers an essential question: Are the differences between means a function of the interventions or are they a function of chance? Analyses, however, can become quite complex when considering logically occurring questions such as: (1) Do intervention effects differ based on gender of the participant? (2) Do effects differ based on age of the participant? (3) Do effects differ based on the baseline assessment of tobacco use? Of course, these questions are vitally important, and each takes the analysis a necessary step farther away from simply comparing means. Chapters Twelve and Thirteen provide a more detailed discussion of data analysis.

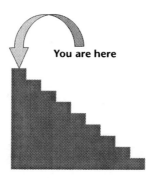

You are here

Step 9: Disseminating the Findings. Rigorous research clearly warrants widespread dissemination. Indeed, this step elevates the project from a work in progress to science. Like each of the previous eight steps shown in this chapter, step 9 is also a process unto itself. The rudimentary starting point in this process is transforming the analytic results (numbers) into carefully articulated findings.

◆ ◆ ◆

In a Nutshell

The rudimentary starting point in this process is transforming the analytic results (numbers) into carefully articulated findings.

◆ ◆ ◆

Findings are answers to the research questions that are generated by the data analysis. Next, the findings must be considered within the context of related research by showing how they strengthen or extend previous work. At this juncture, it is important to know that nonsignificant findings can be just as important

FIGURE 1.2. SCHEMATIC ILLUSTRATION OF THE
NINE-STEP RESEARCH PROCESS.

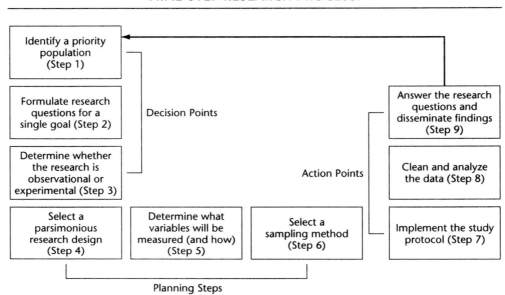

as significant findings with respect to building the research base. The caveat to this statement, however, is that the study should have a high degree of rigor.

Moreover, the findings may raise additional questions that bring the research process back to its origin. Figure 1.2 illustrates this point. Inspection of the figure shows that research is an iterative process. Every time a research question is asked and answered another question (or set of questions) becomes apparent. New researchers should be aware that their research debut (initial entry into this iterative process) is likely to be difficult, but that repeated cycles become progressively less difficult. In fact, this observation may explain why health promotion researchers often tend to specialize in a narrowly defined field of study (such as prevention of adult-onset diabetes, prevention of HIV infection among women, or promoting Pap testing among Latinas).

After the researcher (or research team) has successfully answered the research questions, the remaining task is to prepare written and visual (that is, tables and figures of study results) summaries of the research process (steps 1 through 8). Recall from step 2 that research is a collective process; therefore disseminating the results adds to the larger empirical knowledge base. Fortunately, the preparation of written and visual summaries does not have to be a daunting task. In fact, when rigor is high, this task can be very satisfying and enjoyable. The task is primarily a historical account of the rationale underlying the research questions and the protocols used to answer these questions. Researchers customarily bring the task to a close by suggesting subsequent research questions that could be investigated to further strengthen and expand the research base.

Dissemination of the research findings is widely embraced as a key part of the scientific process. The written and visual records can then be disseminated through multiple channels. Oral presentation of the findings at professional meetings is generally a first step. These presentations create opportunities for informal peer review of the research and study conclusions—peer review is a valued and vital aspect of science. Submission of the written summary to an appropriate professional journal provides opportunity for formal peer review.

◆ ◆ ◆

In a Nutshell

Dissemination of the research findings is widely embraced as a key part of the scientific process.

◆ ◆ ◆

Returning to the vignette, suppose the conclusions have been written and appear as follows:

> In this study of three hundred low-income teens residing in rural, tobacco-producing states, we found that a twelve-hour tobacco-dependence prevention program was equally efficacious compared to a similar program lasting only six hours. The mean number of cigarettes smoked (in one week) for teens in the twelve-hour program and in the six-hour program was significantly lower relative to the number of cigarettes smoked by teens who did not receive either program. Findings suggest that these small-group interventions may be an important strategy for interrupting the formation of tobacco dependence among members of the study population. Further research should continue to investigate the efficacy of this program among teens residing in largely metropolitan states.

Peer review may help identify the strengths and weaknesses of the study and its conclusions. For example, a reviewer might ask, "Do the results truly indicate interruption of dependence?" Another reviewer might ask, "How were rural, tobacco-producing states defined?" Questions derived from the peer-review process can help researchers identify the limitations of the study and its contribution to the health promotion literature base.

When steps 1 through 8 have been thoroughly addressed, and the peer-review process has been successfully navigated, the final product will generally take the form of a published journal article (Chapter Fourteen provides more details related to the publishing of research findings). In health promotion, however, publication of a journal article is *not* the endpoint in the research process. At least two other obligations exist. First, media relations should be cultivated and used to disseminate findings to the public. Second, successful health promotion programs should be made widely available. The process of translating science into practice is ongoing and labor intensive, but is also the cornerstone of health promotion practice.

◆ ◆ ◆

In a Nutshell

The process of translating science into practice is ongoing and labor intensive, but is also the cornerstone of health promotion practice.

◆ ◆ ◆

The Context of Health Promotion Research

The research process occurs in a context characterized by scholarship, grantsmanship, and vigilant attention to ethics. These three principles are highly valued and cherished in the profession. Scholarship implies that the researcher possesses an inherent curiosity regarding the research questions and a dedication to expanding the knowledge base in health promotion. Integrity is a key feature of scholarship. Like rigor in the research process, integrity in the researcher ensures a fair test of the research questions. Integrity implies that any preconceived desire to prove or disprove study hypotheses is not allowed to interfere with the research process. The research process is quite eloquent in that it forces objectivity; however, adherence to the process is based on self-report of the researcher (making integrity vital).

Grantsmanship is also a vital part of the research process. Rigor is often expensive, and obtaining funds for health promotion research is typically a competitive process. In addition to other factors (for example, quality of the research proposal, the importance of the topic and the population, and so on), grant awards, to some extent, are given based on the current degree of engagement in the iterative process shown in Figure 1.2.

Vigilant attention to ethics is the most critical of the three concerns briefly described here (see Chapter Three). Just as practitioners of medicine take the Hippocratic Oath, health promotion researchers must adopt the principle, "First, do no harm." Moreover, health promotion research is highly regulated by local and federal organizations that protect the rights of research participants. The nature of health promotion research demands studies of humans, and these studies are oftentimes directed at very personal (and therefore protected) behaviors.

Applied Example

A study published in the *American Journal of Public Health* provides a good illustration of the nine-step model. Hagan and colleagues (2001) selected a priority population for the prevention of infection with hepatitis C: injection drug users (step 1). Their research question was firmly grounded in the context of previous research. They noted that shared use of drug preparation equipment, in the absence of self-injection with a used syringe, had not been investigated as a source of transmission for the hepatitis C virus (HCV). Their primary research question was to assess the risk of HCV infection incurred by sharing cookers, cotton filters, and water used to rinse drug-injection syringes (step 2).

The study was strictly observational (step 3). A panel study design (with a one-year follow-up) was used. This design is relatively advanced with respect to its location on the trajectory of research shown in Figure 1.1. Only persons initially testing negative for HCV were included in the study. This approach allowed the investigators to compare drug equipment sharing behavior—in the ensuing year—between those who tested positive (seroconverted) and those who tested negative for HCV at the one-year follow-up assessment (step 4). Selected variables included the assessment of race, age, sex, homelessness, sexual behaviors, types of drugs injected, and a battery of measures related to drug equipment sharing behaviors. HCV was assessed through a reliable and valid blood assay (step 5).

The sample comprised a subset of 507 people who were drawn from a larger sample of injection drug users from nine locations in Seattle, Washington. At each location, a random-numbers table was used to select a representative portion of eligible participants (step 6). Unfortunately, procedures used for quality assurance of the data-collection process were not described (step 7). Data were analyzed separately for persons who reported injecting with previously used syringes and those not reporting this form of risk. Among those reporting this risk, persons sharing cookers or cotton were 3.8 times more likely to acquire HCV over the observation period of one year. This difference was significant (that is, not attributable to chance). Significant differences with respect to shared cleaning water were not observed (step 8).

The research team concluded by suggesting that HCV infection may be commonly transmitted by sharing cookers and filtration cotton. This conclusion squarely addressed the research question and provided a valuable extension to the research base. The high degree of rigor, combined with an important research question, yielded findings that contributed to health promotion practice (the initial portion of step 9). From a practice perspective, the finding suggests that injection drug users can benefit from health education efforts that create awareness of HCV risk as a consequence of cooker and cotton sharing. Dissemination of the written report in the *American Journal of Public Health* made this information available to thousands of journal subscribers, untold numbers of media organizations, and (via electronic posting on engines such as Medline) to most anyone with access to the Internet (step 9).

Summary

Health promotion practice and policy should be based on rigorous research. This chapter has provided a thumbnail sketch of the research process as it applies to health promotion. This sketch can be used as a platform to gain competence and proficiency in each of the nine steps described. Competence and proficiency in scholarship, grantsmanship, and ethics should be an equally high priority. The remainder of this volume is devoted to expanding this thumbnail sketch into a more complete primer of health promotion research methods.

Issues to Consider

1. An overriding issue is whether health promotion practice should always be grounded in research. Consider, for example, the emergence of the AIDS epidemic in the United States. By the mid-1980s, the rapid escalation of HIV infection demanded an immediate and escalated public health response (Garrett, 1994). Unfortunately, from a health promotion perspective, research chains specifically pertaining to behavioral intervention of HIV transmission had barely begun to form. In lieu of best practices based on research findings, health promotion programs were created to increase awareness of risk and provide people with essential prevention messages. In retrospect, the efficacy of these initial approaches to prevention may be questionable. Alternatively, the urgency of the epidemic demanded a response. An unfortunate reality of the research process is that it moves slowly. Given the inherent urgency, then, should practice perhaps sometimes proceed without research?

2. The research process as described in this chapter is designed to create objectivity in the investigation of any given research question. Suppose that a study high in rigor (and therefore objectivity) is funded by a drug company (Company Y). The study investigates behavioral compliance with an arthritis medication that typically caused temporary side effects. Furthermore, suppose that the findings indicates that compliance was extremely low due to a nearly universal physical intolerance among study participants for the drug. The research team proceeds to step 9 and is informed by Company Y that dissemination should not occur. Considering the principles of scholarship and ethics, how should the research team respond?

3. The term "publication bias" has often been used to describe a tendency of journals to preferentially accept research reports that find significant results (meaning the data supported a proposition that can add to the quality of health promotion practice). Conversely, studies with nonsignificant findings only provide insight on "things that won't work"; thus, these studies may be less attractive for publication. While nonsignificant findings are admittedly less exciting, they may nonetheless be based on important research questions and stem from rigorously conducted research. Yet, despite a high degree of importance and rigor, nonsignificant findings have very little practical meaning for anyone other than persons investigating questions in the same research chain. How can this seemingly irresolvable problem be addressed?

For Practice and Discussion

A philanthropic organization has asked you to design and conduct a study that can benefit the health of women by promoting regular Pap testing and annual mammography among post-menopausal women. After reviewing the surveillance data relevant to cervical cancer and breast cancer, you conclude that Hispanic women are a priority population for intervention (step 1). Next you develop a single but important research question: What are the cultural and economic barriers that preclude post-menopausal Hispanic women from receiving regular Pap tests and annual mammograms? (step 2). Having resolved steps 1 and 2, you begin to think about the planning phase of the study. Thus, you consider steps 4, 5, and 6. Please think each of these steps through carefully and create a rigorous plan to investigate this research question (if you have trouble with this, please try the exercise again after you have read the remaining chapters in this book).

References

Department of Health and Human Services. (2000). *Healthy people 2010.* Available on-line at www.health.gov/healthypeople. Accessed June 30, 2001.

Garrett, L. (1994). *The coming plague: Newly emerging diseases in a world out of balance.* New York: Farrar, Straus, and Giroux.

Glasgow, R. E., Vogt, T. M., and Boles, S. M. (1999). Evaluating the public health impact of health promotion interventions: The RE-AIM framework. *American Journal of Public Health, 89,* 1322–1327.

Green, L. W., and Kreuter, M. W. (2005). *Health program planning: An educational and ecological approach* (4th ed.). Boston: McGraw Hill.

Hagan, H., Thiede, H., Weiss, N. S., Hopkin, S. G., Duchin, J. S., and Alexander, E. R. (2001). Sharing of drug preparation equipment as a risk factor for hepatitis C. *American Journal of Public Health, 91,* 42–45.

Murray, D. M. (1998). *Design and analysis of group randomized trials.* New York: Oxford University Press.

Smedley, B. D., and Syme, S. L. (Eds.). (2000). *Promoting health: Intervention strategies from social and behavioral research.* Washington, DC: National Academy Press.

CHAPTER TWO

PHILOSOPHY OF SCIENCE AND THEORY CONSTRUCTION

Laura F. Salazar, Ralph J. DiClemente, and Richard A. Crosby

Health promotion research, in general, comprises some or all of the nine steps that were delineated in Chapter One and that are undertaken to investigate health-related behaviors. The overarching goal is to understand better ways in which we can influence health behaviors and ultimately health by first identifying the behavioral risk factors for a particular disease. By first understanding and then affecting behaviors that contribute to health, health promotion researchers can have a substantive impact on the associated morbidity and mortality. When conceptualizing and undertaking health promotion research, however, in addition to knowing the research process, it is also important to understand the underlying philosophy.

Derived from the Latin word *scientia,* the literal meaning of *science* is knowledge. Yet, science can also be viewed as a process. The process entails the systematic gathering of seemingly disparate facts and then organizing them into an interconnected whole. Science is the process of acquiring knowledge for the purpose of having knowledge. Why is science important, and why do we hold science in such reverence? Because science is knowledge, and knowledge is the source of empowerment. Creating a body of knowledge regarding myriad subjects such as the properties of matter and energy (physics), the structure of matter (chemistry), living organisms (biology), human behavior (psychology), or human societies (sociology), to name a few scientific disciplines, can benefit greatly the human experience and provide insight into how nature works and how we as human beings function within nature and with each other. Think of science as an indispensable tool much like the wheel that can take us where we want to go by aiding us in our understanding of, and in our attempt to control, our environment.

◆ ◆ ◆

In a Nutshell

Derived from the Latin word scientia, *the literal meaning of* science *is knowledge. Yet, science can also be viewed as a process. The process entails the systematic gathering of seemingly disparate facts and then organizing them into an interconnected whole.*

◆ ◆ ◆

Health promotion research also involves a process. In Chapter One, we referred to this as a discovery process. Interestingly, if health promotion research is the process through which knowledge on health-related behaviors is "discovered," and science equals knowledge, then health promotion research must be considered a science, right? To answer this question fully and accurately, we first provide an overview of what constitutes science and describe key concepts from its related discipline—the philosophy of science. Philosophy is from the Greek word *philosophia*, meaning love (*philo*) and the pursuit of knowledge (*sophia*). Philosophy of science, therefore, pertains to the structure, principles, and components of the scientific process—the framework lovingly used for the pursuit of knowledge.

Another important and related term used often when discussing the philosophy of science is *epistemology*. Epistemology is the branch of philosophy that studies knowledge and attempts to answer the basic question: what distinguishes true (adequate) knowledge from false (inadequate) knowledge? There are different ways of acquiring knowledge, some of which will be described in more detail later in this chapter. As a health promotion practitioner or researcher you may be called upon to evaluate different types of health information. Learning to distinguish valid health-related information from false information will be an important skill.

Illustration of Key Concepts

The goals of this chapter are to introduce the various epistemological positions taken in pursuit of knowledge, such as authority, tenacity, logic, and, of course, scientific inquiry. Once you have built a solid foundation in epistemology, you may then be in the position to ascertain whether or not specific instances of health promotion research constitute science. Of course, you will also be able to ascertain whether other field's inquiries can be considered science, "junk science," or neither. Consequently, you will also acquire insight about how science generates knowledge.

Epistemology: Ways of Acquiring Knowledge

Given that science is a process in which we gather knowledge and organize that knowledge systematically, does the way or method in which the knowledge is collected determine whether or not the process can be called science? The way in which knowledge is generated determines whether or not it should be deemed science and therefore added to an overall scientific body of knowledge. Just because an effort is conducted "in the name of science" does not necessarily make it science. Second, although *science* literally means knowledge, in the modern sense it refers more to a specific process that adheres to standards and methods of generating knowledge. Thus, it matters greatly indeed, for there are many different ways in which we come by our knowledge regarding the world. Some ways in which we gather knowledge may contribute to science, whereas other ways may appear to be scientific, but, in reality, are not considered science in the technical sense. Regardless of the method, knowledge is conveyed (although it may vary in value). Thus, not all knowledge is created equal. It is most important to know the different ways or methods in which we accrue knowledge so that the quality of the knowledge can be judged appropriately and the implications for choosing one method over another can be determined.

In the following section, we describe various ways of knowing such as authority, tenacity (sometimes called tradition), and logic and reason, which are not considered as science in the modern sense, but nevertheless provide new ideas and suggestions. In addition, we describe scientific inquiry as a way of knowing. The former methods (authority, tenacity, and logic) are ways in which knowledge is derived, so they are important to know. By understanding these alternative epistemologies you will better understand science. Consequently, you may embrace scientific inquiry as the most important way of knowing. As you will see, these ways must be evaluated rather subjectively and contrast sharply with scientific inquiry as a way of knowing because science is able to provide both a body of knowledge and a specific method in which to evaluate that knowledge.

Unfortunately, in some instances, science may not have yet contributed to a specific research goal and thus may not be an available source of knowledge. For example, in the early 1980s before the HIV virus was discovered, researchers did not know what caused the decline in the immune system condition (AIDS) or how it was being transmitted. The other ways of knowing (authority, tenacity, and logic) were the only sources of knowledge available. In essence, scientific inquiry is the only epistemology that requires data-driven conclusions. Other epistemologies exist regardless of whether data are available or whether people choose to consider the data. The challenge in those instances is to examine the underlying source of the knowledge and make the best determination regarding its accuracy.

Authority. Albert Einstein dubbed Galileo "the father of modern physics— indeed of modern science altogether" (Sobel, 1999, p. 326). Most everyone is familiar with the historical account of the renowned mathematician and scientist Galileo and his quest to advance the field of science, which up to that point in history was based mostly on the philosophy of Aristotle. Galileo sought to move beyond an understanding of why *phenomena* occur to how they occur. By phenomena, we mean events or circumstances evident to the senses and possible to describe scientifically. For Galileo, mathematics was one of his scientific tools:

> "Philosophy is written in this grand book the universe, which stands continually open to our gaze. But the book cannot be understood unless one first learns to comprehend the language and to read the alphabet in which it is composed. It is written in the language of mathematics, and its characters are triangles, circles, and other geometric figures, without which it is humanly impossible to understand a single word of it; without these, one wanders about in a dark labyrinth" [quoted in Drake, 1957, p. 237].

Although most scientists concur that Galileo's greatest contribution to science is his application of mathematics to the study of motion, he has been immortalized for his defense of Copernicus's theory that posited the sun rather than the Earth is the center of the cosmos. This sun-as-center-of-the-universe perspective was not only contrary to the Aristotelian perspective (that is, the Earth is the center of the cosmos), but more important, it contradicted the teachings and beliefs espoused by the Catholic Church. Interestingly, the Church also based its views on the Aristotelian perspective.

During this period in history, the Catholic Church was the moral and philosophical authority. If the Catholic Church said it was so, then most people accepted it for fact. Most people did not understand the order of the universe at this time. Thus, it was easier for people to defer to some authority, one who held some degree of knowledge regarding an issue. People during this era mostly obtained their knowledge through authority because there were not many other sources. This approach has a major shortcoming, however; the authority in question can be wrong, as was the case with the Church. Unfortunately, because Galileo went against the most powerful authority of his time, he was tried by the Church in front of the Inquisition. Because he would not recant his beliefs, he was sentenced to life imprisonment, which was later reduced to house arrest (Sobel, 1999).

In his search for knowledge Galileo truly believed that, "the authority of a thousand is not worth the humble reasoning of a single individual" (Redondi, 1987, p. 37). Even in our modern times, this quote should still apply. Yet, many of us still rely upon authority for facts and guidance. For example, many of us look up to our religious leaders as well as our politicians, physicians, and professors. Reliance on authority is not always problematic. Yet, not taking the time to evaluate the validity of an authority's ideas, suggestions, or comments may be problematic. Of course, an evaluation of the knowledge would require knowing what evidence (if any) the authority is using. For example, when a politician describes our current state of the union, we must consider whether or not the description is based on scientific evidence (such as gathering of key economic indicators, scientific surveys, archival data, and so on) or on anecdotal evidence from a few people, or, even worse, is not based on any evidence but is simply rhetoric. Furthermore, when a physician instructs someone to drink eight eight-ounce glasses of water per day, the person can ask if this recommendation is based on scientific evidence or if the recommendation is based on tenacity with no real basis (see Box 2.1, which describes an investigation into the origins of the health recommendation to drink eight glasses of water per day). Even with your professors (including the one teaching this course), you should question knowledge presented in class and inquire about the epistemology. These are only a few ways in which

Box 2.1. The "8 × 8" Recommendation

Valtin (2002) conducted a review of the scientific literature to determine the origin of the advice to "drink at least eight eight-ounce glasses of water per day." He found no scientific studies in support of the "8 × 8" health belief, and he could not find its origins in the scientific literature. In fact, he found evidence to suggest that such large amounts of water are not necessary in *healthy* adults, who live in temperate climates and are largely sedentary. Moreover, his review of a large body of related research suggested that the human body's osmoregulatory system maintains water balance naturally. Thus, it would appear that the ubiquitous "8 × 8" water recommendation is without scientific merit, but persists as a modern myth that is viewed as medically beneficial.

MINCUS TAKES DR. DINCUS'S ADVICE FOR GOOD HEALTH.

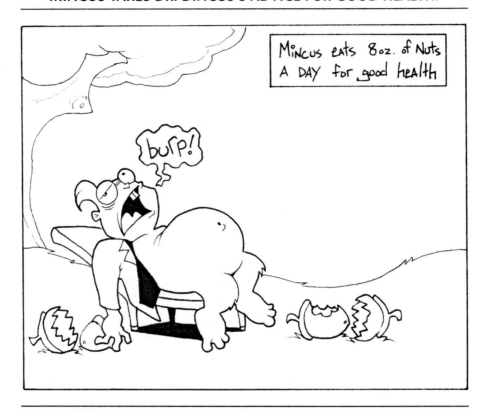

Copyright 2005 by Justin Wagner; reprinted with permission.

to question authority, but as health promotion researchers and purveyors of knowledge, you should learn to question the knowledge that is presented to you. Moreover, you have an obligation to employ scientific inquiry regardless of the prevailing epistemologies. As with Galileo, however, your research may not be popular or readily accepted by society. Yet, as Albert Einstein stated, "A foolish faith in authority is the worst enemy of truth" (quoted in Calaprice, 2000, p. 303).

Tenacity or Tradition. Even in this postmodern age of technology, it is interesting that many health beliefs that have been around for a very long time and are sometimes referred to as "wives' tales" remain firmly entrenched in our minds and culture and continue to influence our health behaviors. For example, were you told that it is dangerous to swim unless you wait an hour after eating? Were you scolded for going outside as a child with wet hair because it would cause you to catch a cold? Did your mother stress to you that you should eat all of your carrots because it will improve your eyesight? Or certainly you have heard the expression, "an apple a day helps keep the doctor away"? Do you still believe that chocolate causes acne? Are you familiar with the notion that oysters are an aphrodisiac? Many young women maintain that they cannot get pregnant while breastfeeding or the very first time they have vaginal intercourse. A more recent health belief that has become somewhat entrenched in modern society is that the flu vaccine will cause you to get the flu. Not surprising, some of these health beliefs may be rooted in truth, which may explain their longevity. For example, eating vegetables high in vitamin A (for example, carrots) is good for maintaining healthy eyesight; however, more than the recommended daily requirement will not improve your eyesight. What is surprising is that some of these health beliefs continue to persist despite the fact they have been proven false—hence the term *tenacity*. For example, many people still believe that going out in cold weather with wet hair will cause them to catch a cold, even though science has shown it is exposure to a virus that causes a cold.

Why do these beliefs persist even though they are false? Many of these beliefs have been handed down from one generation to the next through storytelling, through printed material, and presently through other forms of media. For many cultures, these beliefs become their traditions, and as traditions they tend to provide people with an acceptable way of exerting control over certain unavoidable events. Thus, accepting traditional beliefs as a way of knowing at a very basic level may serve to help people understand and exert control over their environment.

Health beliefs based on tradition, whether true or not, may also contribute to the cohesiveness of a cultural group. For example, unified cultures are grounded in their acceptance of similar beliefs and traditions. It is for these reasons that there may be problems with using only tenacity as a valid way of knowing: if the beliefs are erroneous, then there will be great difficulty in changing or discrediting them once they have been accepted widely and are entrenched within a culture. It may be useful for you to think about different health beliefs you have accepted and consider whether or not they are based on tradition, evidence, or truth.

Logic and Reasoning. The term *logic* is derived from the Greek word *logos,* which traditionally means "word," "thought," "principle," or "speech." *Logos* has been used among both philosophers and theologians and embodies both human reason (that is, intellect, capacity to discern and distinguish) and universal intelligence (that is, the Divine). Although philosophers are undoubtedly concerned with both aspects of *logos,* as health promotion researchers we are concerned mainly with the human-reason aspect for this construct. Reason, along with its cousin term *logic,* is the foundation of philosophy and is still in use today as a way of knowing.

In modern terms, *logic* can be defined as the science of reasoning, proof, thinking, or inference. Logic is useful in that it allows you to analyze arguments or a piece of reasoning and determine whether or not they are accurate or "illogical." Although logic is considered a science, knowing the basics of logic and reasoning can assist you in spotting which arguments are invalid and which conclusions are false.

As previously stated, the Catholic Church based much of its beliefs and knowledge on another authority—Aristotle. Because Aristotle concerned himself with the investigation of natural phenomena, he was able to make many observations about the world. He then used logic and reasoning to define, analyze, and systematize his observations to make sense of what he observed. Logic and reasoning were his tools; thus, in the absence of science, logic and reasoning were the accepted standards of the time.

Specifically, Aristotle used an approach called a *syllogism,* which means an argument of a very specific form consisting of two premises and a conclusion, to amass his knowledge. Generating knowledge regarding the Earth and the cosmos, Aristotle used the following syllogism:

> Again, everything that moves with the circular movement, except the first sphere, is observed to be passed, and to move with more than one motion. The earth, then, also, whether it move about the centre or as stationary at it, must necessarily move with two motions. But if this were so, there would have to be passings and turnings of the fixed stars. Yet no such thing is observed. The same stars always rise and set in the same parts of the earth [Aristotle, 350 B.C. (2004), part 14, paragraph 1].

Using this syllogism, Aristotle concluded that "the earth, spherical in shape, is at rest in the centre of the universe" (Aristotle, 350 B.C. (2004), part 14, paragraph 4). Of course, it was later ascertained that Aristotle's conclusion was inaccurate. His syllogism contained a *fallacy.* In logic, the term *fallacy* has a very specific meaning: a fallacy is a technical flaw which makes an argument unsound or invalid. In this instance, the premises of Aristotle's argument were not true. Although his conclusion was sound, it was based on false premises and was therefore false. There are many other types of fallacies that occur quite frequently, such as a fallacy called *cum hoc ergo propter hoc* ("with this, therefore because of this"), which is to assert that because two events occur together, they must be causally related. An example for this type of fallacy would be

> Teenagers eat a lot of chocolate.
>
> Teenagers have acne.
>
> Therefore, eating chocolate causes acne.

Another fallacy is called *converse accident* or *hasty generalization* and is the reverse of the fallacy of *accident*. The former occurs when you generalize to an entire group based on a few specific cases, which aren't representative of all possible cases. For example, "Professor Dincus is eccentric. Therefore all professors are eccentric."

The latter fallacy (accident) is also referred to as a sweeping generalization and occurs when a general rule is applied to a particular situation, but the features of that particular situation mean an exception to the rule should be made. For example, "College students generally like junk food. *You* are a college student, so you must like junk food." Finally, one last fallacy is called *post hoc ergo propter hoc* (after this, therefore because of this), which occurs when a cause-and-effect relationship is assumed because one factor occurred temporally before the other factor. For example, "After receiving his flu vaccine, Rick came down with the flu. Therefore, we must avoid the flu vaccine because it *caused* him to get the flu."

In present times, people still rely upon information that is derived from logic and reasoning, especially if there are not alternative ways of knowing. Yet, much information derived from logic and reasoning is based on arguments that may contain fallacies. Another issue with this way of knowing is that arguments cannot determine whether a statement is correct. Thus, as a way of knowing, logic and reasoning are useful but only if the arguments presented do not contain fallacies and if there are alternative ways to verify the conclusions. The challenge is to critique any arguments or information presented to you and to attempt to uncover any fallacies.

Scientific Inquiry as Epistemology

Scientific inquiry or research is conducted as a means to test ideas, to evaluate questions, and to determine how things work. Generally speaking, the goal is to generate knowledge regarding the nature of our universe. The nature of our universe can range from knowing and understanding weather patterns to knowing and understanding people's exercise patterns. Scientific inquiry is simply another way of knowing, but as you will discover, it is quite different from the other epistemologies that were described previously. For one thing, "research is a disciplined way we come to know what we know" (Bouma and Atkinson, 1995, p. 9). It involves a process as described in Chapter One, but it also posits certain structures or components to that process. Concepts and structures such as *empiricism, data, theory, hypothetico-deductivism,* and *falsification* are the main building blocks of scientific inquiry and constitute the foundation of modern science. Furthermore, it is because of these concepts and structures that scientific inquiry as an epistemology is considered more reliable and valid than other methods of inquiry.

◆ ◆ ◆

In a Nutshell

Concepts and structures such as empiricism, data, theory, hypothetico-deductivism, *and* falsification *are the main building blocks of scientific inquiry and constitute the foundation of modern science.*

◆ ◆ ◆

Empiricism. From its inception, science began as a process that was viewed as objective and *empirical*. From the Greek word *emperirikós* meaning experienced or skilled, empirical is a concept that denotes observation and experimentation and is therefore linked literally to the concept of scientific inquiry. Moreover, the term *empiricism* represents the philosophical position that true knowledge is a product of sensory perceptions gleaned from observation. The strength of adopting this position is that many important research questions can be answered objectively through the collection of empirical *data*.

Data. Data are essentially concrete facts, records, or collections of information regarding some aspect of our universe that take on meaning when applied to a research question. Data are plural; datum is singular. For example, does Brand X cholesterol-lowering drug reduce LDL cholesterol more effectively than Brand Y drug? is a research question for which there is an answer that can be derived from empirical data. In this instance, empirical data collected to answer this question are the LDL cholesterol levels of people before taking the drugs and after taking the drugs. A limitation of adopting empiricism is that some questions cannot be answered in this manner because the answers cannot be derived from empirical data. For example, is Brand X cholesterol drug's name better than Brand Y cholesterol drug's name? is a question for which there is not empirical data available. Of course, we could modify the question into an empirical question by asking, do women aged forty-five to seventy-five who have high cholesterol judge

Brand X's name to be better than Brand Y's name? We could then survey women in this age category who have high cholesterol and ask them which name they prefer. The survey responses would constitute the empirical data. Thus, when conducting research to answer a health-related question, it is critical that the research question is constructed so that it is an empirical question from the beginning.

◆ ◆ ◆

In a Nutshell

Data are essentially concrete facts, records, or collections of information regarding some aspect of our universe that take on meaning when applied to a research question. Data are plural; datum is singular.

◆ ◆ ◆

Theory. If science were a movie, then theory would be the screenplay. No matter how talented the actors are, a good screenplay is still necessary to provide the framework in which the actors showcase their talents. Without the screenplay, they are simply improvising. For some talented actors, improvisation may work; however, for the majority of actors, a cohesive and intriguing plot coupled with realistic dialogue is critical. In science, theories play a major role as well because they provide an understanding of phenomena. In other words, they organize relationships among "characters" (that is, observations) into a coherent picture of what it all means. They provide a starting point for making future predictions as well. Furthermore, theories guide the research question.

◆ ◆ ◆

In a Nutshell

If science were a movie, then theory would be the screenplay.

◆ ◆ ◆

What exactly constitutes a scientific theory? How are theories generated? And how does a theory contrast with a hypothesis? Many people use the term *theory* interchangeably with *hypothesis,* and you will read instances in textbooks and research articles that use *theory* when they mean *hypothesis;* however, theory expands upon simple hypotheses and considers sets of relationships. *Hypotheses* are statements that specify the nature of the relationships between variables, whereas a *theory* is much more involved and provides order and structure to sets of relationships. For example, "obesity is related to increased risk of breast cancer among postmenopausal women" is a hypothesis that could be tested by comparing incidence of breast cancer among postmenopausal women who are not obese to incidence among postmenopausal women who are obese. A theory, however, would account for differences in breast cancer rates by describing the causative interaction of physiological, environmental, and psychological variables.

It is important to note that the phenomena involved in a theory must also be verifiable, meaning we can measure them or observe them either directly or indirectly. Once phenomena are measured or observed, understanding them translates into two types of theoretical explanations: *phenomenological* and *explanatory*. Phenomenological is when the phenomena are described and generalized, but without specific reference to causal mechanisms. In contrast, an explanatory theory identifies and explains the underling causal mechanisms.

Most theories used in health promotion research are phenomenological theories that specify which variables are involved in health-related behaviors and how the various variables interact to determine the behavior. For example, the Health Belief Model (HBM) is a theory of behavior developed in the 1950s by a group of social psychologists who wanted to better understand the widespread failure of people to participate in programs to prevent or to detect disease (Janz, Champion, and Strecher, 2002). The HBM is depicted in Figure 2.1 and posits that three major components, individual perceptions, modifying factors, and likelihood of action influence behavior. The HBM has been applied to the understanding of health behaviors where much research has generated support for the theory. Such behaviors include flu inoculations, breast self-examination, high blood pressure screening, seatbelt use, exercise, nutrition, smoking, and regular checkups. Other types of behavior that have been tested also include compliance with drug regimens, diabetic regimens, and weight loss regimens.

Given the critical role of theory in science, how are theories generated initially before they are widely implemented? In the case of the HBM, the theory grew out of the academic backgrounds of the theorists and the other theories to which they were exposed. Although there are several strategies for developing theories, such as intuition, previous knowledge, and personal observation, only two main strategies will be described in this section: *Baconian Inductivism* and *hypothetico-deductivism*. Both methods were conceptualized centuries ago and are still in use today. Each has its own strengths and weaknesses, but determining which method to use depends greatly on the domain or scope in which the theory will apply.

If Galileo was the father of modern science, Francis Bacon (1561–1626) was its champion. During the time Galileo was honing new methods to study

FIGURE 2.1. HEALTH BELIEF MODEL COMPONENTS AND LINKAGES.

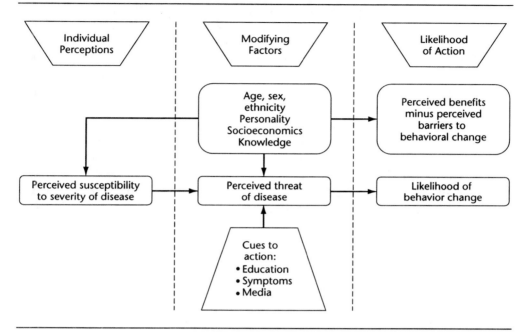

phenomena, Francis Bacon was a philosopher (among other professions) who "proposed an entirely new system based on empirical and inductive principles and the active development of new arts and inventions, a system whose ultimate goal would be the production of practical knowledge for 'the use and benefit of men' and the relief of the human condition" (Internet Encyclopedia of Philosophy, n.d., paragraph 1). His system or method was later called Baconian Inductivism, and it comprised four steps:

- Observation and classification of relevant facts
- Generalization by means of inductive reasoning
- Construction of a theoretical framework that allows one to deduce predictions from its laws and postulates
- Verification of the predictions

Although much improved over other nonscientific methods for generating knowledge, Baconian Inductivism has two major flaws: it cannot be used to derive theories regarding phenomena that are unobservable (for example, gravity), and its validity depends on a large number of observations under varying conditions.

Consequently, it did not emerge as an accepted standard for conducting scientific research and was not embraced widely. In certain instances, however, there may be no other alternative. For example, in the beginning stage of the U.S. AIDS epidemic, two physicians in Los Angeles observed that typically harmless opportunistic bacterial and viral infections among several young, gay male patients were making them extremely sick. Simultaneously, other similar observations were being noted among young, gay men in other cities. It was the emergence of these early anomalous observations that prompted scientists to convene and infer that a serious health issue was looming. From these early irregular observations general hypotheses emerged to explain these data. (See Box 2.2, which describes the various hypotheses that emerged from the data collected during the onset of the AIDS epidemic in the early 1980s.) Of course, many of the early hypotheses were flawed because they were based on a small number of observations and did not consider other varying conditions (e.g., observations from people who contracted the syndrome and were not gay).

Box 2.2. Early AIDS Hypotheses

In the beginning of the epidemic, AIDS was referred to as GRID—Gay-related immunodeficiency disease. The name was not changed to Acquired Immune Deficiency Syndrome until 1982. These are some of the early AIDS "theories" (which actually should be viewed as hypotheses) that were inferred from the available data (Garrett, 1994).

- A virus called "cytomegalovirus" or "CMV superinfection" is the root, where repeated exposures to the virus result in the deadly syndrome.
- Gay men have been exposed to too many microbes and have "microbial overload," causing the immune system to self-destruct.
- The recreation drug called "poppers" (amyl nitrites) plays a critical role in the deadly syndrome along with other gay lifestyle practices such as "fisting," "rimming," or steroid skin creams.
- AIDS is caused by some new variety of the HTLV virus, the virus that causes immune system disruptions and cancer.
- AIDS is an opportunistic infection causing disease only in persons who are already immuno-compromised from other microbes or conditions.
- AIDS is a new manifestation of the hepatitis B virus.
- AIDS is caused by an unknown contaminant of the hepatitis vaccine (early experimental trials of the vaccine had been conducted with gay men).
- AIDS is caused by African swine fever.

Following Bacon in the late 1600s, Sir Isaac Newton (1642–1727) developed a scientific method later termed "hypothetico-deductivism," which was essentially the opposite of Baconian Inductivism. His method entailed beginning with a hypothesis or statement of general principles and then subsequently using deduction to make predictions for a specific event. The predictions could be tested through empirical observation and verified. If the hypothesis is not verified then, it may be modified or rejected.

The strength of hypothetico-deductivism lies in the ability to test any hypothesis and confirm its validity through empirical observation. For example, using this method, Newton was able to test his theory of gravitation. Newton used his theory of gravitation to guide him in deducing specific predictions for which he was then able to make observations that supported or verified his theory. Thus, as a method, hypothetico-deductivism was much improved over inductivism and emerged as the new method for generating reliable and valid knowledge.

However, hypothetico-deductivisim is not without its problems. Research conducted with the main purpose of confirming a theory may, over time, become irrelevant as the theory is modified and perhaps rejected. Moreover, a set of data cannot irrevocably confirm or prove that a theory is valid because different theories can be supported by the same set of data.

◆ ◆ ◆

In a Nutshell

Research conducted with the main purpose of confirming a theory may, over time, become irrelevant as the theory is modified and perhaps rejected. Moreover, a set of data cannot irrevocably confirm or prove that a theory is valid because different theories can be supported by the same set of data.

◆ ◆ ◆

Falsification. Sir Karl Popper (1902–1994), considered one of the most influential twentieth-century philosophers of science, asserted that for a theory to be science, a necessary condition is that the theory consist of hypotheses that could be falsified. According to Popper, *falsification* is the best approach for testing scientific theories and contrasts sharply with the verification approach. The theory must be organized in a way such that its assertions can be refuted. This necessity for a scientific theory to be falsifiable is known as the *demarcation criterion*. Advocating the use of falsifiability as a scientific method to test theories, Popper therefore rejected inductivism, because falsification dictates that you must begin with falsifiable hypotheses before observations are made. Then, you collect data to refute them—not verify them. As noted earlier, it is easy for the same set of data to support or verify many different theories simultaneously. Thus, falsification provides more rigor and confidence in the conclusions.

Integration with the Research Process

Integrating the research process with these underlying scientific principles will provide a better understanding of health phenomena. To accomplish this integration, health promotion research should undertake the nine steps delineated in Chapter One while interjecting scientific structure to those steps. For example, theory should be used to aide in the development of the research question (step 2) and in the choice of variables to be measured (step 5). The research questions should be empirical questions formulated from theory and falsifiable. Moreover, the research design should allow for the falsification of the proposed hypotheses (step 4). The variables chosen also have to allow for empirical measurement. And finally, data analysis (step 8) should go beyond whether or not the data confirm or support the hypotheses to include the falsification of hypotheses. If the research process incorporates these scientific principles, then health promotion as a field will continue to expand and garner the respect of a true scientific discipline.

Summary

Over the centuries, science has revolutionized its sources of knowledge, moving from authority, tenacity, and logic and reason to an elegant arrangement encompassing principles of empiricism, data, theory, deduction, and falsification. As science is considered a process that aids in our understanding of our world, throughout time, numerous scientific disciplines pertaining to specific aspects of our world have emerged. Health promotion can be considered one of the more modern scientific disciplines, but only if it adheres to sound scientific principles. In this chapter, we reviewed the philosophy of science from its origins to better understand the underlying concepts and the importance of science to health promotion research. We noted that one of the most critical scientific principles is the generation and rigorous testing of theory. As health promotion researchers investigating health-related behaviors, most of what we do should be grounded in theory. Theory constitutes the basic structure of our scientific inquiries for two reasons: theory guides the design of basic research studies and theory can be used to design a health promotion program that targets risk factors deemed modifiable and that are related to health-related outcomes.

Issues to Consider

1. In 2001, the Department of Health and Human Services assembled a panel of experts to determine whether condoms are effective in protecting against sexually transmitted diseases. Their conclusion was that the evidence was generally insufficient to support condom effectiveness. The Centers for Disease Control later retracted their fact sheet about condoms from their Website. What are the epistemologies that apply here?

2. Because behavior cannot be isolated (like a pathogen) to determine its causes, what are some scientific issues to consider when generating theories of behavior? Also, given that human behavior, especially health-related behaviors, is complex and multifaceted, how confident would you be in attributing a specific cause to a specific behavior such as smoking?

3. A theory in the scientific sense goes beyond simple hypotheses and provides order and structure to sets of relationships. A theory must also be verifiable either directly or indirectly. Given this definition of theory, what arguments would you present in debating whether or not Creationism should be considered a scientific theory taught in high school science classes?

For Practice and Discussion

You can get a better idea of the different ways we gather knowledge and the implications of choosing one way over another by the following hypothetical example. Say, for instance, that you have been given funds to design a program to prevent heart disease. Before you decide what type of program you would like to conceptualize and implement, you determine there are several possible ways in which you can make your decision. What are all of the different sources you can turn to that will help you conceptualize your program? Will you base your decision on what a cardiologist thinks is the best approach (use authority)? If you are to use logic and reason, what are your premises and conclusion? (for example, men who make more than $100,000 per year are Type A personalities; men with Type A personality will develop heart disease; therefore, men who make more than $100,000 per year are at risk for heart disease). Are there health beliefs related to heart disease that you already know are true? (for example, an apple a day keeps the doctor away). Which approach would you base your decision on and why? How would you examine the underlying sources of the nonscientific approaches?

References

Aristotle. (350 B.C.). *On the heavens.* J. L. Stocks (trans.). Retrieved November 19, 2004, from http://classics.mit.edu/Aristotle/heavens.2.ii.html.

Bouma, G. D., and Atkinson, G.B.J. (1995). *A handbook of social science research.* New York: Oxford University Press.

Calaprice, A. (Ed.). (2000). *The expanded quotable Einstein.* Princeton, NJ: Princeton University Press.

Drake, S. (1957). *Discoveries and opinions of Galileo.* Garden City, NY: Doubleday Anchor Books.

Garrett, L. (1994). *The coming plague: Newly emerging diseases in a world out of balance.* New York: Farrar, Straus, and Giroux.

Internet Encyclopedia of Philosophy. (n.d.). Francis Bacon. Retrieved November 19, 2004, from www.iep.utm.edu/b/bacon.htm.

Janz, N. K., Champion, V. L., and Strecher, V. J. (2002). The health belief model. In K. Glanz, B. K. Rimer, and F. M. Lewis (Eds.), *Health behavior and health education* (3rd ed., pp. 45–66). San Francisco: Jossey-Bass.

Redondi, P. (1987). *Galileo: Heretic.* R. Rosenthal (trans.). Princeton, NJ: Princeton University Press.

Sobel, D. (1999). *Galileo's daughter: A historical memoir of science, faith, and love.* New York: Walker and Co.

Valtin, H. (2002). "Drink at least eight glasses of water a day." Really? Is there scientific evidence for "8 × 8"? *American Journal of Physiology—Regulatory Integrative and Comparative Physiology, 283*(5), R993–R1004.

CHAPTER THREE

ETHICAL ISSUES IN HEALTH PROMOTION RESEARCH

John F. Santelli

Ethical conduct should be intrinsic to health promotion research. Protections for research subjects are essential to prevent harm and maximize benefit. High ethical standards also apply to health promotion practice; however, specific requirements of the federal research regulations do not. Many professional associations have ethical codes of conduct that address the professional practice for the members of the association. Ethical practice in research is guided by core ethical principles including respect for persons, beneficence, and justice. Researchers receiving funds from the U.S. federal government are bound by a specific set of federal regulations designed to protect human subjects, commonly referred to as 45 CFR 46. The federal regulations incorporate special protections for vulnerable populations such as children and prisoners. These research regulations cover all biomedical and behavioral research that is federally funded; however, research institutions commonly extend these protections to participants in non–federally supported research.

I would like to thank Shelly Makleff for her timely assistance with manuscript preparation.

Ethical considerations when designing and implementing health promotion programs and research should be paramount. In fact, one author has questioned the philosophy and corresponding ethical issues underlying the practice of health promotion (Buchanan, 2000). Others have written about ethical concerns in very specific areas of health promotion practice. For example, a recent journal article covers specific ethical issues involved in conducting community-based participatory research (Minkler, 2004) and a book chapter described ethical issues relevant to community-based intervention studies (Glanz, Rimer, and Lerman, 1996). Alternatively, this chapter reviews the essential and most commonly encountered ethical issues related to health promotion research, including the ethical underpinnings of current federal regulations, differences between health promotion research and health promotion practice, regulatory requirements for research, special protections for vulnerable populations, professional codes of conduct, collaboration with communities, and common ethical issues that arise in health promotion research. It concludes with practical suggestions for working with Institutional Review Boards and ensuring that research subjects are protected. Although processes such as ethical review and informed consent are important in the protection of persons involved in health promotion research, ultimately, subjects' protection is dependent upon informed and conscientious investigators.

Illustration of Key Concepts

"Sometimes, with the best intentions, scientists and public officials and others involved in working for the benefit of us all, forget that people are people. They concentrate so totally on plans and programs, experiments, statistics—on abstractions—that people become objects, symbols on paper, figures in a mathematical formula, or impersonal 'subjects' in a study, not human beings."

THE ATLANTA CONSTITUTION, JULY 27, 1972, AS QUOTED IN JONES, 1993.

Research is essential to the advancement of health. Research can provide knowledge that leads to the creation of new health promotion programs (HPPs), and evaluation research can lead to improvement in the practice of health promotion. For specific populations (minorities, women, children, and adolescents) to receive the full benefits of research, it is critical for them to participate in health research. Unfortunately, the story of research ethics begins with episodes of terrible lapses in ethical conduct by researchers (Beecher, 1966; Lederer and Grodin, 1994).

The potential for abuse by researchers became widely understood after World War II with revelations of the atrocities committed by Nazi researchers on unwilling concentration camp inmates. Such abuse was often considered an aberration by the medical community. Yet Beecher, a Boston physician, in 1966 documented twenty-two cases in which investigators endangered "the health or the life of their subjects." All of Beecher's examples included studies that had been published in leading medical journals. One such study involved purposeful infection of severely mentally retarded residents of the Willowbrook State School with the hepatitis virus in order to study the natural history of hepatitis. Abuses have more often been documented in biomedical research, but one of the most notorious examples, the Tuskegee Syphilis Study, involved public health.

The experience of poor, African American men in the Tuskegee Study is especially instructive. The Tuskegee Study was a forty-year (1932–1972) natural history study of untreated syphilis in African American men living in Macon County, Alabama (Jones, 1993; Thomas and Quinn, 1991). It started as a demonstration project for testing and treatment of syphilis, but the Great Depression intervened and resources for treatment became scarce. The U.S. Public Health Service then converted the study into a natural history study. From a research ethics viewpoint, Tuskegee had many problems. Informed consent was not obtained from the men, who were also deceived about the purpose of certain medical procedures conducted for the research. Moreover, when penicillin became widely available for the treatment of syphilis in the mid-1940s, it still was not given to the men. In fact, investigators colluded with the local and state boards of health and with the local draft board so that they would not receive treatment. It was only after the details of the study were highlighted in the press coupled with the resulting Congressional pressure that the Public Health Service halted the study.

The public outrage to the Tuskegee Study along with other serious research abuses led directly to development of the National Commission for the Protection of Human Subjects in Biomedical and Behavioral Research, which wrote the Belmont Report, a key document in research ethics, and created many of the current federal regulations on research. Although the Tuskegee Study was finally stopped in March of 1972, it created profound distrust within the African American community regarding research and researchers. Such distrust has had a negative impact on the current research environment for AIDS, including prevention research in the African American community (Thomas and Quinn, 1991). The Tuskegee Study poignantly demonstrated the potential for initially well-intentioned researchers to fail in their ethical obligations to research subjects.

Researchers should understand this history of research abuse. Such knowledge will help them understand the stringent regulation of research. Understanding this history should motivate them to avoid repeating past mistakes. Finally, a careful understanding of this history teaches that good intentions are not sufficient to protect research subjects.

Ethical Principles from the Belmont Report

The Belmont Report, published in 1979, provides an ethical foundation for the conduct of research in the United States (U.S. Department of Health, Education, and Welfare, 1979). This short document is very readable and is an excellent primer on research ethics. Professional groups have used the ethical principles in the Belmont Report in establishing standards for the proper conduct for researchers and clinicians. The Belmont Report emphasizes three basic ethical principles: respect for persons, beneficence, and justice. Health promotion researchers should understand these principles and incorporate these into their research activities.

Respect for persons means treating people as autonomous beings and not as a means to an end. It also means honoring the capacity of individuals (whose judgment is *not* impaired) to make decisions that are in their own best interests. From the principle of respect for persons flows the notion of full disclosure and free choice for research participants. This means that research participation must be voluntary and given knowing the fundamental goals and aspects of the research. Moreover, freedom from undue persuasion to participate does not end with the start of the research but continues throughout the research study. Respect for persons also demands that special protections be extended to groups with diminished autonomy when they are included in research studies. This includes persons with diminished capacity for informed consent, such as children and those who are cognitively impaired, and those who are unable to exercise free choice such as prisoners. For these groups, certain types of research are not permitted. With children, informed consent processes are tailored to their specific circumstances and abilities. Most children attain adult cognitive capacity during early adolescence. While younger children may not be capable of understanding all the details of an informed consent form, they generally understand salient risks and benefits. Researchers should provide information that is developmentally appropriate and understandable to children. Given that teenagers have cognitive capacity similar to adults, the informed consent process for teenagers should include similar information found in adult consent forms.

Beneficence is the ethical obligation to do good and to avoid harm. In research this means maximizing benefits and minimizing risks. Federal policies to extend the benefits of research to women, minorities, children, and adolescents by promoting their inclusion in research studies are motivated by this principle of beneficence.

Beneficence provides the ethical basis for conducting research that seeks to improve the health and well being of participants. It provides a general guideline that helps determine the acceptability of a research study by creating a balance of the predicted benefits against the predicted risks. Researchers must consider what the potential benefits and risks may be to individual research participants and to groups, and precludes researchers from causing harm to any research participant regardless of the benefit to others.

When considering the benefits of a proposed research study, it is first important to consider *what* the benefits are; however, it may be virtually impossible to truly estimate all the potential benefits. If all the benefits were known, then there would be no point in conducting the research. Nevertheless, an assessment of potential benefits must be made in order to judge the ethics of the proposed research.

The second thing to consider is *who* benefits. The proposed research may have important benefits to individuals, specific groups such as women at risk of HIV infection, specific ethnic communities, or all of the above. For example, research on school-based programs to reduce HIV-related risk behaviors may benefit not only the young people who receive the curriculum but also future generations of teenagers. Thus, there is a concept of benefits accruing directly for the participants involved while also providing indirect benefits for future generations. However, survey research to understand HIV risk behaviors may accrue no direct

MINCUS AGREES TO PARTICIPATE IN DR. DINCUS'S DNA STUDY.

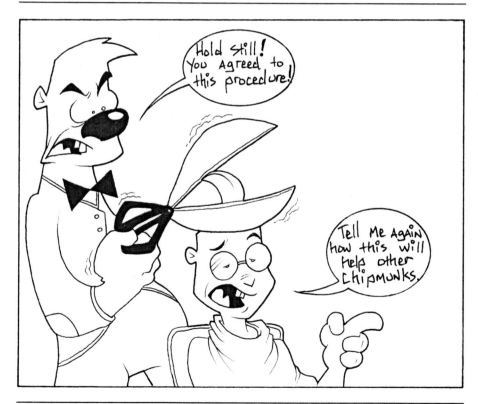

benefit to the participants but may provide significant benefits to others at risk of HIV if the research is applied in the design of targeted and effective intervention programs.

Justice entails a fair distribution of the benefits and burdens of research. The principle of justice demands a fair sharing of both risks and benefits and is important in the selection of research participants. The interests of justice demand that specific communities or specific groups not be exploited for the benefits of others, nor should they be excluded from participation in research that may have direct or indirect benefit to them. Research should not be conducted with groups or communities who are unlikely to benefit from the findings. For example, HIV treatment research conducted overseas by U.S. researchers has been questioned, when citizens of those countries are unlikely to benefit directly from the new treatments that are being tested. Likewise, promoting participation by groups that historically have been excluded from research is founded on the principle of justice. If certain groups of persons are systematically excluded from participation in research, then these groups may not share in the beneficial results of that research. For example, if women are not included in cardiovascular prevention trials, clinicians cannot be sure that interventions that are tested will be effective with women.

◆ ◆ ◆

In a Nutshell

The principle of justice demands a fair sharing of both risks and benefits and is important in the selection of research participants.

◆ ◆ ◆

Federal Inclusion Policies

Federal inclusion policies are motivated by the ethical principles outlined in the Belmont Report. The principles of the Belmont Report, given historical research abuses, are focused on protecting individuals from harmful research. These same principles are also used to weigh the potential benefits with the potential risks of research participation. Such an understanding has fostered the development of policies designed to promote a policy of inclusiveness in research. Such thinking and policies represent a fundamental shift in ethical thinking and federal regulatory approaches, in which the focus is still on *protection* but there is now an added emphasis on *access* (Levine, 1995). Such policies suggest that participation in research is essential if individuals and groups are to accrue the full benefits of research. During the 1990s, children and adolescents, women, and minority groups won rights to increased access to participation in research. AIDS activists, women, and minority health advocates led successful campaigns demanding access to research which led to the enactment of the National Institutes of Health (NIH) Revitalization Act of 1993. The *NIH Policy and Guidelines on the Inclusion of Women and Minorities as Subjects in Clinical Research* (promulgated in 1994 and revised in 2001) were intended "to ensure that all future NIH-supported biomedical and behavioral research involving human subjects will be carried out in a manner sufficient to elicit information about individuals of both genders and the diverse racial and ethnic groups and, in the case of clinical trials, to examine differential effects on such groups" (National Institutes of Health, 2001).

In 1998, given concerns about exclusion of children from research, the NIH issued the *NIH Policy and Guidelines on the Inclusion of Children as Participants in Research Involving Human Subjects* (National Institutes of Health, 1998). The goal of this policy was to increase the participation of children in research so that adequate data will be developed to support the treatment modalities for disorders and conditions that affect adults and may also affect children (National Institutes of Health, 1998). This policy specifies that children must be included in all human subjects' research, conducted or supported by the NIH, unless there are scientific and ethical reasons not to include them. Although much of the impetus for inclusion policies was fair access to clinical trials, notions of inclusion have also been applied to health promotion research.

Policies promoting inclusion in research are rooted in the principle of justice and the concept of nondiscrimination. Research has been "transformed" from being perceived as a fundamentally dangerous activity from which persons must be protected, to being seen as entailing a balance of risk and benefit. Although research may entail risk, it holds the potential of bringing much benefit. Demands for increased participation of women, minorities, and children in research have occurred due to a changing societal understanding about the risks and benefits of participation in research. Health promotion researchers will need to address both inclusion and protection.

◆ ◆ ◆

In a Nutshell

Health promotion researchers will need to address both inclusion and protection.

◆ ◆ ◆

Codes of Ethical Conduct

Although specific federal regulations govern research, professional codes of conduct are designed more broadly to set standards of conduct for both research and practice. A code of ethics is designed to reflect the profession's collective conscience and to promote ethical behaviors based on the collective experiences and traditions of the scientific discipline (Frankel, 1992). A code can be used to evaluate the behavior of individual professionals as well as to create a collective responsibility within a profession. A profession's code of ethics may also contribute to the socialization of new professionals by providing guidance on and standards of expected behavior. Finally, a code of ethics establishes standards that may be used by legislative, administrative, and judicial bodies in adjudicating allegations of misconduct (Frankel, 1992). Thus, the ethical principles found in the Belmont Report, while intended to govern research, also provide a basis for ethical conduct in professional practice.

What Is Health Promotion Research, and What Is Health Promotion Practice?

It is important to understand the distinctions between research and practice within the context of ethical principles and federal regulatory guidelines. The Belmont Report provides guidance on the boundaries between practice and research (U.S. Department of Health, Education, and Welfare, 1979). Similarly, public health researchers have attempted to distinguish between public health practice and public health research (Snider and Stroup, 1997). These documents may be helpful in understanding key differences between health promotion *research* and the *practice* of health promotion. As stated previously, there are ethical standards that apply to health promotion practice; however, it is important to understand that the specific regulatory requirements that apply to *research* do not apply to health promotion *practice*.

Health promotion research includes activities designed or *intended* to contribute to generalizable knowledge. The critical word here is *intended;* research is defined by the intentions of the researchers. Research is often expressed in terms of theory, principles, and statements of relationships (U.S. Department of Health, Education, and Welfare, 1979). Results are often published in research journals. In research, there may be benefits to the individual, but a primary objective is to provide benefits to others via enhanced understanding or knowledge. An experimental evaluation of a new drug prevention curriculum compared to standard health education would generally be considered research. Likewise, a school survey to explore potential new risk factors for drug use among adolescents would be research under this definition. The intention of the survey is to enhance knowledge.

Health promotion practice refers to interventions designed solely to help the individual or group; such interventions are generally recognized as being beneficial or efficacious (U.S. Department of Health, Education, and Welfare, 1979). Health promotion practice may include health education, behavioral interventions such as counseling, and data collection designed to monitor or improve existing programs and policies to enhance health. Publication of results in a research journal is generally not a goal. For example, delivery of a well-evaluated drug prevention curriculum in a public school would generally be considered health promotion practice. Process evaluation to see that the program is well delivered would generally be considered health promotion practice, as the primary benefit is for those receiving the intervention. Likewise, routine, periodic public health surveillance of adolescent drug use via school surveys to assess the need for drug prevention programs and to monitor prevention activities would also be considered practice. There is no intention to contribute to generalizable knowledge; rather the intention is to directly improve prevention practices in these schools.

Practitioners have responsibilities to individual program participants. Researchers have responsibilities to individual participants but also to the integrity of the research. These responsibilities may be in conflict and such conflicts may not be readily apparent to the researcher. Given these dual responsibilities and the potential for harm to research participants, a higher level of scrutiny is required for research than practice. Such scrutiny generally requires review by an Institutional Review Board (IRB).

An IRB is regulated and controlled by the federal government, specifically the Office for Human Research Protections (OHRP). The OHRP provides leadership and oversight on all matters related to the protection of human subjects participating in research conducted or supported by the U.S. Department of Health and Human Services (DHHS). The OHRP helps ensure that such research is carried out in accordance with the highest ethical standards and in an environment where all who are involved in the conduct or oversight of human subjects research understand their primary responsibility for protecting the rights, welfare, and well-being of subjects (U.S. Department of Health and Human Services, 2005).

In addition to human subjects' protection, the regulations also provide standards for the membership of each institution's IRB. An IRB must have at least five members, with varying backgrounds, to ensure adequate ethical review for research activities commonly conducted by the institution. Considerations include the experience and expertise of IRB members, sensitivity to the community, and diversity in terms of race, gender, and cultural backgrounds. The IRB must be capable of reviewing proposed research studies in terms of scientific knowledge, institutional commitments and regulations, applicable law, and standards of professional conduct. IRB members should be knowledgeable in these various aspects of the research endeavor. If an IRB commonly reviews research that involves vulnerable subjects, such as children or prisoners, then the IRB should consider including individuals who are knowledgeable about and experienced in working with these groups. The IRB membership must include at least one scientist member, one nonscientist, and one member not otherwise affiliated with the institution. The regulations require initial review by the IRB and annual review while the research is ongoing.

◆ ◆ ◆

In a Nutshell

An IRB must have at least five members, with varying backgrounds, to ensure adequate ethical review for research activities commonly conducted by the institution.

◆ ◆ ◆

Federal Regulations on Research

U.S. regulations on research (U.S. Department of Health and Human Services, 2005) provide for a nationwide system of IRBs located within specific research institutions and regulated by the OHRP in the DHHS. Institutions conducting research provide an "assurance" to OHRP regarding their capability to comply with the federal regulations by creating a written set of institutional standards on how they will review research in order to protect human subjects. Once the assurance is accepted by the federal government, an assurance number is issued. Federal assurance is contingent on periodic review of the institution's IRB procedures. An institution can lose its federal assurance to conduct research if it fails to meet high standards. OHRP over the past several years has publicly revoked the federal assurances at prominent research universities, stopping all federally funded research (Levine, 2001). Researchers must understand and follow these regulations in all their research activities.

An institution's IRB provides ethical review and approval for all research funded by the U.S. federal government and involving human participants unless the study is determined to be *exempt* (in other words, IRB review is not required). Most institutions in the United States extend the protections of the federal regulations to all research conducted within the institution, including non–federally funded research. For each study, the appropriate IRB must assess the risks and benefits to human participants, ensure proper informed consent procedures, and provide special protections for vulnerable populations. Special safeguards cover pregnant women and the fetus, prisoners, and children. Special sections of the regulations, called subparts, address special protections for specific vulnerable populations. Pregnant women, human fetuses, and neonates are covered under Subpart B; prisoners under Subpart C; and children under Subpart D (U.S. Department of Health and Human Services, 2005). Other populations such as persons who are disabled, who have impaired cognitive capacities, or who are poor and socially disenfranchised do not have special sections in the regulations per se, but nonetheless receive special consideration. The U.S. federal regulations also cover many practical aspects of ethical review including the composition of IRBs, how often research must be reviewed, IRB records, the elements of informed consent, circumstances under which informed consent may be waived, and categories of exempt research.

Certain categories of research are considered exempt from IRB review because they represent little or no risk to human participants (see Table 3.1). Most research institutions require a review by the IRB office to verify an exempt status. As shown in the table, the categories of exempt research that commonly apply to health promotion research are category 2, which involves certain types of interviews and surveys, and category 4, which involves data that are publicly available or where persons cannot be identified. Notably, exemption category 2 does not apply to surveys and interviews with children.

Likewise, certain research requires IRB review that is considered *expedited* (that is, can be reviewed by a single IRB board member such as the chairperson). Expedited research can present no more than minimal risk to human subjects. For a current list of categories of research that can be reviewed in an expedited fashion, see the Department of Health and Human Services Website: www.hhs.gov/ohrp/humansubjects/guidance/expedited98.htm (retrieved March 8, 2005). Expedited categories relevant to health promotion research include certain research employing surveys, interviews, oral histories, focus groups, and program evaluation; and continuing review of research previously approved by the convened IRB.

Consistent with the Belmont Report, the regulatory definition of research is "a systematic investigation, including research development, testing and evaluation, designed to develop or contribute to generalizable knowledge" (U.S. Department of Health and Human Services, 2005, section 46.102). This definition and the federal regulations on research apply no matter what the specific mechanism

TABLE 3.1. CATEGORIES OF EXEMPT RESEARCH
IN THE U.S. FEDERAL REGULATIONS.

Exact Language of the Federal Regulations	Common Interpretations and Examples
(Category 1) Research conducted in established or commonly accepted educational settings, involving normal educational practices, such as (i) research on regular and special education instructional strategies, or (ii) research on the effectiveness of or the comparison among instructional techniques, curricula, or classroom management methods.	This applies to education research. It generally does not include health research conducted in schools.
(Category 2) Research involving the use of educational tests (cognitive, diagnostic, aptitude, achievement), survey procedures, interview procedures or observation of public behavior, unless: (i) information obtained is recorded in such a manner that human subjects can be identified, directly or through identifiers linked to the subjects; and (ii) any disclosure of the human subjects' responses outside the research could reasonably place the subjects at risk of criminal or civil liability or be damaging to the subjects' financial standing, employability, or reputation.	This includes focus groups, health surveys, and interviews if they are not sensitive or conducted anonymously. Importantly, exempt research in this category does not cover research involving children, such as school surveys.
(Category 3) Research involving the use of educational tests (cognitive, diagnostic, aptitude, achievement), survey procedures, interview procedures, or observation of public behavior that is not exempt under paragraph (b)(2) of this section, if: (i) the human subjects are elected or appointed public officials or candidates for public office; or (ii) Federal statute(s) require(s) without exception that the confidentiality of the personally identifiable information will be maintained throughout the research and thereafter.	This is not a commonly used category. It is similar to category 2, but involving public officials or candidates, or federal statutes providing for confidentiality of personally identifiable information.
(Category 4) Research involving the collection or study of existing data, documents, records, pathological specimens, or diagnostic specimens, if these sources are publicly available or if the information is recorded by the investigator in such a manner that subjects cannot be identified, directly or through identifiers linked to the subjects.	This applies generally to research on existing data that is publicly available or where subjects cannot be identified.

TABLE 3.1.   (*Continued*)

Exact Language of the Federal Regulations	Common Interpretations and Examples
(Category 5) Research and demonstration projects which are conducted by or subject to the approval of Department or Agency heads, and which are designed to study, evaluate, or otherwise examine: (i) Public benefit or service programs; (ii) procedures for obtaining benefits or services under those programs; (iii) possible changes in or alternatives to those programs or procedures; or (iv) possible changes in methods or levels of payment for benefits or services under those programs.	This applies to research involving public benefit or service programs that is approved by federal department or agency heads.
(Category 6) Taste and food quality evaluation and consumer acceptance studies, (i) if wholesome foods without additives are consumed or (ii) if a food is consumed that contains a food ingredient at or below the level and for a use found to be safe, or agricultural chemical or environmental contaminant at or below the level found to be safe, by the Food and Drug Administration or approved by the Environmental Protection Agency or the Food Safety and Inspection Service of the U.S. Department of Agriculture.	This applies to certain kinds of research on food preferences.

Source: U.S. Department of Health and Human Services, 2005, section 46.101.

for federal funding. For example, a federally funded public service program (such as Head Start) may be deemed primarily as nonresearch but may practice activities that would be considered research. These activities would then be subject to the U.S. federal regulations.

The purpose of the federal regulations is to protect human subjects participating in research. The federal regulations define *human subject* as "a living individual about whom an investigator (whether professional or student) conducting research obtains (1) data through intervention or interaction with the individual, or (2) identifiable private information" (U.S. Department of Health and Human Services, 2005, Section 46.102). This definition excludes information on deceased persons. Caution should be exercised, however. Health information about a deceased person, such as his or her HIV status, may have important implications for the privacy of living persons.

The federal regulations provide specific criteria for IRB approval of a research protocol. These criteria require that

- Risks to subjects are minimized.
- Risks to subjects are reasonable in relation to anticipated benefits, if any, to subjects, and the importance of the knowledge that may reasonably be expected to result.
- Selection of subjects is equitable.
- Informed consent is sought from each prospective subject or the subject's legally authorized representative.
- Informed consent is appropriately documented.
- When appropriate, the research plan includes adequate provision for monitoring data collection to ensure the safety of subjects.
- When appropriate, adequate provisions are in place to protect the privacy of subjects and to maintain the confidentiality of data.

Informed consent is a central practice for protecting human subjects, and the federal regulations define specific requirements for the process of obtaining informed consent and the specific content of the informed consent document. Informed consent, as described in the Belmont Report, includes three key elements: full information, adequate comprehension, and free choice. Consent is generally obtained from the research subject, although permission may be sought from a guardian or surrogate for individuals or classes of persons, such as children, who are unable to consent for themselves. The criteria for informed consent in the federal regulations are found in Figure 3.1. A sample of an informed consent form is provided in the appendix to this chapter.

◆ ◆ ◆

In a Nutshell

Consent is generally obtained from the research subject, although permission may be sought from a guardian or surrogate for individuals or classes of persons, such as children, who are unable to consent for themselves.

◆ ◆ ◆

Although informed consent and documentation of informed consent by the person's signature on a consent form are general requirements for research, under certain circumstances an IRB may waive requirements for informed consent

FIGURE 3.1.   GENERAL REQUIREMENTS FOR INFORMED CONSENT (45 CFR 46.116).

1. A statement that the study involves research, an explanation of the purposes of the research and the expected duration of the subject's participation, a description of the procedures to be followed, and identification of any procedures which are experimental
2. A description of any reasonably foreseeable risks or discomforts to the subject
3. A description of any benefits to the subject or to others which may reasonably be expected from the research
4. A disclosure of appropriate alternative procedures or courses of treatment, if any, that might be advantageous to the subject
5. A statement describing the extent, if any, to which confidentiality of records identifying the subject will be maintained
6. For research involving more than minimal risk, an explanation as to whether any compensation and an explanation as to whether any medical treatments are available if injury occurs and, if so, what they consist of, or where further information may be obtained
7. An explanation of whom to contact for answers to pertinent questions about the research and research subjects' rights, and whom to contact in the event of a research-related injury to the subject
8. A statement that participation is voluntary, refusal to participate will involve no penalty or loss of benefits to which the subject is otherwise entitled, and the subject may discontinue participation at any time without penalty or loss of benefits to which the subject is otherwise entitled

Additional elements of informed consent. When appropriate, one or more of the following elements of information shall also be provided to each subject.

1. A statement that the particular treatment or procedure may involve risks to the subject (or to the embryo or fetus, if the subject is or may become pregnant) which are currently unforeseeable
2. Anticipated circumstances under which the subject's participation may be terminated by the investigator without regard to the subject's consent
3. Any additional costs to the subject that may result from participation in the research
4. The consequences of a subject's decision to withdraw from the research and procedures for orderly termination of participation by the subject
5. A statement that significant new findings developed during the course of the research which may relate to the subject's willingness to continue participation will be provided to the subject
6. The approximate number of subjects involved in the study

and documentation of informed consent. For example, IRBs commonly waive documentation of written informed consent for telephone interviews when it would be impractical to obtain a signature. Similarly, an IRB may waive informed consent for review of existing health records when obtaining consent would be impractical and the risk is minimal. Criteria for granting these two kinds of waivers are found in sections 46.116 and 46.117 of the federal regulations.

For example, under section 46.117 a signature is not always required. Although this may seem counterintuitive at first, consider a study that is said to be anonymous. Unlike with confidential studies, an anonymous study does not involve the collection of names. The anonymous nature of the study may be important to potential volunteers, and often recruitment efforts will feature the point that "your participation is entirely anonymous." Given such a pledge to volunteers, imagine what their reaction would be if they were asked to sign an informed consent form. Thus, an IRB can grant the study permission to obtain verbal rather than written consent. In this case, volunteers may be provided with formalized, written information about the study. Of course, the informed consent form (minus the signature blanks) can serve this purpose well.

Yet another key point regarding the informed consent document is the question of what qualifies as a potential benefit to the participant. First, it is important not to confuse compensation with benefit. Compensation is typically a cash payment (or its equivalent) that is used to formally recognize that volunteers have given their time to the study. Their time is considered valuable, and thus payment is made to compensate them for this time. It is not a benefit. Second, there may be instances in which there is no direct benefit to the participant, and this should be stated in the consent form. Third, accurately describing the level of potential benefit is important because the level of risk and the level of benefit will ultimately be weighed by the IRB to determine approval or disapproval of the protocol. Thus, the following guidelines are offered to help you think about potential benefit.

- Receipt of an effective education program is a potential benefit.
- A question and answer session following an assessment is a potential benefit of study participation.
- Having free screening tests (for example, tests for a disease) is a potential benefit.
- Any treatment provided in the context of the study, that would not otherwise occur, is a potential benefit.
- Providing referral services to study participants is a potential benefit.

Any explanation of the potential benefits that could reasonably be anticipated must also be accompanied by an explanation of potential risks. Likelihood of risk and magnitude of risk are both important; common risks and potential serious risk should be included in the consent form. Risk can pertain to physical problems or disorders and to a host of emotional, mental, and social problems that could potentially occur as a result of study participation. Guidelines for thinking about risk in health promotion research are provided in the following list.

◆ ◆ ◆

In a Nutshell

Risk can pertain to physical problems or disorders and to a host of emotional, mental, and social problems that could potentially occur as a result of study participation.

◆ ◆ ◆

- Potential risk exists if the study records of the volunteer are identifiable and contain sensitive information.
- If the assessment process could lead to emotional or mental distress then that risk should be disclosed.
- If participation in the intervention could cause emotional, mental, or social distress then that risk should be disclosed.
- For some studies, simply being in the study may cause emotional, mental, or social distress when friends, family members, or sex partners of the volunteer discover that the volunteer is participating. This risk should be anticipated and disclosed.
- Physically invasive procedures, even those that are routine (such as a Pap test), may entail risk, and this risk should be disclosed.

Another critically important aspect of the informed consent document is that it must be written in language that is comprehensible to the study volunteers. This means that the choice of terms and the overall reading level must be appropriate to the people who will compose the sample (Hochhauser, 2003). Many IRBs require that informed consent forms be graded for reading level. For example, typically IRBs require the consent for general U.S. populations to be at an eighth grade reading level. For research presenting significant risk, the research team should check for understanding before consent is obtained.

Regulation of Research Involving Vulnerable Populations

As noted previously, the federal regulations provide special protection for several populations, including children, prisoners, pregnant women, human fetuses, and neonates. These special protections commonly require a higher level of scrutiny by the IRB, restrictions or prohibitions on particular kinds of research (for instance, research involving greater than minimal risk), and alternative procedures for obtaining informed consent, such as requesting the permission of a parent or guardian. Certain research with pregnant women requires the permission of both the pregnant woman and the father of the fetus. In this section we detail some of the specific requirements for research with prisoners and children, including adolescents.

Requirements for Research with Prisoners. Prisoners are afforded special consideration when they are the subjects of research. Some of the worst abuses in the history of human subjects' maltreatment involved Nazi prisoners during World War II. Even where penal systems are not inherently malevolent, incarceration severely limits the ability of prisoners to make voluntary decisions about research participation. The inherently coercive nature of prison implies that full voluntary informed consent may be precluded. Subpart C of the federal regulations describes additional duties of IRBs in reviewing research involving prisoners. When reviewing prisoner research, the IRB must include at least one board member who is a prisoner or a prisoner representative who is sensitive to the circumstances of prisoners. Research involving prisoners may require review by the Secretary of the DHHS and publication in the Federal Register. Research with prisoners is limited to four categories as found in section 46.306 and shown in Box 3.1

Requirements for Research with Children, Including Adolescents. Special protections for children, including minor adolescents, are covered in Subpart D. Within this context, children are defined as persons who have not attained the legal age for consenting to treatments or procedures involved in the research. Under this subpart, a hierarchy of risk and benefit is used in defining the specific protections required. The four categories of research involving children are research that

- Involves no more than minimal risk
- Involves more than minimal risk, but there is a potential for direct benefit to individual research subjects
- Involves a minor increase over minimal risk without direct benefit, but research is likely to yield generalizable knowledge about the subject's disorder or condition
- Is not otherwise approvable but presents an opportunity to understand, prevent, or alleviate a serious problem affecting the health or welfare of children

Minimal risk is defined as follows: "The probability and magnitude of harm or discomfort anticipated . . . are not greater . . . than those ordinarily encountered in daily life or during the performance of routine physical or psychological examinations or tests" (U.S. Department of Health and Human Services, 2005, section 46.102).

___

Box 3.1. Research with Prison Populations, Section 46.306

A. Study of the possible causes, effects, and processes of incarceration, and of criminal behavior, provided that the study presents no more than minimal risk and no more than inconvenience to the subjects

B. Study of prisons as institutional structures or of prisoners as incarcerated persons, provided that the study presents no more than minimal risk and no more than inconvenience to the subjects

C. Research on conditions particularly affecting prisoners as a class (for example, vaccine trials and other research on hepatitis which is much more prevalent in prisons than elsewhere; and research on social and psychological problems such as alcoholism, drug addiction, and sexual assaults) provided that the study may proceed only after the Secretary has consulted with appropriate experts including experts in penology, medicine, and ethics, and published notice, in the Federal Register, of his intent to approve such research

D. Research on practices, both innovative and accepted, which have the intent and reasonable probability of improving the health or well-being of the subject. In cases in which those studies require the assignment of prisoners in a manner consistent with protocols approved by the IRB to control groups which may not benefit from the research, the study may proceed only after the Secretary has consulted with appropriate experts, including experts in penology, medicine, and ethics, and published notice, in the Federal Register, of the intent to approve such research.

___

Source: Department of Health and Human Services, 2005, Section 46.306.

___

Specific requirements exist for each category of risk and benefit. All four categories require the *assent* of the child and the *permission* of one or both parents. Assent is the child's affirmative agreement to participate in research, whereas permission is the agreement of parent(s) or guardians to their child's or ward's participation in research. The federal regulations use the terms *permission* and *assent* to distinguish these processes from the usual informed consent process. Parents are not the research subjects and generally do not experience risks or benefits from the research. Children may lack the intellectual capacity or judgment to make decisions about research, although the concept of assent recognizes the emerging developmental capacity of children to provide informed consent. By the recommendations of the National Commission, assent is commonly obtained from children who are aged seven and older. For minor adolescents who are more cognitively developed (that is, beginning at twelve to fourteen years of age), the content of assent forms may closely resemble that for consent forms used with adults. In some instances, when obtaining parental consent is problematic, the federal regulations governing research dictate that the IRB may waive parental permission.

IRBs may determine that parental permission would not be appropriate because of the nature of the topic under investigation, for example, research involving confidential health care when adolescents may legally receive treatment without parental consent and research involving mature minors, that is, those capable of making a good decision about participation (Society for Adolescent Medicine, 2003). Section 46.408 states

> In addition to the provisions for waiver contained in 46.116 of Subpart A, if an IRB determines that a research protocol is designed for conditions or a subject population for which parental permission is not a reasonable requirement to protect subjects (e.g., neglected or abused children), it may waive consent requirements provided an appropriate mechanism for protecting the children who will participate as research subjects is substituted and provided the waiver is not inconsistent with federal, state, or local law [U.S. Department of Health and Human Services, 2005].

Similar to the protections provided to prisoners, special protections are also provided to children who are wards of the state (for example, those in foster care).

Research in Schools

When health promotion research is conducted in schools additional regulatory requirements are covered by two federal laws: the Family Educational Rights and Privacy Act (FERPA) and the Protection of Pupil Rights Amendment (PPRA). FERPA addresses the privacy of student educational records and the circumstances under which educational records may be accessed, amended, or disclosed. PPRA specifically addresses surveys administered in schools. PPRA requires that written parental permission be obtained for students who are not emancipated prior to participation in surveys or evaluations, funded partially or fully by the U.S. Department of Education (DOE), that collect information about eight specific topics: mental health and psychological problems; sexual behaviors or attitudes; illegal, antisocial, self-incriminating, or demeaning behaviors; critical appraisals of individuals with whom respondents have close family relationships; religious practices, affiliations, or beliefs; political affiliations or beliefs; income; and legally recognized privileged relationships such as those with physicians, lawyers, or ministers. Surveys not funded by the DOE that address any of these eight topics may be conducted after parental notification and after allowing parents an opportunity to opt their child out of participation. Parents have a right to inspect questionnaires and instructional material used in conjunction with surveys, analyses, or evaluations. Local education agencies must notify parents at least annually about school policies regarding these rights and any upcoming surveys. These rights transfer to students when a student becomes an adult or is emancipated. Additional information can be found at www.ed.gov/policy/gen/guid/fpco/ index.html and at www.ed.gov/policy/gen/guid/fpco/hottopics/ht10-28-02.html?exp=0 (retrieved March 4, 2005).

Health Insurance Portability and Accountability Act

The Health Insurance Portability and Accountability Act of 1996, commonly known as HIPAA, is designed to ensure the confidentiality of medical records and private health information. HIPPAA requirements may come into play in health promotion research that is conducted in health care delivery settings. HIPAA provisions also address patients' access to their own medical records and privacy protections that govern both clinical care and research. HIPAA addresses privacy rights of children and adolescents. A full review of HIPAA is beyond the scope of this chapter. Additional information can be found at www.hhs.gov/ocr/hipaa/ (retrieved March 8, 2005).

Risks and Benefits of Health Promotion Research

Health promotion research, like other research, offers the potential for health benefits and presents specific risks. Health promotion research commonly includes intervention programs to reduce harmful behaviors and to increase protective behaviors, as well as projects designed to improve understanding of the factors influencing health-related behaviors. Such research commonly collects data on personal behaviors and behavioral determinants, including sexual practices, alcohol and other drug use, mental health concerns, and perceived support for prevention practices. In contrast to biomedical research, health promotion research generally presents minimal risk to participants. Principal risks may include invasion of privacy, embarrassment, stress and discomfort, loss of self-esteem, and potential loss of confidentiality regarding private information and personal behaviors. Loss of privacy resulting from health promotion research is generally a rare phenomenon. Although the risks of participating in health promotion research may be minimal or even trivial compared to those in biomedical research, the potential risks still must be weighed against the potential benefits to justify the research. Health promotion research may benefit the individuals or groups by improving understanding of adverse health outcomes, by reducing involvement in health risk behaviors, and in the prevention of both. Moreover, completion of surveys may increase self-understanding of one's own risk, and by raising such understanding, survey research may facilitate the process of seeking care. Potential benefits from the informed consent process may include an increased sense of self-control and increased decision-making capacity.

Improving Ethical Practice: Working with Communities

Communities may view the intentions of researchers with skepticism, and these perceptions are not without justification. The legacies of Tuskegee and other abusive research projects have given rise to a mistrust of researchers in many communities (Thomas and Quinn, 1991). Communities may fear direct harm to community members or indirect harm such as when unflattering research findings stigmatize their community.

The involvement of community may enhance human subjects' protection and improve the scientific quality of health promotion research (Melton, Levine, Koocher, Rosenthal, and Thompson, 1988; Quinn, 2004; Society for Adolescent Medicine, 2003; and Sieber and Stanley, 1988). Community consultation provides a context for research findings and may help the researcher to better understand the meaning of behaviors. Community involvement may provide insight into the underlying forces influencing health and may lead to stronger programs that serve to improve health. Community advice on the acceptability and feasibility of study approaches can save resources. Early dissemination of research findings to the community may increase confidence in the research process and help community members understand the potential benefits from research. Likewise, community involvement can assist in the dissemination of health practices and programs shown to be effective. When communities partner with researchers, they learn useful skills and obtain knowledge that can enhance their ability to advocate for community programs and services. Community advisory boards can make communities integral partners in health promotion research.

Practical Guidance

To assist researchers, here is some practical advice for ensuring the ethical conduct of health promotion research:

- The IRB, the informed consent process, and the researcher all have important roles in protecting human subjects. Before submitting a protocol to the IRB, make sure you've considered all potential risks and protections for human subjects. Work with the IRB in helping it understand your research aims, risks and benefits, and your plan to protect human subjects.
- In writing a research protocol for IRB review, explain and justify your plans for human subjects' protection in terms of ethical principles and the specific

requirements of the regulations. For example, if you are requesting an alteration to or waiver of informed consent, provide an ethical rationale for this change and justify this change according to the specific requirements of the federal regulations.

- Strive to understand research involvement from the viewpoint of the research subject. Informed consent documents should address the concerns of the subject and provide them the information needed to make a free and informed decision. Strive to make the informed consent form readable and easily understood.
- IRBs are made up of busy people who have an important mission to protect human subjects. Do your part to create an attitude of mutual respect and openness. Be clear in your written communications to the IRB.
- Make sure that the confidentiality of data is maintained throughout the process of data collection and analysis. Remove identifiers from the data when they are no longer needed.
- Work with the community in preparing the research protocol, conducting the research and disseminating results. Understand community concerns and incorporate these into your research plan.

Remember that the ethical conduct of an informed investigator is the ultimate mechanism for protecting human subjects.

Applied Example

As noted previously in this chapter, Appendix A displays a sample informed consent document. Careful inspection of this document can be quite informative. For example, you will see that the study is a cross-sectional survey designed to assess people's feelings about being screened for colorectal cancer. The survey is estimated to take from forty-five to sixty minutes to complete. The study procedures are outlined for potential volunteers to read. However, it is critically important to remember that the event of obtaining informed consent is viewed as a platform for having a dialogue with potential volunteers about the study procedures.

The informed consent form is intentionally simple. Note that the language used in the form is basic and unsophisticated. It is written at a reading level appropriate for someone in seventh grade. Note also that the sentences are rather short (compound sentences are avoided) and that the document avoids giving potential volunteers an abundance of information. Instead, the document simply provides people with basic information pertaining to the study and describes the likely risks and benefits of participation. It should also be noted that the $20 compensation is mentioned but not emphasized in any way. After reading the form people should have an opportunity to clarify any questions they may have.

Finally, the document shown in Appendix A also provides an example of the principles outlined in the Belmont Report. *Respect for persons*, for example, is demonstrated throughout the document and should be adhered to throughout the informed consent process. The essential spirit of the document and process is to allow people to autonomously decide whether they want to take part in the study. Note that the document specifically informs that such a decision can be revoked at any time, without giving a reason. *Beneficence* is also apparent in the document. The benefits described are benefits to the volunteers. Although the document does state that "we [doctors, researchers and scientists] may learn new things that will help prevent cancer deaths," it does so only after listing personal benefits and then specifically stating that other personal benefits will not occur. Finally, the principle of *justice* may be apparent to students of public health practice. The challenge of promoting colorectal cancer screening has been a long-standing question in health promotion practice and the study apparently seeks data from people who will also ultimately benefit from any applied practice resulting from the brief intervention program.

Integration with the Research Process

Ethical considerations should be at the forefront of your mind from the inception of a research project until the last paper has been published. Thus, each step of the nine-step model shown in Chapter One should be taken in harmony with the ethical considerations described in this chapter. Steps 1 and 2, for example, address the principle of justice. The question must be asked, is this an important research question for this particular population? Unless the answer is clearly "yes," the research may be unlikely to meet the principle of beneficence. In other words, when you tell someone, "Your participation in this study will help others," the statement should be true to form and not simply a vacuous phrase designed to inspire volunteerism.

◆ ◆ ◆

In a Nutshell

Each step of the nine-step model shown in Chapter One should be taken in harmony with the ethical considerations described in this chapter.

◆ ◆ ◆

As you continue to read the remaining twelve chapters of this book, you will begin to see that every aspect of the research process is linked to ethics. This is the case when selecting a study design, conducting program evaluation, or even analyzing data. Thus, you can expect to see the concepts outlined in this chapter implicitly represented within the topics yet to be presented. In many chapters that follow you will find that ethical issues are posed quite frequently. Consequently, you are invited at this juncture to begin thinking with a "critical eye" about research and to thoughtfully deliberate about its obligation to protect volunteers from harm. In addition, Internet resources are available to help you develop a critical eye (see Figure 3.2).

FIGURE 3.2.   INTERNET RESOURCES ON HUMAN SUBJECTS' PROTECTION.

Federal Code of Regulations (45 CFR 46)

Federal Policy for the Protection of Human Subjects (Basic DHHS Policy for Protection of Human Research Subjects). The policy applies to all research involving human subjects conducted and supported by any Federal Department or Agency. www.hhs.gov/ohrp/humansubjects/guidance/45cfr46.htm

The Belmont Report

The document that serves as the basis for the Federal Regulations for protecting human research participants (45 CFR 46). Published in 1979 as a result of the Belmont Commission, this report was the culmination of a presidential commission established to set ethical guidelines for protecting human research subjects in federally funded research.
www.hhs.gov/ohrp//humansubjects/guidance/belmont.htm

National Institutes of Health (NIH), Bioethics Resources of the Web

Resources are available to individuals with an interest in bioethics and the responsible conduct of research, especially when involving human participants in studies. http://www.nih.gov/sigs/bioethics/
NIH Policy and Guidelines on the Inclusion of Children as Participants in Research Involving Human Subjects. http://grants.nih.gov/grants/guide/notice-files/not98-024.html

CDC Guidelines for Defining Public Health Research and Public Health Nonresearch

This document sets forth CDC guidelines on the definition of public health research conducted by CDC staff irrespective of the funding source (in other words, whether provided by the CDC or by another entity). This document provides guidance to state and local health departments and other institutions that conduct collaborative research with CDC staff or that are recipients of CDC funds. The guidelines are intended to ensure both the protection of human subjects and the effective practice of public health. http://www.cdc.gov/od/ads/opspoll1.htm

Public Responsibility in Medicine and Research

A national nonprofit organization dedicated to educating the medical and legal professions, industry, and the public about the ethical, legal, and policy dimensions of appropriate and ethical research. http://www.primr.org/

Summary

Ethical treatment of human subjects is essential in health promotion research. This chapter addressed the general principles used to guide health promotion research. The intent was not to provide an exhaustive review of all the ethical issues involved in conducing health promotion research; however, the most critical issues were presented. Researchers should be knowledgeable about the history of research abuse, core ethical principles, federal inclusion policies, and federal regulations regarding research protections and should incorporate such understanding into their research plans and personal conduct within the research setting. Specific regulations guide research involving children and prisoners and research conducted in schools and involving health care information. Working with communities can improve the quality of health promotion research and the protection of human subjects involved in that research.

Issues to Consider

1. As noted in the Belmont Report, respect for the person is a paramount principle in research ethics. This principle clearly implies that coercion or undue influence to gain assent or consent from potential study volunteers is not ethical. It must be noted, then, that coercion is "in the eye of the potential volunteer" rather than being an objective entity. Thus, an important issue to consider is whether any of the potential volunteers could possibly perceive even minor levels of pressure when making their decision about enrolling in the study. Several factors may contribute to this perception, including
   - Offering compensation amounts that exceed customary payment levels for the people in the population
   - Situations in which the potential volunteer is a student enrolled in a class taught by the investigator
   - Situations in which the potential volunteer's decision may reflect upon the decision of a third party such as a parole board or prison officials
   - Clinical trials that would provide treatment to subjects who could otherwise not afford medical care
   - The perception that the decision to volunteer is somehow linked to the quality of care that people may receive at a given clinic
2. An important issue is the ethics of neglecting to include people from all appropriate populations when conducting research. While it is often easy to limit the study sample to a homogenous population, the cost of excluding populations who otherwise stand to benefit from the research should be carefully

considered. If a research question for a population is truly important then one could make the case that choosing not to include that population in the research constitutes an ethical violation. For example, consider a study designed to investigate the efficacy of a health promotion program aimed at improving the dietary intake of iron, folic acid, and calcium among pregnant women. The proposed study is to be conducted in a community comprising predominantly white, middle-class women. Although African American women and Latinas are not specifically excluded from participation, the selection of the recruitment sites unfortunately will yield a sample that, for all practical purposes, excludes minority participation.

For Practice and Discussion

Box 3.2 provides several realistic scenarios designed to challenge your thinking regarding ethics. Please complete each question in writing. Then, find a colleague who has completed the same exercise and compare your answers to his or hers. For items where there is disagreement, engage in debate until a consensus answer is achieved.

In each of the following ethical case studies, identify risks and benefits, importance of inclusion versus exclusion from the study, specific regulatory requirements, and means of obtaining informed consent

Maria, a fifteen-year-old Hispanic female, is making her first prenatal visit to a university hospital clinic in California and is invited to join a longitudinal study. The study is looking at social and physical environmental exposures during pregnancy and early childhood and the effect of these on child and adolescent health (such as effects on early puberty). She receives a consent form that describes the purposes of the study, the number of follow-up visits, the number of questionnaires and their consents, who to call for questions about the study and who to call at the IRB, and other standard consent language. The research involves several different questionnaires and blood and urine specimens, repeated on a periodic basis. The research assistant also wants to review Maria's medical record. At the first visit, she meets with a clinical social worker who asks her to complete a psychosocial risk assessment. These assessments reveal that she is eighteen weeks pregnant and in generally good health. She has a history of a chlamydia infection a year ago and says that she uses condoms, but not always. She reports that abortion is not an option for her because she could never "kill her baby." She has recently stopped smoking. She is currently repeating ninth grade and getting B's and D's in school. She is living with her parents in an inner city neighborhood. Her parents immigrated from Mexico ten years ago. Maria reports that her father is "very angry" with her about getting pregnant. She initiated intercourse at age

Box 3.2. Scenarios for Ethical Consideration

Is it an ethical violation if

- The amount of financial compensation is so high that people feel they "can't afford" to say no?
- A study is promoting STI prevention but teenagers under the age of 18 are not included?
- The same study includes only African Americans?
- A study is designed in a way that does not provide a fair test of the study hypotheses?
- The data obtained from the study are not disseminated by presentation or publication?
- The data obtained from the study are disseminated but only after a lengthy delay?
- People are recruited in groups (such as in a classroom setting)?
- A member of the research staff urges someone to complete "all" of the questions (even though people have a right to "pass")?
- The intervention program leads people to engage in behaviors that may place them at-risk (for example, a program designed to motivate women to negotiate condom use with men could unintentionally cause negative effects from the male partners including abuse)?
- Participation in the study leads to the diagnosis of conditions or diseases that would otherwise go undetected *and* treatment is not provided?
- Participation in a study is the only way to receive education and treatment about HIV infection?
- Recruitment occurs in a setting where perceptions of coercion may be inherently impossible to avoid (for example, prisons)?
- The control condition is known to be of very little value
- Study participants are led to believe that compensation will not be provided to them unless they complete all aspects of the study?
- Medical records from a local hospital are used to recruit patients with HIV infection into a health promotion study?
- The study concludes by asking people to take part in yet another study?

---

fourteen with her current boyfriend, Ramon, who is eighteen. She denies physical abuse by her family or Ramon. Ramon hopes to join the Army and Maria hopes to finish school, after she has the baby.

Estelle, a sixteen-year-old white female, is visiting an adolescent health clinic for acne. Per clinic routine she is offered a comprehensive biopsychosocial health assessment, based on the AMA's *Guidelines for Adolescent Preventive Services.* Per the clinic routine, she was enrolled in the clinic by her mother but her mother does not always accompany her to the clinic. There is no specific consent-assent form for the health assessment. Per the assessment, Estelle is currently in tenth grade, is getting A's and B's, but doesn't like school sports or clubs. She began smoking at age eleven and reached menarche at age twelve. She has had several boyfriends but has not initiated sexual intercourse; her current boyfriend is eighteen. She likes to drink wine coolers and admits to blacking out a number of times while drinking. She lives with her parents, and says they don't know much about her smoking and drinking. The clinic is conducting a natural history study of HPV and other viral STDs. She is eligible for the study because she has not initiated sexual intercourse. Participants would be randomized to one of two counseling interventions. A risk assessment would be completed on a laptop computer, using headphones. Repeat study visits would occur every three months and involve collection of blood, urine, and vaginal samples. Male partners would be recruited.

APPENDIX A. SAMPLE INFORMED CONSENT DOCUMENT.

Consent to Be a Research Subject

Title: Cancer Screening

Principal Investigator: Dr. Feel Good

Introduction/Purpose:
You are being asked to volunteer for a research study. The purpose of the study is to learn about your feelings toward screening tests for cancer of the colon. If you join, the study will ask you questions about why you might or might not be tested for this type of cancer. The questions ask about side effects, safety, and how good the test is for finding cancer.

Procedures:
You will be asked to take part in a face-to-face interview. A staff member will give the interview. It will last forty-five to sixty minutes. After you are done the staff member will discuss questions you might have. The interview will be taped. The tape will be erased after written versions of the interview have been made. You may refuse to answer any of the questions.

Risks:
Some people may feel a little nervous when thinking about cancer. If the questions cause you a lot of stress, you may end the interview.

Benefits:
Taking part in this study could provide some benefit to you. You will have a chance to discuss cancer with a staff member. Also, the study might increase your awareness of cancer screening. Other benefits to you will not occur. However, we [doctors, researchers, and scientists] may learn new things that will help prevent cancer deaths.

Confidentiality:
The information you give will be kept private. Your name will not appear on any document that also shows the answers you gave. Agencies that make the rules about how research is done, and those that pay for the research, have the right to review records of research subjects. Agencies that have the right to look at records from this research include the Human Investigations Committee at Hip Hop University. If an outside review occurs, your records will be kept private to the extent allowed by the law. Your name will not be used in any report nor will it be used on study records. Only an I.D. number will be used in the study records.

Compensation/Costs:
$20 will be given to you for being in the study for your time and effort. There are no costs to you. If you are injured as a result of this research, medical care will be available. The study will not pay for the cost of this care. If you believe

that you have been injured by this research, please contact Dr. Feel Good at 403-712-5997.

Contact Persons:
If you have any questions about this study, contact Dr. Feel Good at 403-712-5997. If you have any questions or concerns about your rights as a person in this study, contact the Chairman of Human Investigations Committee at 403-783-5649.

Voluntary Participation:
Participation in this study is completely voluntary, and you have the right to refuse to join. You can stop at any time after giving consent, and you can skip any question in the interview. This decision will not affect you in any way nor will you be penalized. The interviewer may stop you from taking part in this study at any time if it is in your best interests or if you do not follow instructions.

New Findings:
If anything new is learned during the study that we believe is important to you, we will tell you about it.

You will be given a copy of this consent form to keep.

I agree to participate for this research study.

Volunteer's signature	Date	Time

Person obtaining consent	Date	Time

References

Beecher, H. K. (1966). Ethics and clinical research. *New England Journal of Medicine, 274*, 1354–1360.

Buchanan, D. R. (2000). *An ethic for health promotion.* New York: Oxford University Press.

Frankel, M. S. (1992). Professional societies and responsible research conduct. In *Responsible science: Ensuring the integrity of the research process.* Vol. II (pp. 26–49). Washington, DC: National Academy of Sciences, National Academy of Engineering, and Institute of Medicine.

Glanz, K., Rimer, B. K., and Lerman, C. (1996). Ethical issues in the design and conduct of community-based intervention studies. In S. S. Coughlin and T. L. Beauchamp (Eds.), *Ethics and epidemiology* (pp. 156–177). New York: Oxford University Press.

Hochhauser, M. (2003). Concepts, categories, and value judgments in informed consent forms. *Institutional Review Board, 25*(5), 7–10.

Jones, H. S. (1993). *Bad blood: The Tuskegee syphilis experiment.* New York: Free Press.

Lederer, S. E., and Grodin, M. A. (1994). Historical overview: Pediatric experimentation. In M. A. Grodin and L. H. Glanz (Eds.), *Children as research subjects: Science, ethics, and law.* New York: Oxford University Press.

Levine, R. J. (1995). Adolescents as research subjects without permission of their parents or guardians: Ethical considerations. *Journal of Adolescent Health, 17*(5), 286–296.

Levine, R. J. (2001). Institutional review boards: A crisis in confidence. *Annals of Internal Medicine, 134,* 161–163.

Melton, G. B., Levine, R. J., Koocher, G. P., Rosenthal, R., and Thompson, W. C. (1988). Community consultation in socially sensitive research. Lessons from clinical trials of treatments for AIDS. *American Psychologist, 43,* 573–81.

Minkler, M. (2004). Ethical challenges for the "outside" researcher in community-based participatory research. *Health Education & Behavior, 31*(6), 684–697.

National Institutes of Health. (1998). *NIH policy and guidelines on the inclusion of children as participants in research involving human subjects.* March 6, 1998. Retrieved April 7, 2005, from grants1.nih.gov/grants/guide/notice-files/not98-024.html. National Institutes of Health.

National Institutes of Health. (2001, October). *NIH policy and guidelines on the inclusion of women and minorities as subjects in clinical research.* Retrieved March 8, 2005, from grants.nih.gov/grants/funding/women_min/guidelines_amended_10_2001.htm.

Quinn, S. C. (2004). Ethics in public health research: Protecting human subjects: The role of community advisory boards. *American Journal of Public Health, 94*(6), 918–922.

Sieber, J. E., and Stanley, B. (1988). Ethical and professional dimensions of socially sensitive research. *American Psychologist, 43,* 49–55.

Snider, D., and Stroup, D. (1997). Defining research when it comes to public health. *Public Health Reports, 112,* 29–32.

Society for Adolescent Medicine. (2003). *Guidelines for adolescent health research.* A position paper of the Society for Adolescent Medicine. Prepared by J. S. Santelli, A. S. Rogers, W. D. Rosenfeld, and others. *Journal of Adolescent Health. 33*(5), 396–409.

Thomas, S. B., and Quinn, S. C. (1991). The Tuskegee syphilis study, 1932 to 1972: Implications for HIV education and AIDS risk education programs in the black community. *American Journal of Public Health, 81,* 1498–1504.

U.S. Department of Health and Human Services, National Institutes of Health, Office for Protection from Research Risks. (2005, June 23). Code of Federal Regulations: Title 45-Public Welfare; Part 46: *Protection of Human Subjects.*

U.S. Department of Health, Education, and Welfare. (1979). *The Belmont report: Ethical principles and guidelines for the protection of human subjects of research.* Washington, DC: U.S. Government Printing Office, DHEW publication no. (OS) 78–0012.

PART TWO

RESEARCH DESIGN

CHAPTER FOUR

CHOOSING A RESEARCH DESIGN

Laura F. Salazar, Richard A. Crosby, and Ralph J. DiClemente

The research design of a study is the *strategy* the investigator chooses for answering the research question. The research question directs the type of design chosen. Other factors may play a significant role as well in deciding what type of research design will be applied. Ethical issues, cost, feasibility, and access to the study population will undoubtedly influence the design of the study in addition to the research question. It is critical for the investigator to choose the most appropriate design as this will have an impact on the success of the research project. Each design has its own strengths and limitations, some of which will determine the conclusions that may be drawn from the research.

Illustration of Key Concepts

In this chapter, we will provide an overview of the research process. This will entail a description of the two overarching stages of research. We will identify general purposes of health promotion research that fall within these two stages, and delineate appropriate research designs that are used to achieve each purpose. Examples from the health promotion research literature will be interjected to illustrate the respective purposes and designs.

FIGURE 4.1. THE CHAIN OF RESEARCH IN HEALTH PROMOTION.

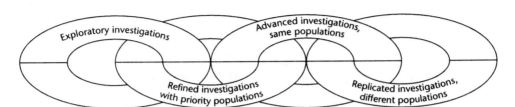

Exploratory investigations generate (rather than test) specific research questions.
Refined studies initially test a given set of research questions, and priority
populations are defined through surveillance and epidemiological studies.
Advanced investigations are built on findings from previous tests of research questions.
After the research questions have been adequately addressed in a priority
population, investigations should be replicated with a second priority population.

Two Stages of the Research Process

In general, scientific inquiry can be conceptualized as an interlocking chain—with
each link being a precursor of the other. The first link in the chain represents *exploratory research,* and the subsequent links represent varying levels of *conclusive research.* The model shown in Figure 4.1 can be applied to health promotion research.

As shown, exploratory research is often conducted because the health issue
has not been clearly defined, or a scientific basis for inquiry has not been established. In other words, hardly anything is known about the topic. In this early stage,
observations are needed to provide investigators with data to define health issues, to begin to understand the etiology of those health issues, to formulate theories, to reveal relevant factors, and to identify potential relationships. The research
conducted in this early stage is regarded as preliminary research and serves as the
basis for future conclusive research efforts. Some examples of exploratory research
questions would include

- Are college students being harassed online?
- What does "using condoms" mean for Latino immigrants?
- What are the factors contributing to obesity among toddlers in the U.S.?
- Does intimate partner violence affect HIV risk for men who have sex with men?
- Is intimate partner violence related to women's health-seeking behaviors?

As these examples indicate, the research question involves investigations that will
describe the issue. Depending on the outcomes, this type of research usually is
viewed as a springboard for further inquiry.

Box 4.1. Prevalence Versus Incidence

Prevalence and incidence are different ways of measuring a disease's occurrence and two very important concepts in health promotion research. *Prevalence* of a condition equates with the total number of people who currently have the condition, whereas *incidence* refers to the annual number of people who have been diagnosed with the condition. These two measures are very different. A chronic incurable disease such as AIDS can have a low incidence but high prevalence. A short-duration curable condition such as a bacterial sexually transmitted disease (STD) can have a high incidence but low prevalence because many people get a STD each year, but few people actually have a bacterial STD at any given time.

Conclusive research, as the term suggests, provides information that is useful for reaching conclusions or in making decisions. Research in this phase generally has five overarching purposes: (1) to document the scope of the issue (see Box 4.1 for common public health indicators of scope), (2) to test causal or etiological theories, (3) to identify the sequelae of disease or health conditions, (4) to evaluate measurement instruments, (5) and to evaluate treatments or interventions (Salazar and Cook, 2002). Take the issue of HIV/AIDS for example; at the onset of the epidemic in the early 1980s, the research conducted was exploratory in nature. Little was known about the issue. Now that we are in the third decade of research and there has been much knowledge generated, most of the research is conclusive research. To glean a better idea of what types of research purposes would be considered as conclusive research, a sample of questions pertaining to HIV/AIDS research from each of these five research purposes is provided:

- How many new cases of HIV infection occurred among men who have sex with men (MSM)?
- How many new cases of AIDS were diagnosed among injection drug users in the Northeastern United States?
- What are the risk factors for HIV infection among African American women?
- What are the psychological and psychosocial effects of HIV diagnosis among adolescents?
- Does social support protect against negative effects of HIV diagnosis among homeless women?
- How well does a sexual risk-reduction program reduce unsafe HIV-related behaviors as compared with an abstinence program?
- What are the long-term side effects of Highly Active Anti-Retroviral Therapy?
- What are the side effects of an HIV vaccine among black men?

As these examples illustrate, conclusive research has clearly defined research questions. In comparison with exploratory research, the process is more formal and structured. Findings inform hypothesis testing and decision making.

Both exploratory and conclusive research can be further subdivided into two major categories of research purpose: *descriptive* and *causal research*. *Descriptive research* provides data describing the "who, what, when, where, and how" of a health issue, not what caused it. Therefore, studies that reveal who either is at risk or has a particular health issue or condition; that document incidence, prevalence, or both; that examine risk factors; that look at the effects of having the health issue; and that assess scale properties designed to measure a construct related to a health issue would be categorized as descriptive research. The main limitation with descriptive research is that it cannot assess what *caused* the health issue. This is where causal research steps in. Determining a cause-and-effect relationship is imperative in situations in which the investigator must reveal the true cause(s) of a particular disease or when evaluating whether or not a program caused the observed changes.

◆ ◆ ◆

In a Nutshell

Determining a cause-and-effect relationship is imperative in situations in which the investigator must reveal the true cause(s) of a particular disease or when evaluating whether or not a program caused the observed changes.

◆ ◆ ◆

Descriptive Research

Descriptive research, whether exploratory or conclusive, uses *observational designs* to achieve its objectives. The term *observational research designs* refers to research in which variables are observed as they exist in nature—no manipulation of variables occurs. Furthermore, observational research can involve both *qualitative* methods and *quantitative* methods. Observational research that uses qualitative methods does not entail the use of specific research designs per se; rather, depending on the research question, different strategies are used (Morse, 1994). A few qualitative strategies are phenomenology, ethnography, and grounded theory. Observational research that uses quantitative methods would entail the use of *cross-sectional designs, successive independent samples design*, and *longitudinal designs* (as noted in Chapter One, these also include prospective cohort designs and panel studies).

Qualitative research methods and strategies are described in greater depth in Chapter Seven; however, in simple terms, qualitative data consists of observations that do not take the form of numbers. For example, conducting interviews with people is one type of qualitative method used. The data collected consist of verbal responses to either structured or semistructured questions. These responses may be audiotaped and then transcribed. The investigator would conduct an analysis by reviewing the transcriptions and identifying themes that emerged. All results are conveyed through description. An example of a qualitative study that used grounded theory as the strategy and face-to-face interviews as the method was conducted by Melville and others (2003). They conducted interviews with twenty-four participants who had a positive herpes simplex virus type 2 (HSV-2) serology by western blot to assess the emotional and psychosocial responses to receiving a positive diagnosis. They identified three categories of themes: short-term emotional responses (for example, denial, surprise), short-term psychosocial responses (for example, fear of telling sex partner, anger at sex partner), and perceived ongoing responses (for example, feeling socially stigmatized, feeling sexually undesirable). The results were used to conceptualize a complex model involving these themes as interrelated constructs that could be tested quantitatively in the future.

Conversely, the nature of quantitative data involves numerical values. Data can be frequency of responses or occurrences, or the data can entail a process whereby participants' verbal or written responses are quantified by transforming them into numerical values. Analyses of quantitative methods require the use of statistical procedures. One example of a quantitative approach would be a surveillance study. For example, the Centers for Disease Control and Prevention (CDC) is interested in knowing how many adolescents engage in certain health risk behaviors. The Youth Risk Behavior Surveillance System (YRBSS) monitors six categories of priority health-risk behaviors among youths and young adults— behaviors that contribute to unintentional injuries and violence; tobacco use; alcohol and other drug use; sexual behaviors that contribute to unintended pregnancy and sexually transmitted diseases (STDs), including human immunodeficiency virus (HIV) infection; unhealthy dietary behaviors; and physical inactivity plus being overweight. Some results from the 2003 national Youth Risk Behavior Survey (YRBS) demonstrated that among the high school students surveyed, 30.2 percent had ridden with a driver who had been drinking alcohol; 17.1 percent had carried a weapon; 44.9 percent had drunk alcohol; and 22.4 percent had used marijuana (Centers for Disease Control and Prevention, 2004).

Observational Research Designs

In Chapter Five, you will find specific details of *how* to conduct observational research. In this section, we describe what is considered observational research by providing an overview of the different types of observational research designs with examples drawn from the published literature.

One of the most commonly used research designs in health promotion is the *cross-sectional design*. The hallmark of this design is that time is fixed (it does not move). One or more samples are drawn from the population at one time point. Most survey-research designs are cross-sectional; however, types of research other than survey research can use cross-sectional designs.

Survey research constitutes a field of scientific inquiry in its own right and is best defined as a scientific method to help understand the characteristics of a population. By *characteristics*, we mean people's thoughts, opinions, feelings, and behaviors. Surveys are conducted for myriad reasons and are used not only by public health professionals, but also by political scientists, psychologists, sociologists, and of course marketing researchers. Moreover, surveys can vary according to their mode of administration. Surveys can be conducted over the telephone or in person. They can be self-administered using paper and pencil in a classroom or using a computer. Some surveys are administered via mail and some are administered via the Internet.

As an example of survey research, consider a study conducted by the Family Violence Prevention Fund. This organization conducted a national telephone survey of a thousand men and women over eighteen years of age living in the United States to investigate public opinion on the issue of domestic violence (Klein, Campbell, Soler, and Ghez, 1997). Respondents were given a fixed set of explanations of why a man would beat a woman (for example, "he gets drunk," or "he wants to control her"). They were then asked to choose which explanation was closest to their own view. The results showed that 20 percent of respondents indicated drinking was involved, 23 percent said that it stemmed from the man being beaten as a child, 34 percent indicated it was to control the woman. In another example, a study conducted by Finn (2004) administered a survey on-line to male and female college students. The goal was to gather data regarding the extent of on-line harassment. Among 339 respondents, 10 to 15 percent reported receiving repeated e-mail or Instant Messenger messages that were threatening, insulting, or harassing; more than half reported receiving unwanted pornography. Although the mode of administration differed, both of these studies sampled the population at one time point and the goal was to describe certain characteristics of the population sampled.

Although there is one criterion to a cross-sectional design (that is, measurement is conducted at one time point), research that uses a cross-sectional design can have more than one purpose. For example, cross-sectional designs can be used to document the prevalence of a health issue. DiClemente and colleagues (2004) used a cross-sectional design to describe the prevalence of sexually transmitted diseases (STDs) among a sample of pregnant African American adolescent females attending a prenatal clinic in the southeast. They found that, overall, approximately

24 percent tested positive for one of four STDs: Chlamydia trachomatis, Neisseria gonorrhoeae, Trichomonas vaginalis, or Treponema pallidum. In another example, Varma and colleagues (2004) also used a cross-sectional design to estimate the prevalence of ocular hypertension and open-angle glaucoma (OAG) in adult Latinos. They found that among 6,142 Latinos, forty years of age or older who lived in the Los Angeles area, and who underwent a complete ophthalmologic examination, approximately 5 percent were diagnosed with OAG and almost 4 percent had ocular hypertension. Moreover, Varma and colleagues made comparisons by age and gender. They found no gender differences, but significantly higher prevalence rates for both conditions were found in older Latinos than in younger Latinos.

In addition to assessing prevalence of disease, cross-sectional designs can be used to estimate levels of knowledge about any given health threat or health protective behavior, and health-related attitudes, beliefs, opinions, and behaviors. For example, Lapidus and colleagues (2002) conducted a mail survey among pediatric primary care physicians to determine rates of screening practices for domestic violence (DV)—the behavioral outcome in this study. Twelve percent of the respondents reported routinely screening for DV at all well-child care visits, 61 percent reported screening only certain patients, and 30 percent said they did not screen for DV at all.

◆ ◆ ◆

In a Nutshell

It is the manner in which you collect the data and not the statistical technique that allows one to make causal inferences.

◆ ◆ ◆

Another function addressed by cross-sectional designs is the ability to assess the relationships among variables for a given population. When investigating relationships among variables, the research is often referred to as *correlational,* but a distinction must be made between the statistical technique and the design. Using a cross-sectional design to investigate the relationship between two variables by applying statistical correlational techniques (for instance, Pearson product moment correlation coefficient) precludes the ability to infer causal relationships. In a correlational relationship, changes in one variable accompany changes in another; however, it cannot be said that one variable influences another when the two variables were measured using observational methods. Conversely, an exception would be made if the data were collected

MINCUS ITERATES THAT CORRELATION DOES NOT MEAN CAUSATION.

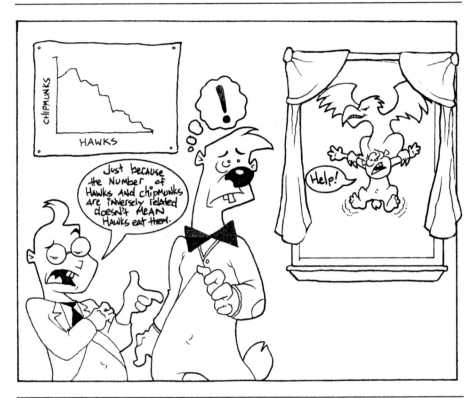

Copyright 2005 by Justin Wagner; reprinted with permission.

using experimental methods. Then, in this scenario, a correlation between two variables may imply a causal relationship. This is an important distinction that needs to be made: **It is the manner in which you collect the data and not the statistical technique that allows one to make causal inferences.** For example, it has been observed that crime rates and ice cream consumption tend to be correlated (because more crimes are committed in warm weather and more ice cream is eaten in warm weather). Yet, you would not conclude that eating more ice cream causes crime rates to increase. This is the classic *third-variable problem,* in which there is another unmeasured variable affecting both of the measured variables and causing the two variables to appear correlated with each other. Although cross-sectional designs are used frequently in correlational research, the design is limited in inferring causation. The design is also unable to establish directionality. Consider the significant inverse correlation (as one variable increases, the other variable decreases) between depression and self-esteem found frequently in the literature as another example. It is unclear whether depression leads to low self-esteem or whether low-esteem leads to depression. In reality, both propositions are equally plausible; thus, a correlational design is incapable of distinguishing cause from effect. An experimental design is necessary for causality to be determined. In an example from the published research, Salazar and others (2004) were able to demonstrate a significant correlation between African American adolescent girls' self-concept (including self-esteem, body image, and ethnic identity) and the frequency in which they refused unsafe sex. However, there was no way of determining with certainty whether or not self-concept *influenced* unsafe sex refusal, or whether the reverse was true. It is also possible that neither variable influenced or caused the other. This is one of the major limitations of conducting correlational research, especially research that uses cross-sectional designs.

◆ ◆ ◆

In a Nutshell

Although cross-sectional designs are used frequently in correlational research, the design is limited in inferring causation. The design is also unable to establish directionality.

◆ ◆ ◆

Nonetheless, we continue to conduct observational research using cross-sectional designs as it provides the necessary foundation for more elaborate studies that improve upon the limitations of a cross-sectional design. Also, in many instances, it is not feasible or ethical to conduct an experimental research study when manipulation of the variable is impossible, or it is unethical to do so (for instance, you cannot assign a person to any condition that entails risk). Furthermore, cross-sectional correlational studies are also useful to identify correlates of behavioral variables, but not necessarily variables that have a cause-and-effect relationship. For example, Hall, Jones, and Saraiya (2001) conducted a cross-sectional study to determine the correlates of sunscreen use among U.S. high school students. They found that among a nationally representative sample ($N = 15,349$) of students, infrequent use of sunscreen was associated with other risky health behaviors such as driving after drinking, riding in a car with a drinking driver, cigarette smoking, being sexually active, and being physically inactive. Clearly, the authors of this study were not attempting to imply a cause-and-effect relationship, but rather, they were trying to reveal a cluster of health risk behaviors to address comprehensively in a health promotion program.

A *successive independent samples design* improves upon the time limitation of cross-sectional designs by incorporating a series of cross-sectional studies conducted over a period of time. Each cross-sectional survey is conducted with an independent sample, which means that a new sample is drawn for each of the successive cross-sectional surveys. This design is used to assess change in a population characteristic (for example, tobacco use, condom use, pregnancy rates) over time and is also referred to as a *trend study*.

As health promotion researchers for example, we may want to document the change in certain health risk behaviors or the prevalence of disease for a given population over a period of time. This would be very important information to have and could inform programs and policy. In fact, this type of design is used quite often in *epidemiology*—the discipline studying the incidence, distribution, and control of disease in a population.

The CDC conducts and sponsors many studies using the successive independent samples design. One example is the CDC's serosurveillance system, which is used to monitor the prevalence of human immunodeficiency virus type 1 (HIV-1) in the United States. In collaboration with state and local health departments, surveys were conducted in selected sites from 1988 through 1999. Populations that were included ranged from low risk (for instance, military, blood donors) to high risk (such as injection drug users and men who have sex with men (MSM)). The objectives of the serosurveillance system are (1) to provide standardized estimates of HIV prevalence among the selected populations, (2) to describe the magnitude and changes over time of HIV infection in these populations, (3) to recognize new or emerging patterns of HIV infection among specific subgroups of the U.S. population, and (4) to assist in directing resources and in targeting programs for HIV prevention and care. The results showed that in general, prevalence was higher among survey participants who were in the older age categories and, with the exception of Job Corps entrants, among those who were male. For most of the surveillance populations included in the report, prevalence by region, race or ethnicity, and age group either decreased or remained stable from 1993–1997. For the MSM population, these results are depicted in graph form and show trends in HIV prevalence by region (Figure 4.2) and race or ethnicity (Figure 4.3).

The CDC also uses this type of design to track changes in behaviors over time. For example, Serdula and others (2004) examined trends in fruit and vegetable consumption among adults living in the United States from 1994 to 2000. Using

FIGURE 4.2.   HIV PREVALENCE AMONG MEN WHO HAVE SEX WITH MEN, AT SEXUALLY TRANSMITTED DISEASE CLINICS, BY REGION (1993–1997).

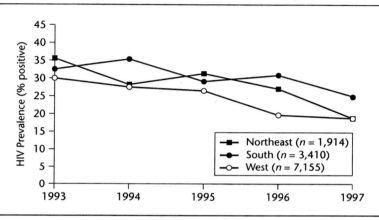

FIGURE 4.3.   HIV PREVALENCE AMONG MEN WHO HAVE SEX WITH MEN, AT SEXUALLY TRANSMITTED DISEASE CLINICS, BY RACE OR ETHNICITY (1993–1997).

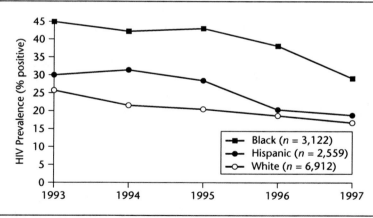

Note: Standardized to 1993 STD clinic population by region and age group.

random-digit-dialing procedures, a method in which each household that has a telephone has an equal probability of being selected, they sampled 434,121 adults in total. Each sample of adults was surveyed at four different time points: 1994, 1996, 1998, and 2000. The results showed that the mean frequency of fruit and vegetable consumption declined over time, although the proportion of respondents who consumed fruit or vegetables five or more times per day remained stable.

Although an improvement over the cross-sectional design, successive independent samples design also suffers from limitations. It is very useful for measuring changes over time for a characteristic such as disease; however, for other characteristics such as behavior, attitudes, or opinions, the researcher cannot determine with certainty the extent to which the population truly changed because the results are based on different samples of people. In order to attribute documented changes to the time factor, the same group of people needs to be followed and surveyed over time.

Longitudinal designs, however, are capable of determining changes in behavior, attitudes, or opinions over time. The defining characteristic of a longitudinal design is that the same participants are followed over a period of time and interviewed more than once during the time period. The time period could range from months to years. In such a study, sometimes referred to as a *cohort study, prospective study,* or *panel study,* the analysis of data usually involves estimation of rates of disease or behavior in the cohort during a defined period of observation. Traditionally, the term *cohort* refers to the part of the population born during a particular period (for instance, baby boomers) and whose characteristics such as causes of death and those still alive can be ascertained as it enters successive time and age periods. The term *cohort study* describes an investigation of any designated group of persons that are followed over a period of time.

The analysis of data typically involves estimation of rates of disease or behavior change during the observation period. Newly diagnosed cases (incidence) of a disease for a cohort would be calculated for an observation period that is measured in years of observation time per person (in other words, person-years). Thus, if you have a cohort of 2000 people who are followed for a period of 30 years, then the incidence of disease would be the ratio of newly diagnosed cases to a denominator equal to 2000×30 years. This ratio would typically be expressed in terms of 100,000 person-years.

Longitudinal designs improve vastly on some of the limitations of cross-sectional designs and of the successive independent samples design. For example, by following the same cohort over a long period of time you may be able to establish the temporal order of occurrences and you may be able to attribute change to the time factor. Also, you may be able to ascertain the effects of naturally occurring events. For example, if within the time frame of your longitudinal study an event such as a natural disaster, a divorce, or heart attack occurs, you could investigate whether or not there were any differences between those in the cohort who experienced the event and those who did not. If significant differences were found, then you could reasonably attribute them to the event. Of course, one major problem with longitudinal studies is *attrition*. Also referred to as *mortality*, attrition is the loss of participants from the research study and can bias the results. Severe attrition can be dealt with statistically by comparing those who returned for follow-up interviews (or completed follow-up questionnaires) with those who did not and determining critical differences between the two groups. For example, in sex research, if those lost to attrition had baseline indicators of more frequent risky sexual activity than those who remained in the study, then the loss to follow-up could bias the study conclusions.

◆ ◆ ◆

In a Nutshell

Longitudinal designs improve vastly on some of the limitations of cross-sectional designs and of the successive independent samples design.

◆ ◆ ◆

An example of a longitudinal study that examined behaviors was conducted by Repetto, Zimmerman, and Caldwell (2004). They were able to determine the correlational relationships between depressive symptoms and alcohol use among a cohort of 456 black high school students. The students were interviewed every year during high school and for three years following the transition to adulthood. The researchers were able to document the temporal order of depressive symptoms, alcohol use, and life changes associated with adulthood.

In another study that used a longitudinal design, Finnish researchers Huurre, Aro, and Jaakkola (2004) identified incidence of asthma and allergic rhinitis. They recruited a cohort of 2,269 that was followed from birth to thirty-two years of age. They estimated the incidence rate of asthma and allergic rhinitis during the full time period, while also estimating the prevalence rates for the diseases at three ages: sixteen, twenty-two, and thirty-two years of age. The overall incidence rate of asthma was 2.1 new cases per 1000 person-years and the overall incidence rate for allergic rhinitis was approximately 12 new cases per 1000 person-years. They found changes in prevalence rates of asthma from 3 percent to 5 percent as the cohort moved from sixteen years of age to thirty-two years old. Prevalence rates of allergic rhinitis also changed significantly from 17.5 percent to 26 percent for the same age ranges.

The *cohort-sequential design* is essentially a hybrid of cross-sectional and longitudinal designs. Starting with an initial cohort and following it over a period of time, another cohort or cohorts are then added at varying intervals within that time period. Changes over time for the first cohort can be assessed while also being able to make cross-sectional comparisons among the different cohorts at specific time points.

An example of cohort-sequential design was conducted by Chassin, Presson, Rose, and Sherman (2001). They reported the results from a study designed to assess age-related changes in health-relevant beliefs from the middle school years through age thirty-seven. Participants were initially recruited between 1980 and 1983, and the sample comprised sixth through twelfth graders in a county school system. Participants completed a survey each year. The final sample included the participation of ten cohorts (that is, the graduating classes of 1980–1989). Follow-up surveys were conducted in 1987, 1993, and 1999 with retention rates of 73 percent, 73 percent, and 71 percent respectively. The results showed systematic age-related changes in the perceived risks of cigarette smoking.

Causal Research

As compared with descriptive research, causal research transcends the natural order of things through manipulation and provides an ability to make cause-effect statements. Thus, causal research employs *experimental designs* so that causal inference can be made with a high degree of certainty, and in some instances *quasi-experimental designs*. Experimental designs entail the manipulation of a variable to test the effects of the manipulation on some outcome. Quasi-experimental designs approximate experimental designs but do not use randomization. Why should we care about making cause-effect statements? Making cause-effect statements provides both theoretical and practical benefits. For example, by isolating the cause of a condition or disease, we may begin work on devising a cure. In addition, causal research allows us to find out if a particular program is helpful in solving a problem. This type of research is usually conducted in controlled settings with small groups of people. If the treatment or program is *efficacious,* meaning it had the ability to produce the desired effect, then it can be applied to a larger group in real-life settings. Within the context of health promotion research, causal research allows us not only to predict, understand, and control behavior, but also to change behavior.

The two main defining characteristics of experimental research designs are the manipulation of an *independent variable* and control over *extraneous variables.* The independent variable is the variable chosen by the investigator to determine its effect on the *dependent variable* and is manipulated or controlled by the investigator. If the investigator is manipulating only one factor, then the design is a single-factor design; if more than one factor, it is called a factorial design. The number of independent variables equates with the number of factors in the design. The dependent variable is the outcome variable of interest and is measured by the investigator. Extraneous variables are not directly related to the hypothesis being tested, but may nevertheless have an effect on the dependent variable. You may *control* the effects of extraneous variables either by holding them constant or by randomizing their effects across treatment levels. To the extent that extraneous variables provide alternative explanations or rival hypotheses for the findings, the *internal validity* of the study will be threatened.

The internal validity of the study is the ability of the design to test the hypothesis it was designed to test. Internal validity can be thought of as the approximate truth about inferences regarding cause-effect or causal relationships. Seven common threats to internal validity have been identified and deserve consideration when designing your study: history, maturation, testing, instrumentation, statistical regression, biased selection of subjects, and experimental mortality (Campbell and Stanley, 1966). These threats to internal validity are defined in Box 4.2. Common threats that may seriously threaten internal validity must be addressed prior to conducting your study so that alternative hypotheses can be ruled out.

Before the different types of experimental designs are discussed, an important and related factor to understand when planning health promotion research is that conducting experiments in a controlled laboratory with pathogens is markedly different from conducting experiments with human subjects in the real world. Although controlling for extraneous variables is critical to the integrity of an experiment, the level of control may vary widely when the experiment takes

---

Box 4.2. Common Threats to Internal Validity

1. History—results might be due to an event that occurred between observations.
2. Maturation—results might be due to participants growing older, wiser, stronger, or more experienced between observations.
3. Testing—results might be due to the number of times responses were measured.
4. Instrumentation—results might be due to a change in the measuring instrument between observations.
5. Statistical regression—results might be due to the selection of participants based on extreme scores, and when measured again, scores move back to an average level.
6. Selection bias—results might be due to differences that existed between participants in groups before treatment occurred.
7. Mortality—results might be due to the differential loss of participants from groups.

place in a real-world setting (such as a classroom or community) as opposed to a laboratory or other "controlled setting" (for instance, an isolated room), and the subjects compose a heterogeneous group. Having a lower level of control over environmental factors and human subjects' factors threatens internal validity and may introduce *error variance*. *Error variance* refers to the variability in the dependent variable that *cannot* be attributed to the independent variable, but rather is attributed to extraneous variables or to variability among human subjects. Thus, reducing or controlling error variance is an important matter to consider as error variance may affect the ability to attribute observable effects to the manipulation of the independent variable. Furthermore, different types of designs handle error variance differently and should be a consideration when choosing an appropriate design.

To illustrate these two main experimental concepts of manipulation and control, consider the research question What are the side effects of a hepatitis vaccine on black men? The independent variable would be the administration of the hepatitis vaccine. There must be at least two levels to an independent variable or it is not a variable. In this instance, manipulation of the independent variable could be using two vaccines qualitatively different, such as a surface antigen vaccine as one and a *placebo* (an inactive substance that may look like medicine but contains no medicine, a "sugar pill" with no treatment value) or a different type of hepatitis vaccine as the second. Moreover, different levels of the independent variable could be quantitatively different when the same vaccine type was used, but in different dosages. The latter scenario is referred to as a dose-ranging study, in which two or more doses (starting at a lower dose and proceeding to higher doses) of a vaccine are tested against each other to determine which dose works best and has acceptable side effects. The dependent variable in this hypothetical study would be the "side effects" and could include measures of fatigue, quality of life, and nausea.

To achieve a high level of control in this study, there are two main issues to consider: first, control related to subject selection and assignment; second, control related to the type of experimental design chosen. Control over extraneous variables through the use of experimental designs increases the confidence that observed outcomes are the result of a given program, treatment, drug, or innovation instead of a function of extraneous variables or events and greatly enhances internal validity. Given these two important issues, the first issue to consider would be the method in which the potential participants will be sampled from the population of black men. A *random selection* procedure such as the use of a random numbers table would ensure a high degree of control in that each potential participant would have an equal chance of being selected. This procedure helps to control variables that could be introduced into the selection process and could cause not only low *generalizability* but also *selection bias*. Generalizability is the degree to which the research findings can be applied to the population under study (for example, black men). Using random selection helps to increase the representativeness of the sample thereby enhancing generalizability. As indicated in Box 4.2, selection bias results when groups differ from each other. Differences could be on either measured or unmeasured characteristics. Selection bias also occurs when the sample is not representative of the population. If random selection is used, then selection bias should not be an issue unless the response rate or the rate in which participants agreed to be in the study was extremely low. Furthermore, if random selection is not possible, then a nonrandom sampling technique such as *convenience sampling* (using individuals who are convenient to access) or *snowball sampling* (using recruited participants to identify others) would have to be used and would not reduce selection bias in the sample. Thus, if participants differ in ways that affect the dependent variable (side effects of HIV vaccine), then the results might be attributed to these differences rather than to the vaccine.

Once the sample is recruited, the next factor to consider is how to assign the subjects into the two groups. Other sources of error variance involving the subjects such as socioeconomic status, age, and education level, to name a few, need to be controlled. One method that would control (in this instance, by "control" we mean hold the effects of these variables constant) these sources of error variance would be to use *random assignment* (a.k.a. randomization) as the method to assign participants into respective groups. Randomization entails assigning participants by chance to one of two or more groups. There are different methods, such as using a random numbers table, using a software program, or even flipping a coin. Randomization minimizes any differences between or among groups by equally distributing subjects with particular characteristics between or among all the trial arms. Randomization rules out many threats to internal validity, but not all of them.

◆ ◆ ◆

In a Nutshell

Randomization entails assigning participants by chance to one of two or more groups. There are different methods, such as using a random numbers table, using a software program, or even flipping a coin. Randomization minimizes any differences between or among groups by equally distributing subjects with particular characteristics between or among all the trial arms.

◆ ◆ ◆

The second and probably the most important issue of control is the specific experimental design chosen. There are different ways in which this specific research question could be answered. The various designs that are used to conduct causal research vary in quality of evidence they provide for making causal inference and in the level of control. Moreover, there are distinctions between experimental designs, "true" experimental designs, and quasi-experimental designs that further influence the level of control and the ability to attribute changes in the dependent variable to the manipulation of the independent variable.

In the remaining section of this chapter, we will describe the various experimental and quasi-experimental research designs that make up causal research along with examples drawn from the scientific literature. We will provide an overview of the related concepts and terminology. Because the focus of this book is on the research methods used in health promotion and practice, we describe designs and methods related to health promotion. For example, research concepts or methods used in the study of pathogen isolation (such as Koch's Postulates), albeit important, are outside the scope of this text and will not be covered.

Experimental Research Designs. In health promotion research, much research can be considered *controlled trial* research, in which human volunteers are recruited to answer specific health questions. For example, controlled trials in health promotion would involve testing the efficacy of prevention programs for reducing health risk behaviors, disease, or the effects of disease. When conceptualizing and evaluating controlled trials, a common experimental design employed is the *between-subjects design*. In this type of experimental design, different groups or *arms* (that is, a group of participants in a clinical trial all of whom receive the same treatment) are exposed to the different levels of the independent variable. Furthermore, if you randomly assign subjects to the different arms, then you have a randomized between groups design. In health promotion research, this type of design is referred to as a randomized controlled trial (RCT) and is considered the "gold standard" of experimental designs.

Although the criteria of an experiment are manipulation and control, there is a distinction between a "true" experimental design and an experimental design. According to Campbell and Stanley (1966), a true experimental design must include more than one group, common measured outcome(s), and random assignment. Thus, because the RCT is a between-subjects design that uses random assignment it is considered a true experiment. The specific details of how to conduct an RCT are provided in Chapter Six. Most health promotion researchers concur that the RCT is the most effective and rigorous design for testing the efficacy of a program or treatment because it allows for causal inference and has the highest level of control possible in a real-world setting.

The number of levels of the independent variable dictates the number of arms to be employed in an RCT. For example, if you were examining the efficacy of an HIV-preventive intervention relative to a general health intervention, then you would require two groups; if you were examining the efficacy of an HIV-preventive intervention and an HIV-preventive intervention with booster sessions relative to the general health intervention, then you would need three groups. An example of a two-arm RCT was a study conducted by Shrier and others (2001), in which they evaluated a theory-driven safer-sex intervention for high-risk girls with cervicitis or pelvic inflammatory disease ($N = 123$). The clinical trial took place in an urban children's hospital adolescent clinic and inpatient service. The intervention was administered by trained female health educators during the time when the adolescents received STD treatment. The adolescent participants were not randomly selected to participate, but they were randomly assigned to the intervention group or to the control group. The intervention included topics such as STD transmission, secondary abstinence, and the female condom. Difference between groups on the behavioral outcomes was not statistically significant at the $P < .05$ level (likely due in part to small sample size).

Another type of between-subjects design, which may be useful in health promotion research, is the *matched groups design*. This design is employed when the researcher is aware of a particular subject characteristic that is strongly associated with the dependent variable. Using randomization, the characteristic may not get equally distributed between groups. Thus, to ensure that the characteristic is distributed equally, subjects are matched on the characteristic prior to random assignment. Depending on the number of groups in the experiment, subjects are matched with other subjects as close as possible to form pairs (two groups), triplets (three groups), or even quadruplets (four groups). Then, taking each set, subjects are assigned at random into groups. The main advantage of this design is significant reduction of the effect of the matched characteristic on the dependent variable. One example would be matching adolescents enrolled in a two-arm sexual-risk-reduction intervention on alcohol and drug use prior to randomization into groups. In this instance, prior to randomization, subjects would be measured on their alcohol and drug use. Subjects who reported similar behavior would be paired together. Each subject would be randomly assigned to one of the two conditions.

Within health promotion research, often the use of this design involves the site versus individual subjects as the unit of assignment (for instance, school, community, workplace, and so on). For example, Emmons, Linnan, Shadel, Marcus, and Abrams (1999) evaluated a multiple-risk-factor health intervention to determine its effectiveness in increasing physical-activity levels, increasing nutritional value of food intake, and smoking cessation among employees. The study employed a randomized matched-pair design in which the worksite was the unit of assignment. Twenty-six manufacturing worksites were matched on characteristics that were thought to be strongly associated with the study outcomes. The matching characteristics were whether or not there was a smoking policy and a cafeteria, size of the worksite, gender distribution, blue or white collar worker status, and the response rate to the baseline survey. Among the final sample of 2,055 participants who completed all three assessments, significant differences in the hypothesized direction were found between treatment conditions in exercise behavior and consumption of fruits, vegetables, and fiber. No differences by condition were found for percentage of calories from fat consumed or smoking cessation. A similar design was used in an evaluation of a community-based health promotion in India (Bhandari and others, 2003). The intervention was an educational program designed to promote exclusive breastfeeding for six months. Eight communities in India were matched on socioeconomic indicators, child mortality rates, recent morbidity, and the prevalence of wasting (the breakdown of body tissue such as muscle and organ for use as a protein source when the diet lacks protein) and stunting prior to randomization into either the intervention or control group. At three-month follow-up, exclusive breastfeeding rates in the intervention condition (79 percent) were significantly higher than the control condition (48 percent). Diarrhea prevalence was also lower in the intervention group than in the control group.

The *within-subjects design,* or *repeated-measures design,* is another experimental design that is also effective in reducing error variance due to human subject differences. In this design, the same subjects are exposed to the different levels of the independent variable. Thus, the same subjects form the different groups for comparisons. For example, if there are two levels of the independent variable, condition one is formed when subjects are exposed to the first level; condition two is formed when subjects are exposed to the second level. Although matching in a between-groups design reduces error variance due to individual differences to a large degree, the within-subjects design is more effective because the same subjects are exposed to the different treatments. Thus, error variance due to subject differences is significantly reduced or eliminated. With this level of reduction in error variance, the ability to detect the effects of the independent variable is greater than in other designs. Although the within-subjects design is classified as an experimental design because of manipulation and control, it is important to note that because this design does not have random assignment, it cannot be considered a true experimental design.

In health promotion research that involves a behavioral intervention, the within-subjects design is rarely used mainly because of *carryover effects,* which occur when exposure to the first treatment (in this instance it could be an educational intervention) affects the subjects' performance during subsequent treatments. Depending on the carryover effect, performance can be enhanced or reduced. For example, subjects may learn a skill in the first treatment that may enhance the observed outcomes after subsequent treatments; however, the observed change in outcome may be from the first treatment and not the second. This effect is called *learning.* Other types of carryover effects include *fatigue* (deterioration in performance due to being tired from the first treatment), *habituation* (repeated exposure to stimulus leads to reduced responsiveness), *sensitization* (stronger responses to stimuli stemming from initial exposure to a different stimulus), and *adaptation* (adaptive changes to a stimulus lead to a change in outcome).

A specific form of the within-subjects design used quite often in drug efficacy trials is called a *crossover trial.* In this type of design, the same group of subjects is exposed to all levels of the independent variable, but the order in which groups of subjects are exposed is varied. Thus, for every possible order combination, there is a group formed. For example, if researchers wanted to examine the efficacy of a drug on reducing pain, then using a crossover trial, they could randomly assign half the subjects to receive the drug first and then the placebo, while the other half receives the placebo first and then the drug. When each group of subjects switches from the first treatment condition to the next, this is the point at which they "crossover." By random assignment into the "groups" in this way, the more simple within-subjects design can be classified as a true experiment.

A randomized crossover trial design was used in a sexual health promotion study conducted among women attending an urban, reproductive health clinic in the southeastern United States to assess their acceptability and use of male and female condoms (Kulczycki, Kim, Duerr, Jamieson, and Macaluso, 2004). The sample of women was randomly assigned to one of two groups: the first group used ten male condoms first followed by a crossover to using ten female condoms; the second group was the reverse order. An intervention was also administered and consisted of a nurse providing instruction in correct condom usage and was given to all women. Overall, the results indicated that regardless of order, women preferred male condoms to female condoms and judged them to be superior.

Many studies in health promotion use *combined* or *mixed designs* in which there are independent groups (that is, an indicator of a between-groups design) that are assessed at multiple time points (in other words, an indicator of a within-subjects design). In this instance, the within-subjects factor is "time" with the number of levels corresponding to the number of time points. This is slightly different from the within-subjects design described previously, in which the within-subjects factor was the administration of all possible levels of the treatment to the same group of subjects. Thus, in a mixed design, comparisons can be made not only between groups and within groups, but also for the interaction of the two factors.

The RCT is considered a mixed design when subjects are assessed at multiple time periods. For example, in simplest terms, implementation of an RCT would involve (1) assessing subjects at baseline, (2) randomizing subjects into groups, (3) exposing subjects to the respective treatment, (4) assessing subjects after completion of the treatment (could be immediately following or at a follow-up period), and (5) assessing them again at subsequent follow-up period(s). Analysis goals for this design could include determining overall differences between groups (main effect for group), overall differences within groups (main effect for time), or whether or not subjects in the treatment group changed differentially over time as compared with subjects in the control group (an interaction of group and time).

St. Lawrence, Wilson, Eldridge, Brasfield, and O'Bannon (2001) applied a mixed design to test the efficacy of an HIV-preventive intervention based on the theory of gender and power, an HIV-preventive intervention based on social learning theory, and an HIV-preventive intervention based on cognitive behavioral principles relative to a wait-list control condition. The population for the evaluation study was disadvantaged African American women, and the sample of 445 was drawn from several community venues. Women were given baseline assessments and then randomly assigned into one of four groups: one of the three theoretically derived programs or the wait list control. Thus, this study had four levels of the first factor. Assessments were also made at postintervention and at a one-year follow-up period indicating three levels of the second factor. The results showed that at one-year follow-up, although there was no difference in condom use among the three treatment groups, in all of the three treatment conditions, condom use increased relative to the wait list control group.

Quasi-Experimental Designs. The word *quasi* means as if or almost; thus, a quasi-experiment approximates a true experiment. Quasi-experiments are similar to true experiments in that there is a treatment of some kind to examine and there are outcome measures; the main difference is that quasi-experiments do not use random assignment to create the groups necessary for comparison on the outcome measures. Many times, conducting health promotion research precludes using random assignment into groups or conditions because it may not be feasible, possible, ethical, or legal. For example, withholding a drug treatment or critical health program from vulnerable populations such as prisoners or pregnant women would be unethical or illegal in some instances if one group benefits and one group is deprived. For school-based health educational programs, resources may dictate that only one designated school receives the program, and it may be cost prohibitive to incorporate another school as a comparison. Although there are myriad reasons underlying the choice to use a quasi-experimental design, especially when conducting field research, it is important to understand that quasi-experiments are considered causal research, but the ability to rule out alternative explanations is much more limited than when using an experimental design. Furthermore, within the category of quasi-experimental designs, there is variability among the different designs as far as level of control and the ability to infer causation.

The *nonequivalent control group design* (NCGD) is used often in health promotion research, as it offers more control than some quasi-experimental designs by including a comparison group. Although similar in concept to the matched-pairs between-groups design, the nonequivalent control group design deviates from the matched-subjects design in that there is no randomization of the matched subjects, sites, workplaces, or communities into respective groups. Because the investigator does not control the assignment to groups through randomization, this design is deemed as having "nonequivalent groups." In the NCGD, a group is matched as closely as possible to the experimental group and is used as a comparison group; however, the groups may be different prior to the study. Because of this nonequivalence of groups at the start, the NCGD is especially susceptible to the selection threat to internal validity. Any prior differences between the groups may affect the outcome of the study. Under the worst circumstances, this can lead us to conclude that our health promotion program did not have an effect, when in fact it did, or that the program did have an effect, when in fact it did not.

◆ ◆ ◆

In a Nutshell

Because of this nonequivalence of groups at the start, the NCGD is especially susceptible to the selection threat to internal validity.

◆ ◆ ◆

Two main types of designs fall under the general category of NCGD: the nonequivalent group, posttest only and the nonequivalent group, pretest-posttest. The nonequivalent, posttest-only design consists of administering an outcome measure to two groups such as a program-treatment group and a comparison group or possibly two program groups, each receiving a different version of the program. For example, one group of students at a high school might receive an abstinence-only program while students at another school receive a comprehensive sexual-risk-reduction program. After twelve weeks, a test measuring sexual debut and risky sexual behaviors can be administered to see which program was more effective. A major problem with this design is that as stated previously the two groups might not be necessarily the same before the program takes place and may differ in important ways that may influence the outcomes. For instance, if it is found that the students in the abstinence-only program reported a delay in sexual debut and less engagement in sexual risk behavior, there is no way of determining if they were less likely to engage in those behaviors even before the program or whether other factors (for example, level of parental monitoring or parental communication about sex) may have influenced their sexual behavior.

The nonequivalent group, pretest-posttest design improves on a major limitation of the nonequivalent group, posttest-only design by allowing the researcher to empirically assess differences in the two groups prior to implementation of the program. If the researcher finds that one group performs better than the other on the posttest, then initial differences (if the groups were in fact similar on the pretest) can be ruled out as explanations for the differences. Furthermore, if in fact the groups did differ on the pretest measure, then the researcher could potentially control for these differences statistically.

Bastani and others (2002) used a longitudinal nonequivalent control group design to evaluate the effects of a systems-level intervention that sought to increase cervical cancer screening among underserved women attending one of several clinics composing the second largest County Health Department in the United States. The intervention consisted of multiple strategies that involved physician education, physician feedback, patient education, policy interventions, and expanding the capacity to serve women better. The authors stated that "logistical constraints, limited resources, and other practical consideration in the County health care system largely dictated the choice of this design. Intervention and control sites were selected in consultation with our partners in the County Health Department. The system did not include sufficient sites to allow for randomization to intervention and control conditions. Likewise, the structure of the health care system made it impossible to randomize the intervention to only a portion of the women receiving care at any one site" (Bastani and others, 2002, p. 893). Intervention sites were a hospital, a comprehensive health center (CHC), and three public health centers (PHCs) and were matched on size, patient characteristics, and a range of services provided to another hospital, a CHC, and three PHCs. Intervention effects were observed at the hospital and the CHC, where there was a significant increase in cervical cancer screening.

The *interrupted time series design* (ITSD) is the strongest quasi-experimental approach for evaluating the longitudinal effects of interventions. It involves collecting data at multiple instances over time before and after a treatment of some kind. The treatment can be a health promotion program, implementation of a new health policy, or a naturally occurring event. Data used in a time series design can range from individual behavior to cumulative incidence of sexually transmitted diseases. It does require knowledge about the specific time in which the program or intervention occurred in the time series. An advantage of collecting a series of observations both before and after the treatment is that a reliable picture regarding the outcome of interest can be gleaned. Thus, the time series design is sensitive to trends in performance. The aim is to determine whether or not the intervention had an effect over and above any trend present in the data. For example, the data collected prior to the treatment may reveal several trends in the data such as a maturational trend (in which observations involve human subjects who are changing their behavior as they age) or a seasonal trend (in which observations are influenced by the season in which data are collected). These trends can be identified and assessed, and treatment effects ascertained. A treatment effect is demonstrated only if the pattern of posttreatment responses differs significantly from the pattern of pretreatment responses. That is, the treatment effect is demonstrated by a discontinuity in the pattern of pretreatment and posttreatment responses. For example, an effect is demonstrated when there is a change in the level or slope of the posttreatment responses as, or both, compared with the pretreatment responses.

The most basic of the ITSDs is the simple interrupted time series, in which there is only one experimental group. This design can be diagrammed as follows:

$$O_1 \quad O_2 \quad O_3 \quad O_4 \quad \text{Treatment} \quad O_5 \quad O_6 \quad O_7 \quad O_8$$

The greatest threat to the internal validity of this design is history, although other threats such as instrumentation and selection can occur.

Adding a nonequivalent control group to the simple interrupted time series will improve on some of the limitations mentioned. This design, called an interrupted time series with a nonequivalent control group time series, is diagrammed as follows:

$$O_1 \quad O_2 \quad O_3 \quad O_4 \quad \text{Treatment} \quad O_5 \quad O_6 \quad O_7 \quad O_8$$

$$O_1 \quad O_2 \quad O_3 \quad O_4 \quad \phantom{\text{Treatment}} \quad O_5 \quad O_6 \quad O_7 \quad O_8$$

As shown, a series of observations are collected both prior to and following the administration of the treatment for the experimental group; during this same time period, a series of observations are also collected for a comparison group. This design allows the researcher to control for history effects, as a historical event would most likely affect both treatment and control groups equally. What may be problematic, however, is when one group experiences a unique set of events. This type of threat is deemed an interaction between selection and history and is called a selection-history effect. It is important to note that for a historical event to pose a threat to internal validity, the event must occur at the same time as the intervention or treatment. Other threats to the internal validity are similar to the basic NCGD, with selection being the greatest threat and the interaction of selection with threats other than history such as selection-maturation, selection-instrumentation, and selection-regression.

Wong, Chan, and Koh (2002) used a simple ITSD to examine the impact of a sexual-risk-reduction program that encouraged condom use for oral sex among female brothel-based sex workers in Singapore. The study observed two outcomes: condom use trends and the pharyngeal gonorrhea trends. Comparisons on the two study outcomes were made across four time periods that corresponded to different phases of the intervention: a preintervention period of two years; an intervention phase of two years; a postintervention phase of one year when activities were withdrawn; and a follow-up period of one year when activities were resumed and incorporated into the brothel's health education policy for its sex workers. The results indicated that for the preintervention phase, consistent condom use for oral sex was stable at below 50 percent. Following the intervention, condom use increased significantly. During the postintervention phase of one year, when activities were withheld from brothels, condom use leveled off and decreased to 79.7 percent. In the last year, when activities were institutionalized, condom use increased significantly to 89.9 percent. The significant changing trend in condom use was mirrored by changes in pharyngeal gonorrhea incidence rates. Preintervention, pharyngeal gonorrhea incidence rates were stable and remained high (12.4 to 16.6 per 1000 person-months). During the two-year intervention phase, the pharyngeal gonorrhea incidence rate significantly decreased to 3.3 per 1000 person-months, but was followed by an increase when program activities were withdrawn. This increase was in tandem with the decrease in condom use during this same phase. During the final phase, when condom use increased significantly, there was also a major decline in the pharyngeal gonorrhea incidence rate, from 14.4 to 4.0 per 1000 person-months.

Integration with the Research Process

Choosing an appropriate research design is a critical part of the overall research process and may depend to a large degree on the nature of the research question; however, there are other issues to consider that may influence the overall process. For example, the stage of the research process, either exploratory or conclusive, will influence greatly many aspects of the research. For example, if a research field is in the exploratory stage, then this may affect the ability to fulfill step 1 (identify a priority population) in the nine-step model described in Chapter One. Consequently, identifying specific populations that require priority because of their risk status may be the goal of the research, especially if previous research has not determined which populations are most at risk. Moreover, the stage of the research process will influence the nature of the research question (step 2). If still the exploratory phase, research questions will be geared toward a better understanding of the phenomena involved or perhaps toward identifying what the problem is. If the field has moved to the conclusive stage, research questions will be more clearly defined involving testable hypotheses with important implications. Once the research question is formulated, it is equally important to identify the main goal or purpose associated with that research question (step 3). That is, is the research purpose to describe salient risk factors associated with a health issue or to determine who is most at risk for a health issue (that is, descriptive purpose), or is it to identify cause-and-effect relationships or test the efficacy of health programs (that is, causal purpose)? The research purpose in turn will affect the selection of a parsimonious research design (step 4). Finally, once an appropriate research design is selected, this defines the appropriate statistical technique to be employed for data analysis (step 8).

Making good decisions in the first three steps of the process will have a positive impact on the latter steps in the process, whereas unwise decisions may negatively affect the latter steps. Specifically, having an understanding of all potential research issues will enhance the planning of the research (steps 4–6). For example, an important practice is to consider whether an HPP might inadvertently produce negative effects of any kind. Indeed, an emerging framework in health promotion suggests that negative, unanticipated outcomes should be measured (Glasgow, Vogt, and Boles, 1999). Also, thinking ahead about research issues may greatly facilitate the implementation of the research (step 7), and, consequently, assist in the testing of the research hypotheses and the dissemination of the results (step 9).

Summary

All of the designs described in this chapter have associated strengths, limitations, and varying levels of rigor. The important thing to know is the strengths and limitations of each research design, and how these may affect the study results and the interpretation of those results. Thus, perhaps the most important decision to make is the selection of a research design. This decision should be examined carefully by every member of the research team, and the pros and cons of each option should be weighed with great attention to rigor. Many of these pros and cons were outlined in this chapter. It may be useful to begin by defining whether the research is exploratory or conclusive, and then asking whether it is descriptive or causal. From that point, it is critical to consider what resources are available to the project so that the selected study design is not only functional but also feasible. In addition, although implicit in this chapter, it is important to remain vigilant regarding your obligation to design research studies that are ethical in nature and that do not violate the rights or well-being of the participants. Finally, it is imperative that your research design optimizes the ability to provide a rigorous and valid test of the research question(s) because your work may have great potential to shape health promotion practice and policy and contribute another link in the chain of research.

Issues to Consider

1. Early in the HIV/AIDS epidemic, researchers wanted to ascertain the effectiveness of giving antiretroviral therapies (ARTs) to HIV-positive women who were pregnant, to prevent the transmission of the virus to their unborn child. At the time, this was considered a risky treatment, and the safety of this drug treatment on the unborn child was not known. Using an experimental design to randomly assign pregnant women who are HIV-positive to receive ART or to receive a placebo would be the most rigorous design with a high degree of control and internal validity. On the one hand, using an experimental design could provide definitive evidence of the effectiveness of the treatment; on the other hand, some women would not receive the treatment, which

could benefit them greatly and prevent HIV infection in their baby. Was there an alternative design that could have been used in this instance? What are the ethical considerations of using an experimental design with a placebo-control group?

2. The value of the cross-sectional study is not always recognized among researchers. At one extreme, researchers might say that "cross-sectional studies are only good for hypothesis generation." At the other extreme, researchers might say that "cross-sectional studies could be very useful, even to the point of supporting causal relationships." Because such a large volume of health promotion research is based on data collected using cross-sectional research designs, this issue of "value" is indeed an important one. Thus, perhaps a critical question to ask is, Under what circumstances can findings from a cross-sectional study be used to test a hypothesis?

3. Earlier in this chapter it was noted that within-subjects designs (also known as the repeated-measures design) actually has less within-subject error variance than a between-groups design. Alternatively, it was noted that the lack of a control group implies that the within-subjects design is not a true experimental design. Given that the use of a control group may not always be feasible (due to limited research funds) or ethical (due to the potentially highly effective nature of the HPP and the lack of any acceptable attention-control condition), could a within-subjects design ever be preferable? If so, under what conditions would this be so? Also, what types of research questions would be the *most* appropriate for this design? Conversely, what types of research questions would be the *least* appropriate for this design?

For Practice and Discussion

1. A research question asks about the relationship of Internet health seeking to the health of infants among first-time parents. The researcher suspects that new parents who vigilantly seek health information on the Internet pertaining to the infants will provide better health care (and preventive care) to their infants as opposed to parents who rarely or never seek this type of information. Assume that sufficient evidence exists to conduct conclusive research. Given that your research funding is only sufficient for an *observational study,* please select the study design you would employ and provide a rationale for your selection to a colleague who is also completing this same exercise. Allow the colleagues to challenge your selection and then "trade places" by asking the colleague to allow you to challenge his or her selection.

2. Please repeat the exercise outlined in number 1, but this time assume that you have sufficient funds to conduct an experimental study.

3. Working with at least one colleague, please consider (and list) the advantages and disadvantages of random assignment. Please rank each advantage on a scale from one to five (with five being the most extreme level of concern). Similarly, please rank each disadvantage on a scale from one to five (with five being the most extreme level of "gain" resulting from randomization). Next, please find another pair of colleagues who have completed this same exercise and compare the two sets of lists and rankings.

4. For each research goal listed below, please select the best research design that could be applied to most effectively address the goal. Parsimony is an important criteria. Be prepared to defend your answer.

   A. To determine the efficacy of a three-session intervention program designed to promote the consumption of a diet low in saturated fats among cardiac rehabilitation patients

   B. To test the hypothesis that childhood activity levels predict obesity in early adulthood

   C. To determine the relationship of sleep to depression in college students

   D. To explore the role of self-efficacy in the decision to enroll in a smoking cessation course

   E. To test the hypothesis that fewer high school students are engaging in sex in 2004, compared with high school students in the 1980s

   F. To assess whether a media program can promote the use of infant car seats

   G. To identify the effectiveness of an alcohol use awareness program (note: you have a strong suspicion that the assessment instrument used for alcohol awareness is also likely to foster awareness—you would like to test this suspicion as well)

References

Bastani, R., and others. (2002). Increasing cervical cancer screening among underserved women in a large urban county health system: Can it be done? What does it take? *Medical Care, 40*(10), 891–907.

Bhandari, N., and others. (2003). Effect of community-based promotion of exclusive breastfeeding on diarrhoeal illness and growth: A cluster randomized controlled trial. *Lancet, 361*(9367), 1418–1423.

Campbell, D. T., and Stanley, J. C. (1966). *Experimental and quasi-experimental designs for research.* Chicago: Rand McNally.

Centers for Disease Control and Prevention. (2004, May 21). Surveillance Summaries. *Morbidity and Mortality Weekly Report, 53*(SS-2).

Chassin, L., Presson, C. C., Rose, J. S., and Sherman, S. J. (2001). From adolescence to adulthood: Age-related changes in beliefs about cigarette smoking in a Midwestern community sample. *Health Psychology, 20*(5), 377–386.

DiClemente, R. J., and others. (2004). A descriptive analysis of STD prevalence among urban pregnant African-American teens: Data from a pilot study. *Journal of Adolescent Health, 34*(5), 376–383.

Emmons, K. M., Linnan, L. A., Shadel, W. G., Marcus, B., and Abrams, D. B. (1999). The Working Healthy Project: A worksite health-promotion trial targeting physical activity, diet, and smoking. *Journal of Occupational & Environmental Medicine, 41*(7), 545–555.

Finn, J. (2004). A survey of online harassment at a university campus. *Journal of Interpersonal Violence, 19*(4), 468–483.

Glasgow, R. E., Vogt T. M., and Boles, S. M. (1999). Evaluating the public health impact of health promotion interventions: The RE-AIM framework. *American Journal of Public Health, 89*, 1322–1327.

Hall, H. I., Jones, S. E., and Saraiya, M. (2001). Prevalence and correlates of sunscreen use among U.S. high school students. *Journal of School Health, 71*(9), 453–457.

Huurre, T. M., Aro, H. M., and Jaakkola, J. J. (2004). Incidence and prevalence of asthma and allergic rhinitis: A cohort study of Finnish adolescents. *Journal of Asthma, 41*(3), 311–317.

Klein, E., Campbell, J., Soler, E., and Ghez, M. (1997). *Ending domestic violence: Changing public perceptions / Halting the epidemic.* Thousand Oaks, CA: Sage.

Kulczycki, A., Kim, D. J., Duerr, A., Jamieson, D. J., and Macaluso, M. (2004). The acceptability of the female and male condom: A randomized crossover trial. *Perspectives on Sexual & Reproductive Health, 36*(3), 114–119.

Lapidus, G., and others. (2002). A statewide survey of domestic violence screening behaviors among pediatricians and family physicians. *Archives of Pediatrics 7 Adolescent Medicine, 156*(4), 332–336.

Melville, J., and others. (2003). Psychosocial impact of serological diagnosis of herpes simplex virus 2: A qualitative assessment. *Sexually Transmitted Infections, 79*, 280–285.

Morse, J. (1994). Designing funded qualitative research. In N. K. Denzin and J. S. Lincoln (Eds.), *Handbook of qualitative research* (pp. 220–235). Thousand Oaks, CA: Sage.

Repetto, P. B., Zimmerman, M. A., and Caldwell, C. H. (2004). A longitudinal study of the relationship between depressive symptoms and alcohol use in a sample of inner-city black youth. *Journal of Studies on Alcohol, 65*(2), 169–178.

Salazar, L. F., and Cook, S. L. (2002). Violence against women: Is psychology part of the problem or the solution? A content analysis of psychological research from 1990 through 1999. *Journal of Community and Applied Social Psychology, 12*, 410–421.

Salazar, L. F., and others. (2004). Self-concept and adolescents' refusal of unsafe sex: A test of mediating mechanisms among African American girls. *Prevention Science, 5*(3), 137–149.

Serdula, M. K., and others. (2004). Trends in fruit and vegetable consumption among adults in the United States: Behavioral risk factor surveillance system, 1994–2000. *American Journal of Public Health, 94*(6), 1014–1018.

Shrier, L., and others. (2001). Randomized controlled trial of a safer sex intervention for high-risk adolescent girls. *Archives of Pediatrics and Adolescent Medicine, 155*(1), 73–79.

St. Lawrence, J. S., Wilson, T. E., Eldridge, G. D., Brasfield, T. L., and O'Bannon, R. E. III. (2001). Community-based interventions to reduce low-income, African American women's risk of sexually transmitted diseases: A randomized controlled trial of three theoretical models. *American Journal of Community Psychology, 29*(6), 937–964.

Varma, R., and others. (2004). Prevalence of open-angle glaucoma and ocular hypertension in Latinos: The Los Angeles Latino Eye Study. *Ophthalmology, 111*(8), 1439–1448.

Wong, M. L., Chan, R. K., and Koh, D. (2002). Promoting condoms for oral sex: Impact on pharyngeal gonorrhea among female brothel-based sex workers. *Sexually Transmitted Diseases, 29*(6), 311–318.

CHAPTER FIVE

CONDUCTING OBSERVATIONAL RESEARCH

Richard A. Crosby, Laura F. Salazar, and Ralph J. DiClemente

As described in Chapter One, observational research is an important link in the chain of research evidence. Whether as a forerunner to randomized controlled trials (RCTs) or as a definitive form of study, observational research is very much the "bread and butter" of evidence in health promotion. Indeed, observational research constitutes the vast majority of early- and mid-level work in any chain of research evidence. Given the low cost and relatively short time commitments of some forms of observational study, graduate students and entry-level researchers are particularly likely to take on a project that is observational rather than experimental.

◆ ◆ ◆

In a Nutshell

Whether as a forerunner to randomized controlled trials or as a definitive form of study, observational research is very much the "bread and butter" of evidence in health promotion.

◆ ◆ ◆

Of course, the ultimate caveat with observational research is that rigor must be high. Several textbooks have provided a litany of conceptual issues that must be addressed to ensure this rigor (for example, Huck and Cormier 1996; Shi, 1997; Sim and Wright, 2000). Unfortunately, the "nuts and bolts" of conducting observational research (that is, the steps that can and should be taken to avoid these conceptual problems) have often been neglected. Indeed, the process of conducting observational research is far from straightforward, and the number of potential pitfalls is endless. Therefore, this chapter will address multiple concerns relevant to the conception, design, and implementation of observational research in health promotion.

Illustration of Key Concepts

Researchers typically confront four distinct types of issues when conducting observational research. The first is gaining access to a sample. Access alone, however, is not enough; thus, effective recruitment strategies are paramount. Next, issues related to assessment are critically important to the preservation reservation of rigor. Finally, studies that follow people over time must have built-in mechanisms to ensure that attrition in the cohort is minimal.

Gaining Access to a Sample

As noted in Chapter One, the first step in the research process is to define the study population. This task, however, is highly dependent on accessibility to the targeted population. For example, imagine that you have identified runaway youths as the study population. You have two options. You could hire staff to recruit youths from various street locations, or you could centralize the process by working in a shelter for runaway youths. The first option may be quite labor intensive, given that you would need to efficiently intercept and screen a massive number of youths on the streets to find even a few (with luck) who are runaways. The second option seems more attractive, yet this option requires something that may be difficult to secure: administrative "buy in" from the shelter. Whether the point of access is a shelter or a public venue, there are *gatekeepers* (in other words, people who are in positions to grant or deny access) who are controlling access. Research ideas may often be looked at with great suspicion among gatekeepers. Thus, gaining their approval to conduct the study may be a challenging (and ongoing) process. The goals of the research and the goals of the gatekeepers may be not only quite different but also incompatible. For example, the shelter for runaway youths may view its primary goal as providing a temporary, safe haven where youths can receive referrals to social services.

Given this mission, concerns about the proposed observational research may arise and could include

- How will kids who take part in this study benefit from participating?
- What assurances do you have to offer that kids will not feel coerced into participating?
- What type of questions will you be asking? Will these questions be personally invasive?
- Will your assessments be anonymous?
- How will your study help us? How will it help the community?

Naturally, addressing these issues in a satisfactory manner is a prerequisite to gaining access to the population; however, this could be a complicated response not addressed easily. For example, in responding to how youths will benefit, one problem is that you are not providing a health promotion program (HPP) (that is, a program that promotes health and well-being). Also, you cannot guarantee that youths will *not* perceive the "offer to participate" as coercive. Furthermore, your research questions necessitate assessing substance abuse and sexual behaviors and may be considered invasive. If your study is prospective, then you will need to ask youths for contact information so you can locate them again in about thirty days (thus, anonymity is not possible). Finally, the expected findings from your study may have very little relevance to the provision of services.

How can these problems be brought to a successful resolution? The answer lies within the second step of the research process (formulating the research question), the fifth step (determining what variables should be measured), and potentially the sixth step (sampling). For example, you may need to include a research question that addresses a unique need of the shelter or the immediate community. This does not diminish your original intent in any way; instead, it simply adds to the magnitude of your project. Next, you may need to either justify or remove planned measures from your assessment. Removing measures may diminish the quality and scope of your research, however.

To illustrate this point further, consider this real-world example. The Centers for Disease Control and Prevention (CDC) conducts a cross-sectional survey of U.S. high school students every two years called the Youth Risk Behavioral Surveillance System (YRBSS) that assesses health risk behaviors. Questions about sexual behaviors, which were to be included in the questionnaire, raised red flags among certain people who had the authority to grant or deny access to the population of high school students. In the 1999 survey year, twenty states either did not participate in the survey or denied the CDC permission to ask questions related to adolescents' sexual risk behavior. Three states (North Dakota, Vermont, and Maine) agreed to ask some of the questions pertaining to sex, but not others (Crosby, Holtgrave, DiClemente, Wingood, and Gayle, 2003). Of note, none of the sexual behavior questions were necessarily "invasive" beyond the level of asking kids if they ever had sex, if they had had sex in the past three months, if they had used a condom or contraceptive at last intercourse, and if they had ever been (or caused) a pregnancy. Questions about oral and anal sex were not included. Thus, in this example, the quality and scope of the research was compromised to gain access to a population. Some states agreed to ask the majority of the questions, but not those related to sex. Other states decided to select which questions they would allow in relationship to assessing sexual behavior.

Based on a delicate balance between gaining access and asking the "right" questions in the assessment, researchers must be prepared to make compromises, but only to a point. The point at which the required compromises jeopardize the ability of the research process to generate rigorous findings is the terminal point of the negotiation. It may be preferable to identify a different population rather than conduct a study that does not meet your needs. Indeed, the search for a population to access may be a time-consuming and labor-intensive task.

◆ ◆ ◆

In a Nutshell

The point at which the required compromises jeopardize the ability of the research process to generate rigorous findings is the terminal point of the negotiation.

◆ ◆ ◆

Finally, gaining access may require compromise in the sampling plan. For example, shelter administrators may insist that youths be recruited into the study only during the daytime hours on Saturday and Sunday (they may feel strongly that other times of the week are "just too busy"). Furthermore, they may insist that only kids aged sixteen and older can participate. Again, the research team needs to respect the negotiation and make every effort to accommodate these requests, but requests that are perceived by the team to jeopardize the rigor and scope of the research should *not* be met. Providing decision makers with a carefully delivered explanation of the sampling needs may go a long way toward achieving a successful resolution.

Recruiting

Chapter One described the importance of rigor. Rigor is lost in small, sometimes seemingly unimportant, aspects of a study. Recruitment is a good example of an opportunity for rigor to decrease substantially. The primary concern is that a low *participation rate* (sometimes called a *cooperation rate*) may lead to *participation bias,* also called *selection bias* (in other words, the sample is not representative of the population). This problem is not a consequence of the selected sampling technique; rather, it stems from poor planning or poor implementation of a recruitment protocol. Incidentally, a criterion for defining "low" participation rate does not exist.

Understanding two key principles can set the stage for successful recruitment in health promotion research: (1) strategies have been devised to promote effective (that is, high participation rate) recruiting, and (2) recruiting efforts should always be systematic. The importance of *effective* and *systematic* recruiting cannot be overstated. Chapter Eleven will describe a number of sampling options that are commonly applied to health promotion research. Sampling plans (also known as sampling protocols) are the direct result of carefully matching a sampling option with the research question(s). Unfortunately, the best laid plans may fall apart if a large number of those eligible (that is, people who were sampled and met the inclusion criteria) do not enroll in the study. This problem may be a direct consequence of ineffective recruiting. Furthermore, plans may fall apart if some of the eligible "would-be" volunteers are recruited more vigorously than others. This problem may be a direct consequence of recruiting efforts that are not systematic.

Effective Recruiting. Although research methods are used to answer health promotion research questions, studies of the various methods employed (that is, research about conducting research) have been neglected. For example, it would be quite enlightening to know the relative importance of three factors involved in the recruitment process: (1) the amount of financial incentive being offered, (2) the effect of timing and the setting on recruitment success, and (3) the effect of the recruitment approach on recruitment success. Unfortunately, empirical evidence addressing these questions is scarcely found in the published literature. In this instance, we rely on anecdotal evidence (from our own studies and studies conducted by colleagues) to provide guidance in effective recruiting.

First, incentives are important. These can take the form of cash, vouchers, gift cards, or tangible goods. The value of the incentive should be commensurate with the amount of time and effort required to fulfill the requirements of the study. For example, spending three to four hours to answer a lengthy questionnaire should have a much larger incentive as compared with taking a fifteen-minute survey. The amount of compensation may be established in part by local standards. In addition to being considered coercive, high-value incentives may create participation bias.

Second, timing is important because it can influence recruitment efforts. For example, people may be more receptive to participating when they are not under stress and when they have "time on their hands." Also, people attending a medical clinic may be more easily recruited while they are in a waiting room and are essentially a "captive audience" rather then when they have finished their appointment. Thus, timing of when people will be approached is everything. In fact, the lead author of this chapter achieved high participation rates (90 percent) in studies of men attending sex resorts by recruiting during the daytime hours (near a swimming pool) rather than in the evenings and nights when a primary concern of the men was engaging in sex (Crosby and DiClemente, 2004).

Third, the recruiting approach can be an important determinant of success. Of course, a "one size fits all" approach does not exist. The best approach is one that matches the needs and perceptions of the potential volunteers. For example, in a CDC-sponsored cross-sectional survey of men who have sex with men, the lead author of this chapter and his colleagues achieved high participation rates, which may be attributable to a recruiting appeal. Men were informed that the study was designed to help researchers learn more about the prevention of HIV and AIDS among men who have sex with men. Given that this population of men has been hit particularly hard by the AIDS epidemic, the study was appealing to men for personal reasons. Indeed, the nature of the study (combined with how it is explained during the recruitment encounter) may be the most important factor in terms of producing a high participation rate.

Recruiting approaches can also be deemed as *active* or *passive*. Active recruiting occurs when investigators seek out participants, whereas passive recruiting is when participants seek out investigators as a result of some advertisement (flyers, radio and television announcements, newspaper ads, newsletters, and Internet banner ads). Box 5.1 displays an example of a recruitment brochure. Active recruiting is necessary when the number of eligible study participants is expected to be low. For example, we collaborated with colleagues to examine the psychological and psychosocial effects of receiving a positive herpes diagnosis among asymptomatic clinic patients. Patients were referred to our study by their health care provider, who had conveyed the diagnosis (Melville and others, 2003). A methodological benefit of this approach is determining a true participation rate and refusal rate, and in some instances, if data are available, then comparisons can be made between those who participate and those who refuse.

Alternatively, passive recruitment relies on the assumption that an ample number of people are eligible, and also that a large number of eligible people will be exposed to the advertisements. A contemporary example of passive recruitment

Box 5.1. Example of a Recruitment Brochure

You're Invited!

You are invited to participate in a study that will investigate concerns people may have about accepting an AIDS vaccine if one ever became available for use in the United States. To be eligible you must

- Be 18 years of age or older
- Be able to read and understand English
- Not knowingly be positive for HIV (the virus that causes AIDS)

Enrollment in the study means that you will agree to participate in a one-hour interview (on the day of enrollment) and another one-hour interview two months after the first. After each interview, you will be provided with $35 to compensate you for your time. All information that you provide will be confidential.

If you would like to learn more about this study, please contact:

Study Director
402 Main Street, Room 390
Washington, MO 30111
Phone: (234) 555-1234

can be found in conjunction with federally funded research designed to test potential AIDS vaccines in human volunteers. Recruitment protocols for these studies require a passive approach (using multiple forms of media to promote the study to massive numbers of people). In contrast to active recruitment, passive recruitment does not allow for the computation of a true participation rate because the total number of people exposed to the solicitation is unknown. Passive recruitment methods also do not allow for making comparisons between participants and those who do not participate.

Systematic Recruiting. A rigorous study will follow a strict recruiting protocol. All potential volunteers should be treated in the same manner. This "sameness" is as equally important as the content of the protocol. One common practice to ensure consistency is to provide research staff with recruitment scripts. Scripts should be short enough that staff can recite the script naturally versus artificially and long

MINCUS AND DINCUS USE PASSIVE RECRUITMENT
FOR THEIR STUDY.

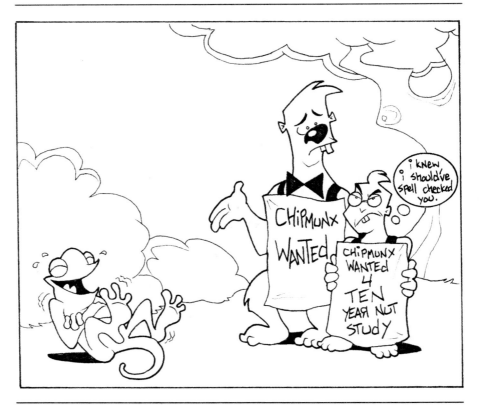

Copyright 2005 by Justin Wagner; reprinted with permission.

enough so that they accurately portray the study. Box 5.2 displays several examples of recruitment scripts applied to health promotion research. One of the best examples of this kind of commitment to a protocol can be found in phone surveys— in these protocols research staff are reciting recruitment lines verbatim. To ensure that staff do not drift from the script, supervisors should intermittently monitor (and correct) staff performance. The importance of this supervision cannot be overstated.

Keeping Recruitment and Retention Records

As described in Chapter Fourteen, a rigorous study will need to document (1) how many people were screened for eligibility, (2) how many were eligible,

Box 5.2. Examples of Recruitment Scripts

"We are conducting a study that will help us learn about the HIV prevention needs of African American women. Would you be willing to provide us with thirty minutes of your time?"

"The Wyoming State Department of Health has commissioned a study of farm injury prevention. Part of that study involves interviewing the teenage children of farm families. You qualify to participate in the study. If you are interested, I can explain the process to you in detail."

"I am recruiting study volunteers who are willing to help me and others who work with me to learn about the reasons why men do not always use condoms. Because you have been diagnosed with an STD today, you qualify to be in the study. Are you interested in helping us? The information you provide could be very useful in the eventual design of an education program."

"To improve the quality of our health care services, we are asking clients to consider volunteering for a two-year study. We would ask you some questions today and then contact you by phone three times during every six months. The questions and phone calls are intended to provide us with data regarding how you make decisions whether or not to be seen by a doctor in our clinic. We are trying to improve our services as much as possible. Would you consider helping us out?"

and (3) how many participated. In prospective studies, it is equally important to include (4) how many returned to the first planned follow-up assessment, and (5) how many returned to the second planned follow-up assessment, and so on. Maintaining these records is, of course, labor intensive. Ideally, a study director (someone who is always "on duty") should keep these records by using a daily diary. However, the records may also require the use of forms. If the local Institutional Review Board (IRB) permits it, documentation could include asking people who refused to participate why they refused and also collecting basic demographic data (age, gender, race) to compare nonvolunteers to volunteers. Some local IRBs, however, may prohibit any data collection among nonvolunteers. The ultimate goal of this data collection is to build a table that empirically addresses the potential for participation bias. Table 5.1 provides an example of this type of evidence.

Notice that the table provides a head-to-head comparison of volunteers and nonvolunteers. The data make clear that volunteers were significantly less likely

TABLE 5.1. A COMPARISON OF VOLUNTEERS AND NONVOLUNTEERS.

Characteristic	Number (%) Volunteers (N = 1,000)	Number (%) Nonvolunteers (N = 400)
Age		
18–29	90 (9.0)	40 (10.0)
30–39	450 (45.0)	160 (40.0)
40–49	410 (41.0)	160 (40.0)
50 and older	50 (5.0)	40 (10.0)
Race		
American Indian or Alaskan Native	12 (1.2)	12 (3.0)
Alaskan or Pacific Islander	95 (9.5)	40 (10.0)
Black or African American	**455 (45.5)**	**200 (50.0)**
White	**438 (43.8)**	**148 (37.0)**
Ethnicity		
Hispanic	290 (29.0)	120 (30.0)
Non-Hispanic	710 (71.0)	280 (70.0)
Employment		
Full-Time	770 (77.0)	320 (80.0)
Part-Time	70 (7.0)	30 (7.5)
Unemployed	**110 (11.0)**	**6 (1.5)**
Retired	**50 (5.0)**	**44 (11.0)**
Sex		
Male	490 (49.0)	210 (52.5)
Female	510 (51.0)	190 (47.5)

Note: Bold entries represent differences that are significant at $P < .05$.

than nonvolunteers to be black or African American and significantly more likely to be white. Also, volunteers were significantly more likely than nonvolunteers to be unemployed and significantly less likely to be retired.

Assessment

Chapter Nine will describe methods of assessment in great detail. For now, it is sufficient to note that the selected assessment method must be implemented with great fidelity. Just as a sampling plan can be foiled by poor recruiting, an assessment method can be compromised by poor implementation. Three key issues are paramount: (1) avoiding response bias, (2) avoiding undue respondent fatigue, and (3) facilitating accurate recall.

◆ ◆ ◆

In a Nutshell

Just as a sampling plan can be foiled by poor recruiting, an assessment method can be compromised by poor implementation.

◆ ◆ ◆

Avoiding Response Bias. Response bias can take on several forms. One common concern is that study participants will "play to" or "play against" their perception of the study hypotheses. For example, if a male participant suspects that the study is designed to test whether people are more likely to be abusive toward a sex partner during periods of intoxication, then his hunch may knowingly or even unknowingly skew his responses to the questions. He may answer in a way that falsely supports the hypothesis or in a way that falsely fails to support the hypothesis. One strategy that is sometimes used to avoid this form of bias is not to provide information to participants about the hypotheses. IRBs will occasionally approve consent forms that do not fully disclose the purpose of the study. Of course, the recruitment script and even the questions being asked should be constructed to avoid bias. Most important, however, research staff must be skilled in the art of responding to any questions volunteers may ask without appearing impolite or unconcerned when they do not directly answer questions that would betray the hypotheses.

Another common form of bias stems from social desirability. This form of bias is easy to understand for anyone that has ever been sitting in a dental chair and been asked, "How often do you floss?" Most people are tempted to inflate their answer to "please" the hygienist or dentist and to create the impression that they practice excellent dental hygiene. In observational research that addresses health behavior, study volunteers may experience a similar need to please the person conducting the interview. Fortunately, this problem can be addressed by informing participants that the "best answer" is an honest answer. Although this seems simple enough, it requires a completely nonjudgmental atmosphere (especially in face-to-face interviews). For example, if someone is asked, "How many sex partners have you had in the past three months" and the answer provided is "about three dozen," then the person conducting the interview must not react any differently to this response than if the response had been "two."

Avoiding Undue Respondent Fatigue. Although research is the backbone of science, conducting research with people also requires simple attention to their needs. One important principle to keep in mind is that the research and the questions are probably not as interesting to the study participants as they are to the researchers. In fact, the questions may be perceived as tedious. Apart from constructing clear questions and devising interesting response formats (see Chapters Nine and Ten), the people conducting the assessment must be attuned to the energy and interest-level of the respondents. Are people attentive during the entire assessment period or does their attention wane after the first ten minutes? If their attention does wane, then what can be done to get them back on track? Do people need a break at some point during the process? Does providing food help? Attending to these questions is the responsibility of the research staff and is similar to being a good host who ensures the comfort and enjoyment of his or her guests. The goal is to create an environment that is comfortable and ask people to complete a reasonable task without undue constraints.

Simultaneous with the process of alleviating fatigue, the research staff also must engage in a form of quality assurance. One of the worst fates suffered by a data set is the absence of answers—to any number of questions—from a substantial proportion of the participants. Depending on the arrangements agreed upon in the consent process, members of the research staff may, for example, review completed questionnaires before respondents leave the setting. A polite request to "please consider providing responses to questions 76 through 89 on the last page" (for example) may be met with cooperation. This small task may make the difference between including and excluding the participant's data from the final analysis. Less forward strategies include asking participants—before they leave—to please be sure they have answered all of the questions except for those that don't apply or those they purposefully chose not to answer. Of course, participants should also be informed (perhaps at several points in the assessment process) that the research staff would be happy to clarify any of the questions that may be confusing or problematic to answer. This offer, though, must never be taken lightly by the research staff because "clarification" can easily become a source of bias if the staff member strays from the written, spoken, or recorded question. Defining words and modestly paraphrasing questions are two practices that may be safe.

◆ ◆ ◆

In a Nutshell

A polite request to "please consider providing responses to questions 76 through 89 on the last page" (for example) may be met with cooperation. This small task may make the difference between including and excluding the participant's data from the final analysis.

◆ ◆ ◆

Facilitating Accurate Recall. Health promotion research often asks people to recall past events. Infrequent events that have high salience generally do not pose a problem (for example, events that occurred on September 11, 2001). Generally it can be expected that events with high saliency and low frequency facilitate the most accurate recall. As an example in health promotion, consider someone who has had sex (high salience) twice in the past six months. Recalling the details of these two events may be relatively easy. Conversely, someone who has had more than a hundred sexual events in the past six months may be challenged to recall with a high degree of accuracy any details of these one hundred events. Other events may be frequent but lack salience, leading to low accuracy in recall. For example, asking study participants who regularly eat eggs to recall the number of eggs they have consumed (low salience) in the past thirty days would probably lead to inaccuracies in recall. The most challenging scenario occurs when the behavior under study is low in salience and is relatively frequent. Such a challenge may require the use of shortened recall periods, calendars marked with key dates, and verbal "probes" if the assessment is given in a face-to-face format.

◆ ◆ ◆

In a Nutshell

The most challenging scenario occurs when the behavior under study is low in salience and is relatively frequent.

◆ ◆ ◆

Short recall periods may be extremely useful. It is not at all unusual for health promotion research studies to use a one-day recall period (for example, "what are the foods that you consumed yesterday?") or a last-event recall period (for example, "the last time you ate out at a restaurant, what did you order?"). Of course, the risk of this truncated assessment period is that the "one day" or "last event" may not represent the true nature of the health behavior of the person being assessed.

Research staff might also increase accurate recall by starting each assessment with a large calendar. In settings where the staff member can interface with participants individually, the session can begin by helping participants fill in key dates. To illustrate, imagine asking questions designed to assess how many alcoholic beverages people consume in a typical month. To facilitate accurate recall, a staff member might ask, "Have you had any special events in the past month that were celebrated by having a party?" Another question might be, "In the past month, there were four weekends (show these by pointing at the calendar). On any of these weekends (if so, which ones) did any sporting events occur that you watched while drinking?" Another example might be, "In the past month, was there a time in your life when you were extremely stressed or depressed? Can you please indicate those days on the calendar for me?" Any affirmative answer can be followed up to elicit a date which is then recorded on the calendar. This entry may serve as a benchmark for the person when asked to recall how many drinks had been consumed. Notice that the questions are not the issue here; instead, the goal is to train research staff in the "art" of conducting an assessment that will maximize the odds of accurate recall from the participants.

◆ ◆ ◆

In a Nutshell

The goal is to train research staff in the "art" of conducting an assessment that will maximize the odds of accurate recall from the participants.

◆ ◆ ◆

Finally, in face-to-face interviews, verbal probes can greatly facilitate accurate recall. For example, to assess how many sex partners someone had over the past six months, the interview would begin with the basic question and proceed with probes if the initial answer is somewhat unclear. A hypothetical example follows:

Interviewer: In the past six months, how many different people have engaged in sexual intercourse with you? (Sexual intercourse means that the penis is placed into the mouth, vagina, or rectum of another person.)

Participant: Uhhh, umhh, I would have to say between ten and twelve people. On second thought, umhh, make that fifteen.

Interviewer: This kind of counting can be difficult—I noticed you initially said "ten" and finally said "fifteen." Please think about why you raised your answer—did you raise it too much—or perhaps not enough?

Maintaining the Cohort

The advanced version of recruitment is retention. In prospective observational studies, retention is so vital that complete failure of the study may easily occur if the rate is low. Prospective data are complete only when at least two time points have been covered by the study. A baseline assessment alone will not answer research questions that are prospective in nature. Thus, the attrition of any one participant negates the value of his or her baseline assessment. Of course (as described previously in this chapter and elsewhere in this book), as attrition rates grow, rigor shrinks.

◆ ◆ ◆

In a Nutshell

In prospective observational studies, retention is so vital that complete failure of the study may easily occur if the rate is low.

◆ ◆ ◆

Unfortunately, attrition is inevitable: in general, the longer the follow-up period the greater attrition. To minimize attrition, a number of tracking procedures have proven effective. These procedures include (1) hiring a full-time recruitment-retention coordinator to track participants; (2) requesting friendship contacts—participants are required to provide the name, telephone numbers, and addresses of two confidants; (3) providing monetary compensation for completing follow-up assessments; (4) ensuring confidentiality of data and identifying information (in other words, all data will be maintained, offsite, in a locked cabinet that is limited to access by key staff only, with only code numbers used on data forms); (5) providing appointment cards indicating the time and date of the follow-up assessments; (6) providing reminder phone contacts a week before as well as forty-eight hours prior to their scheduled follow-up assessment; (7) mailing "thank you" cards to participants for attending their follow-up assessments; and (8) mailing "touching-base cards" such as birthday cards and holiday cards (there are many holidays throughout the year that provide an opportunity to maintain contact with participants). There are a range of strategies designed to maintain the study cohort. Implementing them in a timely fashion, treating participants with courtesy and respect, providing assurances of confidentiality, and maintaining frequent contact to identify changes in locator information will enhance retention. We will discuss two of these strategies in greater detail.

Phone Contacts. The type of "maintenance contact" that occurs between research staff and study participants will be a function of the agreement with the IRB. The telephone is an essential tool for contact; therefore, gaining permission from the IRB to ask volunteers for a reliable phone number is clearly important in prospective studies. After the baseline assessment is complete, research staff members have two essential obligations: (1) collect accurate contact information and (2) provide any promised incentives for study participation. Both tasks can be performed with one goal in mind: to establish a rapport with participants in order to inspire them to come back! Merely asking for a phone number would be wasting an opportunity to build rapport. The occasion should, instead, be used to learn when and how to contact participants. An example follows.

◆ ◆ ◆

In a Nutshell

The telephone is an essential tool for contact; therefore, gaining permission from the IRB to ask volunteers for a reliable phone number is clearly important in prospective studies.

◆ ◆ ◆

Staff Member: I would like to call you a few times before we meet again in three months. It would be very helpful to me if you would let me know what time of day is good for me to call you.

Participant: I work the night shift so the best time is just before I leave for work, usually around ten P.M.

Staff Member: Great, thanks. Is that every weeknight or do you have to work on weekends sometimes?

Participant: Luckily, I never have to work on weekends—just Monday through Friday.

Staff Member: Okay, thanks. What phone number should I use when I call you around ten o'clock?

Participant: My home number, 345-1733, would be fine, but the problem is I don't want my spouse or anyone else that may be at my house to know that I'm in this study.

Staff Member: I understand—I will ask for you by name, and I will not leave a message if you are not home. If someone else answers and that person asks who I am, what would you like me to say?

Participant: Just tell them that you are trying to sell me something and hang up after that.

Staff Member: Sounds fair—I will be polite if that happens.

When making phone contact with a participant it is important to "talk" rather than run through a scripted agenda. The staff member should have and show a genuine interest in the person. This interest may result in potentially important information being conveyed. For example, the staff member might ask, "When we talked last you were living an apartment that you hated; have you had any luck getting a better one?" This question may yield a new address (information that may also be critical to keeping the retention rate high).

Mail Contacts. Birthday cards, holiday cards, and postcards can all be efficient ways to keep the study and the staff member relatively "fresh" on the minds of participants. Sending cards requires thoughtful use of the time between when participants complete the baseline assessment and when participants are given their promised incentive. If the birth date was not collected in the assessment, then it can be requested during this time. Honesty is important—simply tell participants that you want to send them a birthday card! Similarly, it easy enough to think about upcoming holidays and then to ask participants whether or not they celebrate these.

Although birthday and holiday cards may be hit or miss, every participant should be sent a postcard if possible. Postcards are an informal way of keeping in touch with someone, and their use can be casual—almost anonymous. The word "anonymous" is important because it may be that the study involves a sensitive topic (sex, drugs, disease) and the participant does not want his or her involvement disclosed. Thus, the postcard should be from a place not a person, and the "place" should be generic rather than specific. For example, it may come from "The Greater Chicago Board of Health" rather than from the "Substance Abuse Prevention Center of Greater Chicago." To promote recognition of this communication, the staff member could actually show a blank postcard to the respondent and say, "I would like to send one of these to you before we meet again—if that is okay with you, then what address should I use?" The postcard should only be a greeting—it should not be personalized to the point where the participants' involvement in the study is disclosed in any way. Postage for this card should include a guarantee that it will be returned to the sender if needed. This is an important way for a staff member to know that someone in the cohort has moved without leaving a forwarding address. This event necessitates immediate attempts to make phone contact.

A critical aspect of promoting retention is to assign one staff member only to "track" any given participant. This should be the same staff member who performs the baseline assessment and, more important, interfaces with the participant to collect contact information (phone and address) and provides the incentive payment. At this time, the assigned staff member should make it clear that he or she will be the only person making the interim contact, and that one purpose of the contact is to ensure that the follow-up assessment occurs on the day and time planned. Naturally, planning this day and time should be a very deliberate process—one that is guided by the needs of the participant only (research staff *should not* be under the illusion that data collection must occur between nine A.M. and five P.M. Monday through Friday). Once the day and time are planned, a brightly colored appointment card should be provided to the participant. The card should also clearly indicate how the participant can contact the staff member. If time allows, then the staff member should run the card through a lamination machine to give it some durability and to make it stand out. Reminding participants about their appointment should occur only by phone, and it should occur close in time to the agreed-upon date.

Attrition bias is naturally a prime concern. If, for example, people who drop out do so for a variety of practical reasons (for example, change of residence, employment schedule conflicts with appointment times, lack of transportation to the appointment) then odds of developing a biased final sample are relatively low. Alternatively, if people drop out based on lack of interest in the study or personal conflicts with the nature of the research questions, then odds of developing a biased final sample go up substantially. Indeed, the final sample might comprise people who really like the study topic and who are not in conflict with the topic in any way. In health promotion research, this "one-sided" sample may rarely reflect reality. Here are just a few of many possible examples of topics that may create this problem:

- Sex and sexuality research
- Research on eating disorders
- Vaccine-acceptance research
- Substance abuse prevention research
- Drunk driving prevention research
- Cancer prevention research
- Research on compliance with exercise and diets to improve cardiovascular health

Experimental Studies

These key concepts apply to observational studies; however, each concept also applies to the larger and more challenging task of conducting experimental studies. Chapter Six will use the material covered in this chapter as a starting point for a detailed description of planning and implementing experimental research from a "nuts and bolts" perspective.

Applied Example

A study published in *Cancer Nursing* provides a good example of recruitment and retention strategies applied to a difficult-to-reach population: women diagnosed with lung cancer. Cooley and colleagues (2003) conducted a prospective study of women with lung cancer to assess their quality of life. Sites in five cities participated in the study. To be eligible, women had to have been diagnosed with lung cancer at least six months previous to the potential enrollment date, but the diagnosis also had to be less than five years old.

Three of the five sites reached agreement with their IRBs to use active as well as passive recruitment methods. In this case, a member of the research team made direct contact with potential participants by phone or in person. The contact was initiated by the researcher. Passive approaches (used at all five sites) included distributing brochures, mailing letters, hanging up flyers and posters in key locations, and advertising in newspapers or by radio. The researchers also used the media to promote community awareness of the study. Once potential study participants initiated contact, a member of the research team used a phone script to recruit these individuals into the study.

Screening and enrollment rates were monitored on a monthly basis. Overall, 435 women were screened and 364 were deemed eligible. Of these 364 women, 230 (63 percent) were enrolled. Enrollment success rates varied by site (this could be due to differences in populations by site or to different practices by recruiters at each site). Of great interest, the success rate for passive recruitment was 92 percent compared to 61 percent for active recruitment. The finding is quite logical given that passive recruitment begins with people who already have enough interest in the study to initiate contact, whereas active recruitment does not "screen out" the people who are clearly disinterested.

The article displayed a table enumerating reasons for attrition from the prospective study. Attrition rates varied by site and by method of recruitment (active versus passive). The overall attrition rate was 24 percent. Again, passive recruitment produced better results in that attrition was more likely (33 percent) among those recruited actively as opposed to passively (22 percent). Detailing the reasons for attrition was clearly important, especially given that a substantial number of women experienced severe relapse (with some deaths). Efforts to keep attrition low included the provision of a pleasant baseline assessment (including breaks during the interview) and measures designed to promote contact between the research staff and participants between the first and second assessments. These methods included birthday cards, holiday cards, periodic phone calls, and a $25 cash incentive provided after each interview.

Integration with the Research Process

Just as one defective O-ring can cause an entire space shuttle to come crashing back to earth, a study designed without adequate attention to the daily activities of the project director and research staff is likely to fall apart. Thus, the planning steps (steps 4 through 6) in the nine-step model of Chapter One should always be pursued with great attention to detail. Major barriers to effective recruitment, retention, and assessment (for example) can sometimes be averted through the exercise of foresight and caution when selecting a study design (step 4), crafting an assessment plan (step 5), and choosing a sampling method (step 6). However, implementing the research protocol (step 7) is ultimately the last chance a study has to permanently gain or lose rigor. Note that data analysis can be repeated over and over again, but planning and implementation steps occur at discrete points in time and cannot be "reversed."

◆ ◆ ◆

In a Nutshell

Data analysis can be repeated over and over again, but planning and implementation steps occur at discrete points in time and cannot be "reversed."

◆ ◆ ◆

Summary

Although observational research is often a forerunner to experimental research, it may also constitute the terminal point of evidence in the research chain. Either way, rigor in observational research is essential. This chapter has described some of the key concepts that ensure this rigor. An initial concern is gaining access to the desired population followed by the creation and implementation of a successful recruitment protocol. Assessment, the main activity in observational research, is important in its own right and is also related to whether volunteers return for scheduled follow-up interview sessions. Given the importance of using prospective designs in health promotion research, multiple steps can and should be taken to ensure an optimally high retention rate. Ultimately, constant attention to the everyday operation of observational research is vital to ensuring a high degree of rigor. This attention includes careful record keeping, thorough training of research staff, and periodic monitoring of all recruitment and retention procedures. The successful study will be one that is planned in great detail and implemented with fidelity.

◆ ◆ ◆

In a Nutshell

The successful study will be one that is planned in great detail and implemented with fidelity.

◆ ◆ ◆

Issues to Consider

1. In observational studies, it is not uncommon for researchers to differentiate between refusal rates and dropouts before the first assessment. In essence, people may be recruited (and agree to enroll) at a discrete point in time that precedes the first scheduled assessment. This may be particularly likely when assessments are conducted in groups rather than on an individual basis. Thus, people who agree to participate may not "show up" for assessment. For example, imagine that 900 people were eligible. Of these, 810 (90 percent) agreed to enroll in the study with the understanding that an initial assessment would occur during the first Saturday of the following month. Of the 810 who agreed, 630 (70 percent of those eligible) showed up on the appointed Saturday. Is the participation rate 90 percent or is it just 70 percent? Also, when does enrollment occur? Does it occur upon agreement to participate or when the person actually provides data? (Please keep in mind that the researcher has discretion over when informed consent will be provided—the only requirement is that it must occur before assessment.)

2. The relationship of the research question(s) to the design implementation of the observational research study protocol should also be considered. Without question, the research question should be the sole driving force behind the design of any study. During planning, any level of compromise that impinges on the scope of the research question should be avoided. However, it may become sadly apparent during this phase that the logistical complications of implementing the necessary protocol will unfortunately produce low participation and retention rates. Upon reaching this conclusion, should the researcher abandon the project? Would your answer be different if the study had been federally funded and money would have to be returned to the federal treasury?

3. Given that active recruitment is sometimes a necessity, it is important to keep in mind that this procedure may yield lower success rates than a passive procedure. However, active recruitment may actually provide more information about the relationship of the sample to the population. For example, imagine that the research question involves the study of people newly diagnosed with genital herpes. In a relatively small community it might be logical to assume that only a few health care providers perform this test and therefore these providers could (conceivably) provide a fairly complete count of the number of community residents diagnosed with genital herpes during any given period of time. Developing these relationships with the providers would easily lead to the next step—active recruitment of those testing positive during a given time frame. Conversely, passive recruitment techniques would be "blind" to the number of potentially eligible participants. Thus, an important issue to consider is whether active or passive recruitment is better suited for any particular study.

For Practice and Discussion

1. A search to find standards for acceptable participation rates and acceptable retention rates would be endless and produce multiple answers. Two explanations for this problem are apparent. First, as noted earlier in this chapter, research about conducting research has been neglected. Although having a defensible number (for example, 70 percent) available for judging the likelihood of participation bias (or attrition bias) would be ideal, an empirically derived value does not exist. Second, it can be argued that a universal standard for participation and attrition rates should not be applied to health promotion research. The argument would be based on the concept that these rates are inevitably a function of (1) the selected population and (2) the nature of research. Please consider each of these explanations and then select one to defend in conversation with a colleague who is completing the same exercise.

2. Much of the material contained in this chapter is intimately connected with ethical issues and principles as described in Chapter Three. Due to this intimacy, several conflicts could occur. For example, a perceived need to have a high participation rate may lead research staff to present skewed versions of the consent process—leaving out or under-emphasizing aspects of the study that may be less appealing. Working with a colleague who is completing this same exercise, please identify at least two additional conflicts between ethical principles and achieving goals described by the key concepts outlined in this chapter. Take a position on each conflict that you identify (for instance, what is the solution?).

References

Cooley, M. E., and others. (2003). Challenges of recruitment and retention in multisite clinical research. *Cancer Nursing, 26,* 376–386.

Crosby, R. A., and DiClemente, R. J. (2004). Use of recreational Viagra among men having sex with men. *Sexually Transmitted Infections, 80,* 466–468.

Crosby, R. A., Holtgrave, D. R., DiClemente, R. J., Wingood, G. M., and Gayle, J. (2003). Social capital as a predictor of adolescents' sexual risk behavior: A state-level exploratory study. *AIDS and Behavior, 7,* 245–252.

Huck, S. W., and Cormier, W. H. (1996). *Reading statistics and research.* New York: Longman.

Melville, J., and others. (2003). Psychological impact of a serological diagnosis of herpes simplex virus type 2: A qualitative assessment. *Sexually Transmitted Infections, 79,* 280–285.

Shi, L. (1997). *Health services research.* Albany, NY: Delmar Publishers.

Sim, J., and Wright, C. (2000). *Research in health care: Concepts, designs, and methods.* Salisbury, Wiltshire, UK: Stanley Thrones (Publishers) Ltd.

CHAPTER SIX

DESIGNING RANDOMIZED CONTROLLED TRIALS IN HEALTH PROMOTION RESEARCH

Ralph J. DiClemente, Laura F. Salazar, and Richard A. Crosby

As noted in Chapter Five, much of the research in health promotion has been observational in nature. However, the very definition and, indeed, the identity of the discipline of health promotion are predicated on the premise of designing programs that "promote health." As such, a mainstay of health promotion is the development and implementation of programs that have as their expressed purpose enhancing the health of human populations.

At this juncture, perhaps it would be useful to define health promotion programs (HPPs). By HPPs, we imply any intervention, whether it's a new school smoking-cessation curriculum, a new exercise-enhancement class at a community-based organization, or an HIV-prevention program. Broadly defined, an HPP can be any intervention that has as its expressed purpose changing a person's health-related attitudes, beliefs, intentions, and behavior so as to enhance his or her health.

The focus of this chapter will be on describing how to design and conduct experimental research. Although experimental research is used in many fields, in health promotion we focus mainly on evaluating whether HPPs are effective in enhancing health-protective behaviors (or health-protective attitudes, beliefs,

knowledge, and intentions). There are many different types of evaluation strategies applicable for these assessments (see Chapter Eight); however, in this chapter
we focus on a *true experimental research design* because it is the optimal research design
in health promotion and indeed, in any discipline involving human populations.

Illustration of Key Concepts

This chapter describes key concepts in the design of the randomized controlled
trial. This is not an exhaustive treatment of this area of methodology. We do, however, describe the essential concepts that form the cornerstone of the randomized
trial design and discuss the importance of these concepts in enhancing the validity of health promotion research.

What Is an Experiment in Health Promotion Research?

An experiment in health promotion research involves the manipulation of an *independent variable* (something that is intentionally altered by the research team). In
this case, the HPP would be the independent variable. It is altered by randomly
allocating some people to receive the HPP and others not to receive the HPP. Then
the effects of this manipulation can be measured by assessing the designated
outcome variables (for example, weight, blood pressure, depressive symptoms,
and so on) over some specified period of time. In the parlance of experimental
research, the outcome measure is called the *dependent variable.*

To illustrate, an investigator (you, for example) has developed an innovative
approach designed to motivate adolescents to increase their consumption of vegetables. Essentially, the HPP comprises five group sessions that describe the health
benefits associated with higher vegetable consumption. You have decided to
develop this program based on evidence derived from numerous studies, which
observed significant decreases in adverse health outcomes (such as heart disease
and some cancers) for people with higher vegetable consumption.

You recruit about two hundred teens from the local Boys and Girls Club. You
ask them to complete a baseline questionnaire that assesses their consumption of
vegetables. Then you randomly assign them to either your innovative HPP or to
a group that does not receive any health promotion intervention (this could be
some other program that does not include any focus on enhancing vegetable intake). Next, you present the program comprising five sessions and then follow all
the teens (from both groups) over time, let's say twelve months. You ask them to
return and complete a follow-up questionnaire that again assesses their intake of
vegetables. This time, however, you ask them about their vegetable consumption

over the past twelve months. You hypothesize (and hope) that the teens in the HPP report more consumption of vegetables over the past twelve months relative to the teens in the control. This would be an indication that the program was successful (effective) in enhancing vegetable consumption. You have just conducted an experimental research study! This is a simplified illustration; of course, there are other design nuances that need to be considered in your study.

The Advantages of Experimental Research

The major advantage of experimental research over observational research is the strength of *causal inference* it offers. *Causal inference* implies that a fair conclusion can be made regarding the effect of an independent variable on a dependent variable (for example, a change in X will create a corresponding change in Y). It is the best research design for controlling potential confounding influences. As we'll see in more detail later in this chapter, in experimental research casual inference is based on comparing the outcomes observed among the teens in the HPP (for instance, the amount of their vegetable consumption) relative to the teens not in the program. Thus, in this example, manipulating the independent variable, randomization into groups, and then observing differences in outcomes for those exposed to the HPP and those who were not exposed represent a "true" experiment.

Types of Experimental Research Designs

Experimental research designs, like ice cream, come in multiple flavors. There are a number of choices. We suggest you see Campbell and Stanley (1963) for a more detailed discussion. Rather than try to review all the available designs (see Chapter Four), this chapter will focus on what is commonly referred to as *between-groups experimental research design*. Between-groups research design compares the outcomes observed in two or more groups of people that receive different interventions. Between-groups designs are commonly used in health promotion research. One between-group design, the *randomized controlled trial* (RCT) is often described as the "gold standard" for evaluating HPPs (or, for that matter, any intervention). In this experimental design participants are assigned, by chance alone, to either receive or not receive the HPP. This is not to say that other experimental designs are methodologically weak, just that the RCT is considered the optimal design.

Given the importance of methodological rigor for accurately evaluating HPPs, this chapter will focus exclusively on the RCT. There are, of course, numerous variations of this design. We will, however, restrict our discussion to describing the basic research structure of the RCT. Readers interested in more detailed presentations are referred to Piantadosi (1997) and Pocock (1993).

FIGURE 6.1.   A SCHEMATIC ILLUSTRATION OF A RANDOMIZED CONTROLLED TRIAL (RCT).

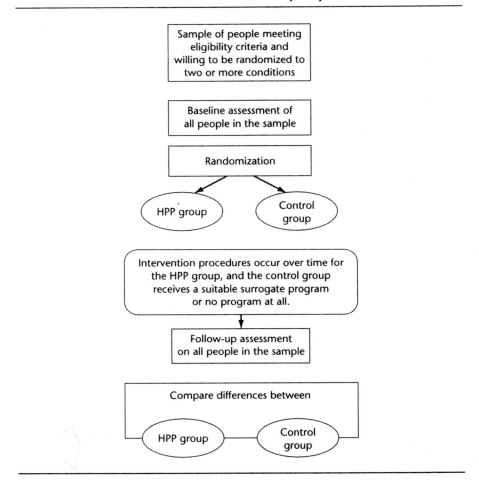

Conceptualizing a Randomized Controlled Trial

We have graphically represented a basic RCT in Figure 6.1. Although the research design shown may appear basic, do not be fooled. This is a very powerful evaluation design.

There are a number of key steps that are necessary to consider when designing and implementing any RCT. We provide a step-by-step approach to designing an RCT. These steps include

1. Defining the sample
2. Conducting a baseline assessment
3. Randomizing participants
4. Implementing the health promotion program
5. Following the sample over time

Step 1: Defining the Sample

The first step is to decide who will be in the study and how best to recruit them to participate. There are numerous sampling strategies that can be used to identify a target sample. (See greater detail about sampling in Chapter Eleven.) There are also a number of effective strategies that can be used to recruit the sample into the study (see Chapter Five). Whatever the sampling and recruitment strategy employed, it is important when defining the sample to establish a set of inclusion and exclusion criteria that specify the target population and are appropriate to the research question the study purports to answer. These criteria, sometimes referred to as *eligibility criteria,* establish the parameters for determining who is able to participate (*inclusion*) and who is not able to participate in the study (*exclusion*).

For example, consider an HPP for preventing dating violence among adolescents. First, it is important to define the characteristics of those adolescents who will be selected and recruited to participate in the study. The HPP to be implemented will be tailored by gender (that is, designed for young men) and will focus on preventing perpetration (the key outcome). Thus, inclusion criteria would be that participants have to be male, between fourteen and eighteen, and actively dating. Because this is a primary prevention program, the exclusion criterion would be previous perpetration. There is no magic formula for defining the inclusion and exclusion criteria. It is based on understanding the HPP that is to be evaluated: understanding the key outcomes of interest, and weighing the competing concerns of *internal validity* (the extent to which the study evaluates the hypotheses) and *external validity* (the extent to which the results of the study can be extended beyond the sample used in the study). Once the sample is defined, selection of the sample and recruitment can begin.

Step 2: Conducting a Baseline Assessment

Once the sample has been selected and recruited, the next step is to "characterize" the sample. This involves assessing the characteristics of the sample at baseline (before they are randomized to either receive or not receive the HPP). The purpose of characterizing the sample is to obtain measurements of key outcome variables prior to the HPP that will provide a baseline for measuring anticipated change in those key outcomes for those randomized to the HPP condition relative to those in the control condition. Another important aspect of characterizing the sample is to test for group differences after randomization. The groups should theoretically be identical, implying that randomization worked. This is a critical step to ensuring the internal validity of the study. If there are significant differences, for example, on sociodemographic characteristics (age, gender, race, SES, and so on) or outcome variables (behaviors, attitudes and beliefs), then these differences may confound the results. Significant differences between groups on these characteristics should be further explored and possibly controlled for in statistical analyses.

DINCUS'S SIMPLE RANDOMIZATION PROCEDURE.

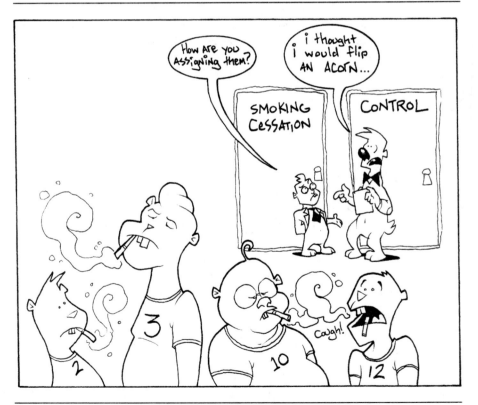

Copyright 2005 by Justin Wagner; reprinted with permission.

Step 3: Randomizing Participants

Once participants have completed baseline assessments, the next step is to randomize them to either receive or not receive the HPP. Randomization is one of the most critical aspects of the RCT. By randomization, we mean that participants are assigned to receive or not receive the HPP by chance alone. Randomization has a number of advantages in experimental research. Foremost, randomization comparably distributes subject characteristics that were assessed at baseline across groups. Moreover, randomization provides an efficient strategy for also distributing characteristics that were not measured. Often, for a variety of reasons (such as prohibitive cost, time, participant burden) the baseline assessment cannot reasonably measure all variables that may potentially affect the relation between exposure to the HPP and key outcomes.

◆ ◆ ◆

In a Nutshell

Foremost, randomization comparably distributes subject characteristics that were assessed at baseline across groups. Moreover, randomization provides an efficient strategy for also distributing characteristics that were not measured.

◆ ◆ ◆

How to Randomize Participants. Because randomization is so critical to an RCT, it is important that it be conducted properly. In general, there are two main features to consider when randomizing participants to study conditions; first, implementing a valid randomization procedure, and second, establishing procedures to safeguard the integrity of the randomization procedure so that unintentional or intentional biases do not influence the allocation process. We discuss both aspects in turn in this section.

◆ ◆ ◆

In a Nutshell

There are two main features to consider when randomizing participants to study conditions; first, implementing a valid randomization procedure, and second, establishing procedures to safeguard the integrity of the randomization procedure so that unintentional or intentional biases do not influence the allocation process.

◆ ◆ ◆

Implementing randomization requires reliable procedures that create comparability between groups. As with many other aspects of research, there are numerous randomization procedures that could be effectively and efficiently employed in an RCT. One common way is to manually use a table of random numbers to assign participants to groups. In this case, the investigator could consult a statistics textbook or even the Internet. How exactly does this work? Participant 1 (P_1) has just completed the baseline assessment and is now ready to be randomized. Opening a random numbers table, begin reading down the column of numbers, paying particular attention to the last digit in the sequence. Read down the column until you come to a number sequence that has either a "1" or a "0" as the last digit. If the number has a "1," then P_1 would be assigned to the HPP group. Now, the next participant completes the baseline assessment (P_2). Starting from where you ended, again read down the column of numbers until you come to a number sequence that has a "1" or "0" as the last digit. This time, suppose the next number has a "0" as the last digit. Then P_2 would be assigned to the control group. Continue this process until all participants have been assigned to either the HPP or the control group. Although this randomization strategy is effective, it can be time-intensive and does not guarantee an equal number of participants in each group. Fortunately, computer programs are now available to conduct randomization. These programs provide an equivalent randomization process, and they may be more efficient for larger numbers of participants.

Safeguarding the Integrity of the Randomization Procedure. The second concern in implementing randomization is to safeguard the integrity of the randomization procedure so that unintentional or intentional biases are avoided. This is essential to reduce potential confounding effects associated with bias. In terms of health promotion research, this means designing randomization procedures so that members of the research team who have contact with the participant cannot influence the assignment of the participant to the HPP or the control group. Sometimes, given the nature of the HPP, a team member involved in the randomization procedure may tacitly decide that a particular participant could benefit from being in the HPP group. This person may assign that participant to the HPP group without adhering to the established randomization procedure. In this instance, the participant did not have an equal chance of being in either the HPP or control group. In effect, the randomization procedure has been subverted.

To avoid subverting the randomization procedure, participants could be assigned to study conditions using *concealment of allocation procedures*. (See Schulz, 1995, Schulz and Grimes, 2002, and Schulz, Chalmers, Hayes, and Altman, 1995, for a thoughtful discussion of concealment of allocation in randomized controlled trials and for a more detailed account of subverting randomization.) Essentially, prior to beginning study enrollment, an investigator could generate the allocation sequence using a random numbers table. Thus, all the participants who are to be randomized would adhere to this pregenerated sequence. In practice, this procedure would operate as follows. The randomization sequence (that is, 0 or 1) is written on a piece of paper and placed in sealed opaque envelopes. As participants are ready to be randomized they are either given or asked to draw the envelope from the top of the stack of envelopes containing the randomization sequence. The investigator (or the participant if he or she drew the envelope) opens the envelope and displays the group to which the participant has been allocated. Although this is an effective procedure to protect the randomization process, it is critical that the randomization sequence be determined beforehand, and that only the principal investigator or the project statistician be involved in constructing the stack of envelopes. Minimizing the involvement of other staff and having a predetermined randomization sequence that is concealed from other research team members will guard the integrity of the randomization procedure.

◆ ◆ ◆

In a Nutshell

Although this is an effective procedure to protect the randomization process, it is critical that the randomization sequence be determined beforehand, and that only the principal investigator or the project statistician be involved in constructing the stack of envelopes.

◆ ◆ ◆

Step 4: Implementing the Health Promotion Program

Implementing an RCT requires particular attention to a number of methodological issues that revolve around the HPP. Four key issues to consider are (1) blinding, (2) designing the control condition, (3) ensuring fidelity of HPP implementation, and (4) enhancing participation in the HPP.

Blinding. Blinding is a research procedure that prevents participants from knowing whether they have been assigned to the experimental or control condition. This procedure effectively avoids problems known collectively as *demand characteristics*. Demand characteristics occur when participants behave differently as a consequence of knowing they are being "studied." In essence, they may selectively change their behaviors or distort their reports of behaviors upon assessment.

◆ ◆ ◆

In a Nutshell

Demand characteristics occur when participants behave differently as a consequence of knowing they are being "studied." In essence, they may selectively change their behaviors or distort their reports of behaviors upon assessment.

◆ ◆ ◆

Furthermore, if the research staff is aware of the study hypothesis, their behavior could affect study outcomes. This phenomenon is called *experimenter bias*. To control for this bias, a *double-blind* procedure can be implemented. For example, in medical trials, particularly studies designed to evaluate the differential effectiveness of medication, double-blind trials are often designed. In a double-blind trial, neither the investigator nor the participant is aware of whether the assigned condition is experimental or control.

Finally, the person conducting data analysis could be biased by knowing which participants' data come from experimental and control conditions. Thus, a study could be *triple-blinded*. In this case, the participants, investigators, and persons conducting data analysis are all unaware of whether the assigned condition is experimental or control.

Although an effective procedure, blinding is difficult to implement in the context of HPP. Typically, participants and group facilitators are aware of (or surmise) what program they have been assigned. For example, in a dating-violence-prevention program, it would be difficult (if not impossible) to adequately blind the participants and group facilitators who are, respectively, receiving and administering the intervention. Indeed, the facilitators are often involved in developing the HPP and thus blinding on this level would be impractical.

Not all forms of bias are remedied by blinding. For example, one common form of a demand characteristic is known as the *Hawthorne effect*. This effect was named after a study conducted in the town of Hawthorne, Illinois. The study assessed changes in employee productivity as a hypothesized consequence of additional lighting. Productivity increased when lights were made brighter, but also when they were dimmed! The conclusion was that simply knowing they were being observed caused employees to increase their productivity. This form of bias can be minimized by the use of a *structurally comparable control group* (in other words,

Box 6.1. A Control Group Is Not the Same as a Comparison Group

A simple and important rule to keep in mind is that a control group can only be formed through random assignment. Because people are randomly assigned to the control group, it is reasonable to anticipate equivalence between groups before the intervention begins. Often, however, forming a control group is not feasible. For example, imagine that the research question asks, "Does a community-level intervention, designed to reduce risk of cardiovascular disease, produce behavior change that is maintained for at least five years?" The question implies that the HPP is delivered to an entire community (perhaps using mass media and working with local health agencies). Thus, one key step in the planning process will be gaining support from key members of the community. Given that this process can be quite time consuming, it may not be feasible to garner support from several communities and then randomly allocate only half of these to receive the HPP. Instead, it makes sense to assign all of the communities to receive the HPP and to carefully select communities that "match" the HPP communities with respect to basic demographic profiles. Because the communities are not selected randomly, they are termed a comparison group rather than a control group. This difference is used to classify experimental designs apart from quasi-experimental designs. Thus, random assignment produces a control group, making the design experimental. Alternatively, nonrandom assignment produces a comparison group, making the design quasi-experimental.

a randomly assigned group of people who do not receive the HPP). See Box 6.1 for a full discussion. The control group would be similar to the HPP with respect to time, frequency of meetings, intensity of activities, and enjoyment of intervention activities. In the dating violence example, the experimental intervention could be four hours in duration (time) and four sessions (frequency), and could use interactive role-play techniques to enhance learning. A comparable control condition would therefore have to mirror these same conditions. This provides a suitable remedy to the Hawthorne effect, although this increases the cost of conducting the study, as additional staff is needed to develop and implement the comparable control group.

Designing the Control Condition. There are three types of control groups. One type is to have the control condition receive no intervention or attention. This is referred to as a "true control" group. Essentially, participants who are assigned to the control group following baseline assessment would return to complete follow-up assessments roughly on the same time schedule as participants randomized to the HPP group. Participants in a true control group would not receive any additional intervention. Sometimes, if the study is conducted in a clinical setting that routinely offers treatment and counseling, the control group would receive the "usual care or standard-of-care treatment or counseling" that would normally be provided. A second type is to have the participants assigned to the control group enter into the HPP following a wait period. There may be ethical issues involved that require every participant to receive the HPP. (See Chapter Three for more details.) In this type of control group, referred to as a *wait-list control group,* participants follow the same schedule of assessments as the HPP group. After all assessments are completed, they enter the HPP. The third type has been discussed and involves having a structurally similar attention control group that does not receive information or education hypothesized to affect the study outcome variables but does receive different health promotion messages (sometimes this is referred to as a "comparison group" because they are receiving some form of intervention, although the intervention selected is not thought to affect the study outcomes).

When using a structurally similar attention control condition, create a program that can be relevant and valuable to the participants. Be careful that the control program does not provide information or skills that are relevant to the goals of the HPP (sometimes referred to as "bleeding"). This could potentially compromise the validity of the RCT and produce artificial null findings.

◆ ◆ ◆

In a Nutshell

Be careful that the control program does not provide information or skills that are relevant to the goals of the HPP.

◆ ◆ ◆

Ensuring Fidelity of HPP Implementation. In any RCT it is imperative that implementation of the HPP be monitored regularly to safeguard against *drift* (that is, deviation from the established protocol). Drift can occur when persons delivering the intervention unintentionally or intentionally deviate from the intervention protocol. At times, they may interject personal experiences or anecdotes into a given HPP that clearly deviate from the HPP curriculum. In addition, they may perceive that the situation or circumstances in a particular group necessitate presenting information that is not included in the scripted curriculum.

Implementation drift can affect the internal validity of the RCT and reduce the ability to detect effects of the HPP on study outcomes. Internal validity may be compromised because the intervention is delivered differently by different staff members, or may be delivered differently by the same staff member throughout the course of the study. Thus, evaluation of the "HPP" is problematic because it may have assumed several forms throughout the trial.

To minimize implementation drift it is always critical to develop an implementation monitoring or assurance protocol. This is the protocol that governs what can and cannot be done in delivering the HPP. The protocol should be sufficiently detailed, and include (1) specification of each activity, (2) the goal and objectives for each activity, (3) who will implement the activity, and (4) the time allocated to each activity. Investigators and research staff need to be acutely aware of all aspects of the protocol and taught to adhere to it diligently. Although a detailed training program can be useful, continual monitoring of implementation is also needed to ensure that drift is avoided. And, if drift does occur, then it can be promptly detected and rectified.

Detecting drift requires constant monitoring by HPP implementation staff. To this end a number of procedures have proven useful. In our own research, we use a *dual-assurance methodology*. First, we ask participants to rate the health educators after each HPP group session. The health educators are blind to the participants' ratings, as these are collected by other staff members and placed in unmarked envelopes. Identifying information is not requested on the rating forms. The form asks participants to check off all the activities that were covered in the HPP group session that day. Thus, the investigators have an objective determination of the HPP activities that participants report being exposed to during the group session. This record is then checked against the implementation manual. Inconsistencies can then be addressed in meetings with the health educators.

Our second method of assessing fidelity of implementation is to have a rater assigned to each and every HPP intervention group session and also to each and every comparison group session. The rater completes a checklist much like the participants' rating form. The rater's checklist is significantly more detailed and requests not only whether particular HPP activities were implemented but also the amount of time spent on each activity and whether they were correctly implemented. These assurance methods can be used to quickly identify a health educator who is not compliant with the HPP manual and help to minimize the adverse effects of poor implementation fidelity.

Enhancing Participation in the HPP. In any multisession HPP there exists the potential that some proportion of participants will not complete the full HPP program. It is critical to develop strategies designed to minimize participant loss during the implementation of the HPP. For example, consider a study designed to test whether yoga exercises, conducted during a one-hour session for thirty consecutive days, help reduce blood pressure. Unfortunately, nearly 36 percent of the participants in the HPP (yoga) group do not attend all thirty sessions. Thus, they have not received the "full dose" of the HPP.

Dropping out before completing the full HPP can result in reducing the likelihood that HPP effects will be detected. To remedy the situation, it may be tempting to discard or eliminate data from participants who do not complete the full intervention. To do so would be inappropriate. Once participants have been randomized to their respective treatment groups, they are analyzed within those groups, regardless of whether they complete all required procedures. A common phrase that captures this rule is, "once randomized, always analyzed." This is referred to as an *intent-to-treat analysis*. This approach is critically important because it avoids what would otherwise result in a *self-selected sample*. In essence, eliminating those with incomplete attendance to the HPP changes what had initially been a randomized group. A second aspect of the intent-to-treat analysis is that it should be applied when issues arise relative to missing follow-up assessments (or key items within those assessments). Again, the initial temptation may be to delete people from the analysis. Doing so, however, would introduce further bias into the findings. A substantial number of techniques have been devised to deal with missing data and should be used when appropriate. For a discussion of these techniques please consult Graham and others, 1997, or Schafer, 1999.

◆ ◆ ◆

In a Nutshell

Once participants have been randomized to their respective treatment groups, they are analyzed within those groups, regardless of whether they complete all required procedures. A common phrase that captures this rule is, "once randomized, always analyzed."

◆ ◆ ◆

Because statistical solutions to missing data are not as desirable as design-based solutions, it is important to consider how best to ensure full participation in the HPP and follow-up assessments. A number of strategies have been designed to reduce barriers to attending health promotion interventions. First, although compensation to participants for attending HPP may not be permissible by certain funding agencies, it is permissible to provide compensation for completing assessments. Typically, assessments are administered at baseline and subsequent follow-up time points, which occur after the completion of HPP activities. Thus, it is important to build in brief assessments that coincide with HPP intervention sessions. One example would be to provide compensation to participants for completing the rating form of each HPP session. Another example would be to provide compensation for child care, if necessary. Also, providing compensation for transportation to and from the HPP sessions could be effective in reducing barriers to accessing the HPP and enhancing participation. Finally, designing an HPP that is perceived by participants as valuable, enjoyable, and engaging, and having health educators (that is, group facilitators) who are perceived as caring, knowledgeable, and dedicated are critical features of any HPP.

Step 5: Following the Sample over Time

Maintaining the cohort over protracted periods of time may be one of the most formidable challenges in conducting an RCT. Several problems can easily occur. Here we describe some of the problems that are unique to RCTs. Chapter Five provides more detail about procedures that can be used to maintain cohorts over time.

Conducting the Follow-Up Assessment.
Follow-up is critical to capturing data assessing the effectiveness of the HPP. After participants complete an HPP, we need to follow them over time and ask them to return for another assessment (follow-up assessment), so that we can measure any changes in attitudes, beliefs, intentions, behaviors, or health indices. A number of issues are related to participant follow-up.

One issue associated with the follow-up assessment is to decide who will collect the follow-up data. Health educators involved in administering the HPP should not be involved in conducting the follow-up assessments. Health educators have established a relationship with participants, which may influence the way in which participants respond to questions. Likewise, health educators may subtly influence participants' responses. Thus, using a person not known to the participants may reduce this form of bias. A related issue involves the mode of administration of the assessment instrument. Face-to-face interviews may create greater potential for bias, as participants may respond in socially desirable ways (in other words, providing answers they think the assessor wants to hear). Furthermore, this bias may be even greater if the assessor is also the facilitator who administered their HPP. This potential for bias may be minimized, although not entirely eliminated, with computer-assisted techniques to administer the assessments (Turner and others, 1998). The most effective strategy to reduce this potential bias is to maintain a strict distinction between HPP implementation staff (interveners) and the data collection staff (assessors).

◆ ◆ ◆

In a Nutshell

Health educators involved in administering the HPP should not be involved in conducting the follow-up. Health educators have established a relationship with participants, which may influence the way in which participants respond to questions. Likewise, health educators may subtly influence participant responses.

◆ ◆ ◆

Blinding of Data Collectors. Though it is difficult to blind the participants and interveners, it is not as difficult to blind the data collectors so that they are unaware of the participants' group assignment (that is, whether participants are in the HPP group or the control group). Unblinded assessors, knowledgeable about the participants' group assignment, may differentially probe or assess participants during the follow-up interview, thus resulting in interviewer bias. Again, new advances in technology, such as computer-assisted and audio-computer-assisted data collection procedures are available that avoid this potential bias. Self-administered surveys are also less susceptible to this bias.

Applied Example

In this section we describe a recently published RCT that was designed to test an HPP. Our aim is to use this example as a heuristic strategy to illustrate some of the key concepts previous described and discussed.

A Health Promotion Program for Stroke Survivors

A study published in the *American Journal of Preventive Medicine* provides an example of an RCT designed to test an HPP for recent survivors of stroke (Rimmer and others, 2000). The HPP comprised thirty-six sessions delivered over twelve weeks (three sessions per week). The HPP was designed to achieve multiple goals:

- Improve lipid profiles
- Increase peak oxygen uptake
- Increase muscular strength and flexibility
- Reduce obesity

- Increase physical activity
- Reduce dietary fat intake
- Increase life satisfaction
- Reduce depression

To test the efficacy of this HPP the research team employed a pretest, posttest design using a wait-list control group. Recruitment occurred by provider referrals. Sixty-two people met the following eligibility criteria: (1) the person was thirty to seventy years of age, (2) the person was able to walk at least fifty feet without a mechanical aid, (3) at least six months had elapsed since the person had had a stroke, (4) the person served as his or her own guardian, (5) the person resided within a one-hour commute of the intervention site, and (6) the person's primary care physician provided written medical permission for the person to participate. Thirty-eight of these sixty-two people were then randomly selected to enroll in the study. Of these, thirty-five agreed to participate.

The HPP was described in detail. Each session included fitness instruction, exercising, nutrition education (including cooking instruction), and education designed to improve health behaviors. Persons performing the education were well qualified, including an exercise physiologist, psychologists, a social worker, and postdoctoral research assistants.

Of interest, the research team identified several barriers (for instance, lack of transportation) that might have precluded participation in the thirty-six-session HPP. Efforts were then made to eliminate these barriers (for example, providing free transportation to and from the intervention site). The overall attendance rate for the thirty-six sessions was 93 percent.

Eighteen persons were randomly assigned to receive the HPP, with the remainder being placed in the wait-list control group. Findings included (1) a significant decrease in total cholesterol serum levels for HPP group members versus an increase for those in the control group, (2) a significant loss of weight for HPP group members but not for the control group, (3) a significant improvement in "time to exhaustion" among HPP group members but not the control group, and (4) improvement in several indicators of life satisfaction and depression for HPP members but not for the control group.

Several points deserve mention. For example, the research team was quite successful in ensuring optimal attendance to the thirty-six sessions. In addition to eliminating barriers, such as transportation issues, the HPP actively involved participants in learning (for example, cooking classes, exercise sessions, group discussions), and this high level of interaction may have inspired people to return. (Note: people were not financially compensated to participate in this study.) Also, the wait-list control group was used for ethical reasons, as the research team did not want to withhold a potentially beneficial program from any of the study volunteers. It should also be noted that the small sample size should not be counted as a "strike" against the study. Indeed, the authors provided evidence suggesting that the statistical power for the study was adequate to detect a medium effect size. (See Chapter Eleven for a more in-depth discussion of power and effect size.) Most important, it should be noted that (with some exceptions) the HPP was effective (it worked!). Without conducting the RCT, evidence to support the efficacy of the HPP would not exist; thus, the RCT served as a way to validate and justify the continuation of the HPP for stroke survivors.

Integration with the Research Process

This chapter has focused on a single but highly important research design, namely, the randomized controlled trial. Recall that in step 3 of the nine-step research process (Figure 1.2), the task is to determine whether the research question necessitates the use of observational or experimental research designs. Although other types of experimental designs exist (see Chapter Four), the RCT provides evidence that is widely accepted as rigorous and valid. As a tool, the RCT is an indispensable part of research in health promotion practice. The design requires attention to two distinctly different activities. First, all of the rules and procedures of conducting an RCT (as described in this chapter) must be followed. Equally important, however, is that an HPP must be developed and implemented with great fidelity in order to create a "treatment." Unlike drugs that are tested by RCTs, the HPP is not a tangible entity and therefore it cannot be easily or readily dispensed. To the contrary, the HPP requires constant attention to ensure consistent delivery of a treatment throughout the course of the study.

A final note is offered as a word of caution. Findings from even the most rigorous RCT should never be generalized beyond the population in which it was conducted. For example, in the study of stroke survivors the majority of participants were low-income African Americans residing in an urban area. Whether the HPP would be comparably effective for a population of middle-class Caucasians can only be determined by repeating the RCT with an entirely different sample. This cautionary note speaks to a general principle of the RCT: internal validity does not guarantee external validity.

Summary

The aim of this chapter was to provide fundamental information to help guide the design of randomized controlled trials assessing the effectiveness of HPPs. One limitation of this chapter is its inability to cover all aspects of RCT design.

A second limitation is the inability to provide an in-depth discussion of the issues presented. Notwithstanding these limitations, the chapter has provided a broad overview of key issues to be considered in designing and implementing an RCT. In addition, we emphasized how these issues affect the validity of the study and the interpretation of the findings. And finally, we proposed practical solutions. Given the importance of HPPs and the cost and time associated with designing and implementing these programs, it is critical that we also consider how best to evaluate their effectiveness. The RCT, carefully designed and implemented, represents a rigorous methodological approach to assessing the effectiveness of health promotion interventions.

Issues to Consider

1. As noted in this chapter, deciding what kind of "treatment" will be provided to control group participants is often a difficult task. The research team must weigh two competing concerns. On one hand, it is imperative that the control condition does not provide participants with information, motivation, or skills that could predispose them to improvement on the outcome measure(s). On the other hand, an ethical and moral responsibility exists to help people at risk of any negative health outcome to avoid continued or escalated risk. Thus, several questions arise. Is a wait-list control group an ethical alternative to a do-nothing control group? If so, will the quality of the HPP be equal and highly monitored when delivered to the wait-list control group even though the study has ended? If a placebo-attention control group is used, what constitutes a reasonably interesting and valuable HPP that does not confound the study design?

2. An unresolved issue in RCTs involves the provision of monetary compensation to study participants. From a research perspective, the core issue becomes whether the amount of compensation creates an artificial incentive to participate in the HPP. Stated differently, would people attend the HPP if they were not being paid? Would they be equally motivated to learn if they were not being paid? In essence, any suspicions that answer either question with a "no" should lead to doubts about the external validity of the RCT. Thus, in an "ideal" RCT, compensation would not be provided. We suspect, however, that an RCT without participant compensation would be very difficult to conduct, given the potentially low participation rate and (in all likelihood) a high attrition rate. Not providing compensation to study participants for their time and effort also presents an ethical issue in that the intervention is "experimental" and, thus, of unproven value.

3. Finally, an important question to consider is "Are RCTs always the logical endpoint of the research chain?" Do some research questions require evidence that cannot be provided using an RCT? We feel compelled at this juncture to refer you to a recent commentary published in the *British Medical Journal*. The authors suggested (with a great deal of wit) that the protective value of parachutes has never been established by an RCT (Gordon and Pell, 2003). The satire of this work is as informative as it is entertaining.

For Practice and Discussion

1. Imagine that you accessed a population of low-income Hispanic women who are at high risk of cervical and breast cancer. Your intent is to test an HPP designed to promote regular Pap testing and mammography. The HPP is a nine-hour program delivered in three sessions. Women will be paid $50 to complete a baseline assessment and another $50 to complete a follow-up assessment. All women will be asked to provide permission for study investigators to track their medical records for the next five years. Because these women would not otherwise have any education designed to promote Pap testing or mammography use, you decide to use a do-nothing control group for your RCT. Provide a defense of this decision. Then assume that the defense is not sufficient and provide an alternative plan that can be defended on the basis of rigor alone (excluding ethical concerns from your argument).

2. This chapter emphasized the importance of using an intent-to-treat analysis for RCTs. Unfortunately, a rather large number of articles reporting RCTs have been published that do not employ the intent-to-treat principle. Consider a hypothetical scenario in which 140 women were randomized to the HPP condition and 110 women were randomized to an attention control condition. Baseline measures were collected on all 250 women. In the ensuing six weeks, women were expected to attend a two-hour intervention on each Saturday afternoon. By the end of the sixth week, 90 percent ($n = 126$) of the women in HPP condition remained in the study (that is, they attended the sessions as required). By contrast, only 50 percent of the women in the control group ($n = 55$) remained in the study. How might failure to use an intent-to-treat analysis influence the study findings? Keep in mind that the influence is a form of bias, and that bias can favor the null hypothesis (the HPP did not work) or the alternative hypothesis (the program worked). Provide and be prepared to defend an answer that takes all of the possibilities into account.

References

Campbell, D. T., and Stanley, J. C. (1963). *Experimental and quasi-experimental designs for research.* Chicago: Rand McNally College Publishing Company.

Gordon, C. S., and Pell, J. P. (2003). Parachute use to prevent death and major trauma related to gravitational challenge: Systematic review of randomized controlled trials. *British Medical Journal, 327,* 1459–1461.

Graham, J. W., Hofer S. M., Donaldson, S. I., MacKinnon, D. P., and Schafer J. L. (1997). Analysis with missing data in prevention research. In K. Bryant, M. Windle, and S. West (Eds.), *The science of prevention: Methodological advances from alcohol and substance abuse research* (pp. 325–366). Washington, DC: American Psychological Association.

Piantadosi, S. (1997). *Clinical trials: A methodologic perspective.* New York: John Wiley & Sons.

Pocock, S. J. (1993). *Clinical trials.* New York: John Wiley & Sons.

Rimmer, J. H., Branschweig, C., Silverman, K., Riley, B., Creviston, T., and Nicola, T. (2000). Effects of a short-term health promotion intervention for a predominately African-American group of stroke survivors. *American Journal of Preventive Medicine, 18,* 332–338.

Schafer, J. L. (1999). Multiple imputation: A primer. *Statistical Methods in Medical Research, 8,* 3–15.

Schulz, K. F. (1995). Subverting randomization in controlled trials. *Journal of the American Medical Association, 274,* 1456–1458.

Schulz, K. F., and Grimes, D. A. (2002). Blinding in randomized trials: Hiding who got what. *Lancet, 359,* 696–700.

Schulz, K. F., Chalmers, I., Hayes, R. J., and Altman, D. G. (1995). Empirical evidence of bias: Dimensions of methodological quality associated with treatment effects in controlled trials. *Journal of the American Medical Association, 273,* 408–412.

Turner, C. F., Ku, L., Rogers, S. M., Lindberg, L. D., Pleck, J. H., and Sonenstein, F. L. (1998). Adolescent sexual behavior, drug use and violence: Increased reporting with computer survey technology. *Science, 280,* 867–873.

CHAPTER SEVEN

QUALITATIVE RESEARCH STRATEGIES AND METHODS FOR HEALTH PROMOTION

Laura F. Salazar, Richard A. Crosby, and Ralph J. DiClemente

As iterated throughout this book, the overarching purpose of scientific inquiry is to generate knowledge. In the context of health promotion, scientific inquiries are undertaken to generate knowledge specifically regarding prevalence and incidence of disease, risk factors for disease and health-risk behaviors, etiologic factors, theoretical perspectives, and effectiveness of health promotion programs, to name a few. The long-term goal of these scientific inquiries is to prevent morbidity and premature mortality. Conceptualizing and implementing these scientific inquiries entails embarking on a journey through a nine-step research process (see Figure 1.2).

As with any journey, however, there are always many decisions to make and myriad options from which to choose. To some degree, each leg of this research journey will have consequences (both good and bad), and, depending on the path taken, may result in reaching a crossroad or even reaching a dead end. Thus, it is important to consider each decision point and plan your journey carefully. Of course, because you may not have been on this type of journey before, we don't expect you to travel alone. We have attempted to be your tour guide for this journey, walking you through the research process, helping to identify salient points of interest, and issuing warnings of any potential dangers. In the spirit of being the best tour guides possible, however, we must acknowledge that so far we have taken you on this journey using only one mode of transportation. Let's assume that for this analogy you have been primarily traveling by plane. As you can imagine, traveling cross-country by plane will provide quite a different experience than going by train. Therefore, because we want you to have the fullest experience possible, it is time to deplane and see how the countryside looks from the seat of a passenger train.

In this journey analogy, the mode of transportation refers to the methodological *paradigm* applied to the research process. From the Greek word *paradeigma*, *paradigm* literally means model, pattern, or example; however, this rather simple definition can be expanded to encompass a "worldview" that may be influential in shaping the development of a discipline. A methodological paradigm is a discipline's view of which research techniques and practices are promoted and should be practiced. A discipline's methodological paradigm has strong implications for how the discipline as a whole will progress. Thomas Kuhn, a twentieth-century professor in philosophy and history of science, is credited with popularizing the term *paradigm*. He wrote a provocative book titled *The Structure of Scientific Revolutions*. In it, he describes science as "a series of peaceful interludes punctuated by intellectually violent revolutions" (Kuhn, 1970, p. 10), which can change profoundly the existing view and result in a paradigm shift. He articulated the importance of paradigms in shaping and guiding a scientific discipline:

> A shared commitment to a paradigm ensures that its practitioners engage in the paradigmatic observations that its own paradigm can do most to explain. Paradigms help scientific communities to bind their discipline, in that they help the scientist create avenues of inquiry, formulate questions, select methods with which to examine questions, define areas of relevance, and establish or create meaning. A paradigm is essential to scientific inquiry [Kuhn, 1970, p. 142].

◆ ◆ ◆

In a Nutshell

A methodological paradigm is a discipline's view of which research techniques and practices are promoted and should be practiced. A discipline's methodological paradigm has strong implications for how the discipline as a whole will progress.

◆ ◆ ◆

The approaches, methods, designs, and perspectives described thus far mostly fall under a paradigm termed *positivism*. Positivism is the view that serious scientific inquiry should not search for ultimate causes deriving from some outside or unidentifiable source, but rather must confine itself to the study of relations existing between facts, which are directly accessible to observation. Science or knowledge is based on the exploration of natural phenomena, in which properties and relations are observed and are verifiable. Consequently, positivism involves the use of methods that should be objective and involves testing theories through the generation and falsification of hypotheses in order to assemble "facts" (see Chapter Two for more details). In the end, relations can be supported, disconfirmed, or falsified. As you can extrapolate from this description of positivism, positivistic inquiries lend themselves to the use of quantitative modes of inquiry.

Given that the research questions, designs, and methods described thus far can be labeled as positivistic, if we stopped and did not go any further, then we would have presented a skewed view of health promotion's paradigm. It would ostensibly appear that health promotion research was ideologically bound by research methods (for example, experimental designs, random sampling, quantitative data, inferential statistics) that many of us have been conditioned to view as the epitome of rigor and as "real" research (Glesne and Peshkin, 1992). Although much health promotion research uses these methods, designs, and data justifiably, as a discipline we are not *bound* by them. Indeed, much health promotion research uses epistemologies that are supported by an *interpretivist* paradigm (Glesne and Peshkin, 1992).

In contrast to positivism, interpretivism views the world as a multiplicity of realities where each individual perceives, understands experiences, and makes meaning of that reality in different ways; thus, reality is socially constructed. Research in this paradigm focuses on studying individuals' lives and their significance. The overall aim within this paradigm is to understand others' experiences and relate them to one's own reality (Colangelo, Domel, Kelly, Peirce, and Sullivan, 1999). Thus, an interpretivist paradigm is supported through the use of qualitative modes of inquiry. Just as positivism and interpretivism differ, because they are supported mainly through two different modes of inquiry, their modes of inquiry also differ. Quantitative and qualitative modes of inquiry differ in the assumptions made about the generation of facts, in their purposes, in their approaches, and in the role of the researcher. These differences are highlighted in Table 7.1.

In viewing Table 7.1, is it important to note that there is no judgment attached to the underlying assumptions of the two modes and there shouldn't be; rather, differences are illuminated to assist in making decisions regarding the research process. One approach is not necessarily better than the other in this instance, and one approach should not be considered more scientific or more rigorous than the

TABLE 7.1. PREDISPOSITIONS OF QUANTITATIVE AND QUALITATIVE MODES OF INQUIRY.

Quantitative Mode	Qualitative Mode
Assumptions	
Social facts have an objective reality	Reality is socially constructed
Primacy of method	Primacy of subject matter
Variables can be identified and relationships measured	Variables are complex, interwoven, and difficult to measure
Etic (outsider's point of view)	Emic (insider's point of view)
Purpose	
Generalizability	Contextualization
Prediction	Interpretation
Causal explanations	Understanding of perspectives
Approach	
Begins with hypotheses and theories	Ends with hypotheses and grounded theory
Manipulation and control	Emergence and portrayal
Uses formal instruments	Researcher as instrument
Experimental	Naturalistic
Deductive	Inductive
Component analysis	Searches for patterns
Seeks consensus, the norm	Seeks pluralism, complexity
Reduces data to numerical indices	Makes minor use of numerical indices
Abstract language in write-up	Descriptive write-up
Researcher Role	
Detachment and impartiality	Personal involvement and partiality
Objective portrayal	Empathic understanding

Source: From C. Glesne and A. Peshkin, *Becoming Qualitative Researchers: An Introduction,* copyright © 1992. Published by Allyn & Bacon, Boston. Copyright © by Pearson Education. Reprinted by permission of the publisher.

other—just different. There are some similarities as well. We strongly advocate that both are compatible and that each approach provides a different perspective and reveals additional information that allows us to gain a fuller understanding of whatever it is we are trying to know. Nevertheless, it is important to learn how the two modes differ along the dimensions presented in Table 7.1.

Illustration of Key Concepts

In this chapter, we will provide an overview of several qualitative research strategies, methods, and analyses so that you can glean a better understanding of how to conduct a qualitative inquiry. We will describe what constitutes qualitative research and several major purposes within health promotion for which qualitative inquiry is conducive. We also identify the methods most appropriate for health promotion research. Last, we provide a basic approach to data analysis. Keep in mind as you read through this chapter that unlike traveling by plane, this train trip requires no seat belt. So, relax and enjoy your trip!

What Constitutes a Qualitative Mode of Inquiry?

Essentially, there are five aspects of qualitative research that make it "qualitative": it is naturalistic, the data are descriptive, there is concern with process, it is inductive, and meaning is the goal (Bogdan and Biklen, 1998). In any one given qualitative research study it is not necessary to have all five features weighted evenly to signify that the research is qualitative, or to even have all five of the features. For example, imagine that a qualitative researcher studying homeless women wants to understand the circumstances of their lives and what led them to become homeless. He or she may collect descriptive data, be concerned with the process, and be focused on revealing the meaning of the participants' experiences. Yet, he or she may conduct in-depth interviews with the women in a coffee shop rarely visited by homeless women. Some qualitative research will emphasize certain features more so than others, but for practical purposes, ideally, qualitative research should attempt to encompass all five features.

◆ ◆ ◆

In a Nutshell

Essentially, there are five aspects of qualitative research that make it "qualitative": it is naturalistic, the data are descriptive, there is concern with process, it is inductive, and meaning is the goal.

Naturalistic. Qualitative research is *naturalistic* as opposed to observational or experimental. Naturalistic and experimental differences can be quite distinct; however, distinctions between naturalistic and observational are more subtle. Although both designs involve a lack of manipulation or control, naturalistic signifies that the data are collected in the natural setting such as a person's home or school, whereas observational research can occur in an artificial setting. Furthermore, it is the setting in which the research takes place that provides the data, and it is the researcher who serves as the mode for data collection. Thus, the data are collected in a manner that is also natural (such as observing or conversing). Because qualitative research is concerned with contextualizaton, naturalistic approaches provide a high level of context. In a study of women seeking drug treatment, for example, one researcher went to a methadone clinic where he observed women in various areas of the clinic and interviewed them onsite (Fraser, 1997). Although we cannot say for certain, had the researcher attempted to bring the women into a different setting such as a university, conducting the interviews in an artificial setting could have had an impact on the results.

Descriptive Data. Qualitative research uses data that are descriptive (Bogdan and Biklen, 1998). Qualitative data can take several different forms such as words, pictures, video, notes, charts or records, and narratives. Data are not represented in numerical terms. If some numerical interpretation is provided, it is usually minor and may be presented to emphasize a pattern in the data. Written results may contain participants' quotes, interview transcripts, field notes, photos, and so on and provide a rich, in-depth analysis centering on interpretation. This approach, of course, contrasts with a quantitative mode in which data are expressed in numerical forms and statistical analyses are performed to describe the data and to test hypotheses. The results are then presented in statistical terms with little or no context.

Melville and colleagues conducted a qualitative research study of patients visiting a sexually transmitted disease clinic to determine the emotional and psychosocial impact of receiving a positive genital herpes diagnosis (Melville and others, 2003). In-depth interviews were conducted with twenty-four clinical patients onsite. A sample of the "data" is provided in Box 7.1 and a sample of the write-up from the published article is provided in Box 7.2. As shown, the data are words composing the transcription of the interview, and the results represent the researchers' interpretations and understanding of the participants' words.

Process-Focused. Qualitative research entails a focus on the process rather than on the outcomes (Bogdan and Biklen, 1998). Again using the research study of homeless women as an example, one focus of the research could be to understand the process through which women came to be homeless. How did these women become homeless? What happened in their lives that brought them to this point? Other examples from health promotion could be, how do young women negotiate condom use with their partners? What processes do they go through to protect themselves? And, why do some young women think they are overweight? How do they come to view themselves in this way? What is the impact of thinking they are overweight? Yu-Jen, Yiing-Mei, Shuh-Jen, and Mei-Yen (2004) conducted semistructured interviews with five young women to investigate their experiences with body image and weight control, and other researchers (Johnson, Kalaw,

Box 7.1. Text Transcribed Verbatim from an Interview with a Patient from an STD Clinic

I: Thinking back to when you first found out you had genital herpes, how did you feel at the time? This would have been not when you and I talked the other day, but when you first heard your results. And I'm assuming you talked to them on the phone, is that correct?

P: Yeah, I called in. How did I feel? Uh . . . I don't . . . can you stop this for a second?

I: Sure.

P: Okay.

(Tape stops.)

I: So you're not even sure how you actually felt?

P: I knew I had something, but in a way I was relieved to find out what it was, because as bad as it could be . . .

I: Right, I understand that.

P: And I guess a part of me could move on now. I could figure out what I needed to do.

I: As opposed to someone saying, "No no you don't have anything." And yet you know you have these weird symptoms?

P: Yeah.

I: Okay. So part of you was relieved and part of you was . . . ?

(Pause)

P: You know I think I had a little bit of anger too, because I think I know who it was. I remembered back to this whole incident and I'm pretty sure, so I had a little bit of anger with that. So relief and I don't know . . .

I: Herpes is a source of stress for some people but not for others. Did your discovering that you had herpes cause you enough stress to affect your daily behavior, for example your work, friends, and relationships? If so could you please explain in as much detail as possible?

P: No it hasn't really. It hasn't changed. The relationship a little bit. I'm putting off . . . I have a girlfriend but I'm putting off going over to her house. I know I need to tell her, but I'm not sure exactly how to go about that. So that's stressful, that could be classified as stressful. But as far as work goes, no.

I: But it sounds like from what you said before though that part of it was confirming and a relief to hear that you had something. That would be a relief of some kind of stress as opposed to creating stress. And having to tell someone about it—that's a whole different category that needs to be addressed at some point.

P: And as far as my life goes, I've been through a lot and I'm used to rolling with what comes at me. So I don't really feel all that much stress.

I: Maybe this is minor compared to some other things?

P: Yeah.

I: Self-concept is broadly defined as how you view yourself as a person. Did any of the feelings you experienced when you first discovered you had herpes change your self-concept in any way?

P: Wow. I think it makes me feel like, How am I going to get something going in a relationship as far as being with somebody? I don't understand how I could talk to someone about this, I really don't. I think in a way it's closed me—I'm already pretty closed as it is—but I think it's closed me a little bit more. Out of fear—I guess bottom-line rejection.

I: Do you recall if the discovery affected your daily moods at all?

P: I don't really recall. Maybe it'd be better if you had a list of questions—I'd get a chance to think about them before I came in.

(Laughter)

No. I don't think so.

I: Did it affect your feelings of body image and sexual attractiveness?

P: Maybe body image. I'm not sure about sexual attractiveness. That's really a mind thing I think. I think attractiveness is really a mind thing. I think it's the same.

I: Has it affected your sex drive?

P: No.

I: Has it affected your desire for long-term sexual relationships?

P: Has it affected my desire for long-term sexual relationships? I don't know. I still have that desire, it's just what am I going to do with this?

I: After the tape is off, we can talk more about this and your sex partners.

P: Okay.

I: Has it affected your ability to relate to your partner?

P: Yes.

I: Yeah, you mentioned that you haven't gone to her house.

P: Yeah, I'm staying away. I have to tell her, I can't just . . .

I: How long have you been with her?

P: Uh, two months, three months.

I: Some of the initial affects experienced by people who newly discover they have herpes change with the passage of time. Can you compare the answers that you just gave me to the feeling you have today? For example, how do you feel about learning that you were positive for herpes type 2?

P: How do I feel?

I: Well for example when you first heard your results part of you felt relieved because you suspected and now it was confirmed. And another part of you was angry because you were thinking who gave it to you and it brought that up. So now that you've had some time since you first heard your results what are your feelings now? Are they different from that day?

P: Yeah, I think now I'm more, not resigned but like resigned to move on. There's not really anything I can do about that now. It's water under the bridge. But I need to move on.

I: That's the impression I have too. So in terms of stress affecting your daily behavior, that sounds like it's still just affecting your relationship with your girlfriend?

P: Yeah work is going, it's really going well.

I: Has there been any change in your self-concept in any way?

P: Well I have a pretty good self-concept for someone who just did a lot of time. But I think as far as—I don't understand the question. I'm trying to ramble on.

I: Since finding out that you have herpes you talked about how initially it did affect your self-concept a little bit. But I'm hearing from the way you are talking about things, it's probably not affecting you as much anymore. In fact if I could put forth what I'm picking up is that maybe in the beginning it was something you thought about a lot, but now it's on the back burner and it comes up when you think about seeing your girlfriend because then you have to talk about it. But otherwise it's not really bothering you.

P: Very good, very good!

I: Is that where you are?

(Laughter)

P: Yeah. Part of me puts it off into the back and then when the opportunity arises when she'll call me up and I'll make excuses.

I: Oh good. We're going to have a lot to talk about when the tape is off.

P: Okay okay.

I: For many people, having herpes causes problems at some points in life but not at other times. After you knew you had herpes up till now, do you recall specific situations that may have intensified any negative feelings attached to your having herpes?

P: Something negative that is attached?

I: Yes.

P: I would think that outbreaks would be negative. That would be a hard time to deal with it. But I can't really think of anything else.

Box 7.2. Sample Results Write-Up

"Fear of telling a current partner was a frequent psychosocial response associated often with fear of rejection, present even for participants who knew that their current sex partner had herpes. One man (32, STD) said, 'I thought she was going to freak out and run away from me. Scared that she was going to run off and leave me forever.' Another man (37, STD) reported that his initial thought was, 'Oh my gosh, I'm positive, and if I tell him, he probably, you know, might reject me for this. Then I thought, oh no he's had herpes so he's certainly not going to do this to me. But there's always the possibility. So there was this little thinking that went on subconsciously. . . . I waited a couple of days and then told him, because I think I had to go through my own little process of dealing with that.'"

Source: From Melville and others (2003). "Psychosocial Impact of Serological Diagnosis of Herpes Simplex Virus Type 2: A Qualitative Assessment," *Sexually Transmitted Infections, 79,* p. 282.

Lovato, Baillie, and Chambers, 2004) have used a qualitative approach to examine the process youths undergo to regain control over their smoking. In each instance, the focus was on the process rather than the outcome of "being overweight" or "smoking."

Inductive Approach. Qualitative research is inductive. As you may recall from Chapter Two, inductive logic involves deriving general patterns from your observations that may eventually become hypotheses or that may constitute a theory. This approach contrasts with deductive logic, which involves testing specific hypotheses that were derived from general ideas and is the approach most often used in quantitative inquiries. The process underlying qualitative research is considered inductive because in very simple terms you begin by making observations and gathering data, then you describe the data, and finally, an attempt is made to interpret the data. The interpretation typically involves putting the pieces together so that they make an understandable "whole." This process is ongoing, dynamic, and emerging. After making initial observations and deriving initial patterns, you might go back and gather more observations, and you might even revise your initial conclusions. In this sense, the process is inductive, but you may at times use deduction within this process. Not surprisingly, considering this type of research process, qualitative research has been compared to patchwork quiltmaking and filmmaking (Sterk and Elifson, 2004).

Finding Meaning Is the Goal. Essentially, the task of qualitative research is to find meaning in the observations and experiences of the participants, which brings us to the fifth feature of qualitative research. The perspective of the participants is the main concern. For example, Miller-García (2004) wanted to understand the *meaning* of condoms for Mexican couples. Through in-depth interviews with five couples, she found that condoms meant "preventing pregnancy" and "being responsible." Her interpretation of the data is provided in Box 7.3.

Box 7.3. Meaning of Condom Use

Condoms as Contraception

All participants were asked what using a condom means to them. The overwhelming response among both women and men is that using a condom means preventing pregnancy. In fact, four of the five couples were in agreement that this was the primary meaning that condom use has for them. The fifth couple also said that using condoms means prevention of pregnancies to them, but only second to the prevention of illnesses and infections—this couple, however, has never used condoms.

For one woman, using condoms to prevent pregnancy is very important to her. She explained that while she is here in Atlanta working with her husband to save money and pay off debt, their two small children live in Mexico with her mother-in-law: "No, I can't get pregnant. Supposedly, one comes here to work, and so I am the one who says, 'I don't want to get pregnant because I don't want my children to feel betrayed . . . if I go back to Mexico with another baby in my arms.'" Another woman, in addition to the primary meaning of pregnancy prevention, expressed that condom use has a more global meaning for her: "To me, using condoms means fewer unwanted children in the world, fewer abortions, fewer illnesses, and fewer submissive women."

Condoms as Responsibility

Several men's explanation of what condom use means to them extended beyond contraception. For one man, using condoms means taking precautions, and for another, using condoms is "something special, something necessary." Another explained that for him, using condoms means being responsible: "It means being responsible. As a responsible person, I prefer to have to wrinkle up my nose a little so that, well, you have to use a condom to be together for a while or else you get the surprise of another baby."

Source: Miller-García, 2004. *Gender, Power, and the Meaning of Condom Use: A Qualitative Assessment of Condom Use Among Latino Couples.* Unpublished master's thesis, Rollins School of Public Health, Emory University, Atlanta.

Understanding the perspective of the participants in their natural surroundings in some way that is meaningful is the main goal of qualitative research. Although ostensibly this may seem like an easy task, interpreting the experiences of other people is rather difficult. As with any research, qualitative or quantitative, researchers bring their own experiences, values, and biases with them that may color or influence the interpretation. The main difference (refer to Table 7.1), however, between providing meaning to qualitative research and quantitative research is that in the former, the researcher typically acknowledges his or her values and biases and also understands that the process is subjective. Conversely, in quantitative research, an assumption of objectivity is made by the researcher when collecting and interpreting the data. This implies that the researcher is detached and impartial for all aspects of the research including the interpretation. You may want to consider whether or not researchers truly detach themselves from the process just because they are implementing an experimental design, administering quantitative measures, and performing statistical analyses.

Purposes for Which Qualitative Mode of Inquiry Can Be Used

Although there may be an infinite number of purposes for which qualitative inquiry can be used and should be used in health promotion research, we shall focus on four major purposes. Qualitative inquiry is useful for conducting exploratory research where little is known about a particular health issue. Qualitative inquiry should also be used when conducting formative research to develop a health promotion program (HPP). In this instance, qualitative inquiry can be combined with quantitative approaches. Qualitative research should also be viewed in certain instances as a complement or supplement to quantitative inquiries. Program evaluation is one such instance. Finally, qualitative inquiry can be used as an alternative when other methods are precluded.

Exploratory Research. As you may recall from Chapter Four, investigations of certain health phenomena generally evolve through a two-stage process, exploratory and conclusive. The exploratory stage entails research questions that will shed light on an issue for which little is known. "In this early stage [of the process], observations are needed to provide investigators with data to define health issues, to begin to understand the etiology of those health issues, to formulate theories, to reveal relevant factors, and to identify potential relationships." Thus, there is purpose to exploratory research, and its purpose corresponds highly with a qualitative mode of inquiry.

Because not much is known yet during the exploratory stage, it would be difficult to develop any hypotheses a priori that warrant testing. It may not be prudent at this stage to launch a large-scale research study using large samples and geographically diverse locations. Thus, exploratory research lends itself quite nicely to a qualitative mode in which you could begin to gather observations using a naturalistic approach within a limited geographical context, and data collected are not structured and formalized but descriptive. Interpretation of the data would center on defining the patterns grounded in the data and making sense of it all. Perhaps preliminary hypotheses or even a theory could emerge from the data at this point. Let's illustrate this point by referring back to the research study involving patients with herpes who were asymptomatic. At the time the study was conceptualized there was little known about how varied asymptomatic people's reactions would be to receiving a positive herpes diagnosis. Also, the serological test (western blot) used to detect antibodies to herpes simplex virus was becoming readily available and was emerging as a useful screening tool for diagnosing large numbers of people. The researchers felt that it was important to understand the emotional and potential psychosocial responses people may have to receiving a diagnosis, so that counseling strategies could be devised that would address these responses. Thus, a qualitative study was conducted to ascertain a relatively small number (twenty-four) of people's responses to receiving a positive diagnosis. The results suggested a theory of both short-term and ongoing responses and their relations as well as the influence of other factors (such as social support or knowledge about herpes) on those responses—both negatively and positively. The theory that Melville and others (2003) generated from the data is graphically depicted as a model in Figure 7.1. In viewing the model one can see the nature of the relationships between the variables and that the variables are such that measurements could be derived; thus, a quantitative mode could be employed to test the model on a larger scale. Thus, this example of exploratory research helped to advance the field to the next stage so that conclusive research could be conducted.

Referring back to Table 7.1, we can see that qualitative inquiry's purposes, which are parallel to that of exploratory research's, are contextualization, interpretation, and understanding of perspectives. Contextualization means that the research seeks to provide an understanding based on the experiences of the participants in a *particular* social setting. Whether or not the interpretation of those experiences will generalize to others is not the goal. Once an understanding of perspectives is reached, depending on the situation, future research can use other modes of inquiry to see whether these experiences generalize to others. Suppose, for example, that you are interested in understanding better the role parents may play, beyond the genetic component, in contributing to the obesity of their children. You could choose a setting such as small, rural town or even a particular school district that may have unusually high rates of obesity for the inquiry. Your approach in understanding the daily lives of the families who reside in the setting could entail not only observing, interviewing, and interacting with them

FIGURE 7.1.   MODEL OF PSYCHOLOGICAL RESPONSES
TO A SEROLOGICAL HSV-2 DIAGNOSIS.

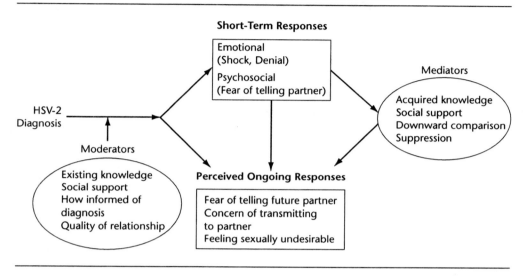

and trying to determine how they view their lives, but also identifying the histor-ical, social, political, and environmental influences that interact and shape their reality. Once meaning is derived and a complex picture of the phenomena is obtained, then perhaps a larger-scale study that is more on the "conclusive" side can be justified and implemented.

When using a qualitative mode of inquiry, another caveat may be in order: this process is one of complexity, and trying to reduce or simplify the complexity of people's lives is not the goal. The researcher must "do justice to that com-plexity, to respect it in its own right" (Glesne and Peshkin, 1992, p. 7). Thus, for researchers using qualitative mode of inquiry, it helps if they immerse themselves and take an insider's point of view (that is, emic) and use multiple methods such as interviewing, observation, focus groups, and so on. The end result will reveal the complex nature of the phenomena in question and help to identify relevant qualities, interactions, and relationships. Consequently, new theories may result, hypotheses may develop, and hopefully the field will advance to the next stage in the process. Similar to quantitative inquiries, qualitative inquiries can also add yet another link to the research chain.

As Formative Research to Designing and Implementing HPPs. There may be some instances when it will be the research stage or the specific research question that dictates the decision to use either a quantitative or qualitative mode; other times, either mode may be plausible. In these instances, the researcher may have to choose. The decision that the researcher makes more than likely will rest on the personal perspective of the researcher. Each researcher holds a worldview that is shaped by his or her discipline's paradigm, personal experiences, and other socialization processes; thus as researchers our own ideals and values shape our research. More important, however, is that regardless of how or why the decision is made to adopt a certain approach, we do not want to present this decision as a conflict. The two approaches are not necessarily incompatible, and choosing which approach to use in your research does not have to be viewed as an "either-or" decision.

◆ ◆ ◆

In a Nutshell

As researchers our own ideals and values shape our research.

◆ ◆ ◆

Many times in health promotion research both modes are useful, compatible and, indeed, desirable. In fact, as opposed to endorsing or adopting only one approach, researchers should aspire to *triangulation* when planning any research study. Triangulation is a way for researchers to obtain a multidimensional view of phenomena of interest and involves multiplicities in data sources, methods, investigators, or theoretical frameworks (Denzin, 1978). It does not mean that you are limited to "three" types of each, however. Thus, the literal meaning of the word is not used in this context. It does imply that by incorporating both quantitative and qualitative approaches and data sources into any one research study, you can provide a more thorough understanding of phenomena.

◆ ◆ ◆

In a Nutshell

Triangulation is a way for researchers to obtain a multidimensional view of phenomena of interest and involves multiplicities in data sources, methods, investigators, or theoretical frameworks.

◆ ◆ ◆

Designing HPPs is a major goal of health promotion researchers and practitioners. Before programs can be designed, however, we must garner a thorough and complex understanding of the factors contributing to a particular health behavior or disease occurrence. One way is to conduct observational research as described in Chapter Five. For example, observational research using quantitative modes of inquiry is an effective way to document the prevalence and incidence of disease and to identify measurable risk factors; however, qualitative modes of inquiry may be used as an effective way of knowing both *why* a particular disease is prevalent, and also *how* to begin to prevent it. Thus, triangulation is a comprehensive way for health promotion researchers to know as much as possible, so that more effective programs can be derived. Nakkash and others (2003) used triangulation of methods (quantitative and qualitative) and data sources (community members and coalition members) in their development of a cardiovascular disease prevention program. They first conducted a household survey (a quantitative method) using a representative sample from the community (the first data source) in which the program was to be implemented. The survey was designed to assess knowledge, attitudes, and behaviors related to cardiovascular disease and to identify risk factor levels. They also asked participants from the household survey to participate in focus groups (a qualitative method) to identify the facilitators and barriers to achieving healthy lifestyles as well as intervention ideas. A coalition consisting of key informal and formal community leaders (the second data source) was assembled. The researchers conducted natural group discussions (a qualitative method) with the coalition members to understand the relevancy, feasibility, affordability, acceptability, and sustainability of proposed intervention activities. The researchers made the following comments regarding their use of triangulation in developing the community-based program:

> The advantages far outweigh the disadvantages. The intervention activities developed as a result of the triangulation of data methods and sources are community specific, relevant, and affordable. As a result, they are more effective and sustainable. This combination of intervention activities could not have been developed in the absence of any one piece of information. Effective and sustainable interventions are, in fact, cost-effective. Thus, the cost-intense disadvantage is ultimately diminished in an assessment of efficiency. Practitioners are encouraged to obtain information from a variety of methods and sources in the development of community-specific interventions [Nakkash and others, 2003, p. 738].

Although some researchers may admit that carrying out a sophisticated quantitative study while also conducting in-depth qualitative research is rife with challenges and may be difficult for many; essentially all research is rife with challenges. Thus, given the breadth of experiences described by Nakkash and others (2003) and their subsequent endorsement of combining approaches in retrospect, it would be hard to argue that using a combination of approaches should not be attempted or at least considered. If the researcher's perspective endorses more of a quantitative view, then he or she could use triangulation of data sources. Furthermore, if multiple methods are desired, the researcher could use triangulation of investigators (that is, a multidisciplinary approach) and collaborate with researchers who are experts in qualitative methods thereby expanding the methods used. There are myriad ways to use triangulation, but you may have to be creative.

Another way in which qualitative research may be useful is before the HPP is implemented. Methodological issues related to the implementation of the program are best determined beforehand through the use of qualitative research. These include issues such as

- Recruitment strategies (for example, what the best way is to recruit)
- Participants' perceptions of randomization (for example, thoughts of being in a control group)
- Retention of participants (for example, strategies to stay in contact with participants)
- Compensation (for example, the amounts or the type that are appropriate)
- Logistical issues (for example, what the most convenient time is to have the HPP)

Given the time and resources involved in developing an HPP, it would be judicious to conduct some qualitative research to ensure that the program will be well-received and that the research to evaluate it can be conducted successfully. For example, Salazar, Holtgrave, Crosby, Frew, and Peterson (2005) conducted a qualitative research study to examine the attitudes and beliefs toward obtaining a hypothetical AIDS vaccine (in this instance, the vaccine would be considered an HPP) among men who have sex with men (MSM). The purpose of the research was to understand their perceptions and opinions toward vaccination given the commercial availability of an AIDS vaccine, and also to understand the salient issues critical to their decision-making process. Because several AIDS vaccines are currently undergoing Phase II and Phase III clinical trials, understanding the barriers to and facilitators toward getting vaccinated is necessary to ensure widespread uptake of a vaccine that may be approved in the future. For a vaccine to truly protect people there must be widespread acceptance of the vaccine. Limited motivation to obtain vaccination would have a great impact on the success of a vaccine program. Thus, the qualitative inquiry was conducted with twenty-four MSM to better understand their motivation to participate in an AIDS vaccine program. The interviews were transcribed and analyzed. The main issues that emerged from the data are shown in Table 7.2.

TABLE 7.2. EMERGENT THEMES RELATED TO GETTING A FUTURE AIDS VACCINE.

Factors and Description	Illustration
Knowledge Factors	
Vaccine strategy	"Is it made with a piece of the HIV virus?" "Do they actually inject you with HIV?" "What symptoms or damage would it prevent?"
Clinical trial research	"First of all that it's solid and that it works 100 percent." "Very little side effects where it would not affect our daily lives." "How many people were in the study; what was the make of the study as far as males, females; different ethnic groups; what were their sexual practices, were they straight or gay (sexual orientation); and how the long does the study last?" "How does this drug work on different ethnic groups?"
Vaccine attributes	"We have to realize that medicine costs money, and our health has an economic consequence." "Is it something that I would only need to take once?" "Can it be put into a pill?" "I'd like to know who sponsored it and who stands to make a profit." "Does the vaccine have FDA approval?"
Racial differences	"It makes a big difference to me if it was tested in Acorra, Cameroon, where it's all black people, with high HIV percentage rate, or if it was tested on white gay males in Chelsea, in New York."
Encouraging Factors	
Knowledge about AIDS vaccine	"I would be cool with it if there were no side effects."
Perceived high risk	"If I were dating someone who was HIV positive, I may take the vaccine."
Cost	"If all the research states that it works fine, no adverse reactions, I don't see why I would not take it as long as I could afford it."
Discouraging Factors	
Harsh side effects	"I can't really think of a reason why I would not want to take this vaccine other than side effects that would affect my body that would stifle my daily progress or my daily functions in my life."
Low perceived risk	"If I have sex, which might be rarely, it is safe sex and I don't put myself in the situation where I would need the vaccine."
Backlash effect	"Because our people take it and think 'Oh God, it's a cure and let me go throw my rubbers away, I can get back out there and do whatever I want.'"
Cost prohibitive	"Something that was really expensive . . . like $1,500 or $5,000."

Numerous studies have been conducted that have examined patient characteristics such as race, marital status, and age as influencers of enrollment in cancer trials (Roberts, 2002), while other studies have examined barriers to participation such as lack of social support, availability of child care, and transportation concerns (for example, Richardson, Post-White, Singletary, and Justice, 1998), uncertainty of side effects (for example, Barofsky and Sugarbaker, 1979), and even physicians' communication style (for example, Grant, Cissna, and Rosenfeld, 2000). Although these studies have provided much-needed information that is helpful for researchers implementing a randomized controlled trial (RCT) of cancer treatments, Roberts (2002) felt that a clear understanding of *how* trials were being presented to potential volunteers was lacking. She wanted to understand the process that oncologists went through in their presentation of options to potential study volunteers. In other words, she wanted to know what type of information was being presented as well as how it was being presented. She audiotaped interactions between oncologists and their patients who had been diagnosed with breast cancer. The interaction represented the communication between the oncologists and their patients as they discussed the patient's options for adjuvant therapy. She analyzed the transcripts and found much variation in the way oncologists presented information regarding the clinical trial option. Her qualitative analysis suggests that differences in the way physicians present information for the same clinical trial can lead to differential response rates. This information could not have been gleaned using a quantitative mode of inquiry.

When implementing an RCT, equally important to understanding the physician's perspective is understanding the potential volunteer's perspective. How do certain people perceive the details of participating in a trial? Knowing and understanding this viewpoint may provide information needed to ensure adequate enrollment and reduce participation bias. Moreover, ethical guidelines stipulate that patients who participate must be adequately informed, but how do you gauge or measure whether participants have been adequately informed? Not surprisingly, we advocate that qualitative research methods are an appropriate way to answer some of these methodological and ethical questions. Ferguson (2002) used a qualitative approach to explore seventy-eight trial participants' views on the amount of information provided and of their own understanding of that information. The participants' perceptions were that they felt they had been given adequate amounts of information and that they were able to understand the information presented to them.

Featherstone and Donovan (1998) wanted to understand participants' perspective of one of the most critical aspects of the RCT—the randomization process. They conducted in-depth interviews with twenty clinical trial participants and found that they had recalled and were able to describe aspects of the process such as "chance," "comparison of treatments," and "concealed allocation," but relayed some confusion in terminology (for instance, "trial" and "random") and held some misgivings about the procedures used. These results suggest that potential volunteers may need more information regarding the rationale for the RCT and specific terms used by the researchers. Thus, their qualitative study provided information that is useful for implementers of RCTs but most likely could not have been ascertained using a quantitative approach.

Complement or Supplement to Quantitative Inquiry. With the advent of new treatment modalities for combating disease and the need for new behavioral programs to modify a spectrum of high-risk behaviors, trials to evaluate these regimens are critical to moving the field forward and to determining what works and what doesn't. In Chapter Eight, on program evaluation, you will learn the importance of program evaluation and specifically how triangulation (in other words, multiple data sources, methods, and investigators) is often used when designing and conducting a program evaluation. As you may have been able to glean from the phrase "program evaluation," it basically involves some type of HPP and a research plan to evaluate it. Whether it is a large-scale phase III clinical trial involving thousands of participants or a smaller scale pilot study, these evaluation investigations can only benefit from including qualitative research as an adjunct to the methods and data sources constituting the quantitative component.

A specific type of quantitative mode, namely the experimental design, is used quite often to evaluate HPPs and is described in detail in Chapter Six. Thus, the quantitative approach answers whether the HPP was effective. Yet, a quantitative approach may be limited in answering *how* or *why*. Because qualitative research is about the process, it is an excellent mode to use for researchers to learn *how* the intervention worked. What activities resonated to the participants, and what activities did not? Why did the participants change their attitudes or alter their behavior? If the program was not effective, then why did participants think it didn't work? What about the intervention evoked the observed changes? Even if the program was effective, what did they like about it? All of these questions could be asked of the participants and their responses could reveal patterns that would provide researchers with a much more in-depth understanding of their intervention. In fact, a recent textbook has been dedicated to describing various process evaluations that have used qualitative methods and strategies for answering many of these questions (see Steckler and Linnan, 2002). Clearly, it is critical to know whether the program worked, but equally important is to know why and how it worked. Thus, incorporating a qualitative approach into an evaluation will help to supplement, validate, explain, and illuminate or possibly reinterpret the quantitative data gathered from the participants. The result will be more comprehensive and have a multidimensionality that could not otherwise have been achieved without triangulation (Miles and Huberman, 1994).

◆ ◆ ◆

In a Nutshell

Incorporating a qualitative approach into an evaluation will help to supplement, validate, explain, and illuminate or possibly reinterpret the quantitative data gathered from the participants.

◆ ◆ ◆

An Alternative Method When Other Methods Are Precluded. In certain jurisdictions of the United States there are laws that restrict the type and nature of educational programs and subsequent inquiries to evaluate those programs. For example, Box 7.4 highlights a specific piece of legislation from the state of Louisiana that dictates the type of sex education programs that can be implemented in the schools and proscribes the nature of questions students can be asked. As you can see from the bolded text, "Students shall not be tested, quizzed, or surveyed about their personal or family beliefs or practices in sex, morality, or religion." Thus, for health promotion researchers who are interested in prevention of pregnancy and STDs among adolescents in Louisiana, not only must they adhere to abstinence-only education, but also they must restrict their evaluations of these programs to content other than sexual beliefs and behavior.

Clearly, this presents a challenge to program evaluators who are seeking to determine the effectiveness of abstinence-only educational programs in this jurisdiction. Thus, alternative ways of investigating students' experiences with the program must be devised. Of course, this legislation does not preclude the use of surveys or quantitative instruments per se; however, it does limit to a large degree what *can* be surveyed. One alternative in this instance would be for program evaluators to query participants' about their experiences with the program and what value the program had for them. Moreover, they could ask participants their opinions of how the program could be improved. Thus, in this context, a qualitative mode of inquiry may be the best method and even perhaps the only method for gathering these types of information related to the program.

Yoo, Johnson, Rice, and Manuel (2004) implemented a qualitative evaluation of a sexual abstinence program that was implemented in southern Louisiana. They conducted semistructured interviews with principals, teachers, and peer mentors. In addition, they conducted eight gender-stratified focus groups of students who received the program. By using qualitative methods, they were able to garner

Box 7.4. Louisiana State Legislation

RS 17:281 SUBPART D-1. PERMITTED COURSES OF STUDY

281. Instruction in sex education

A.(1) (a) Any public elementary or secondary school in Louisiana may, but is not required to, offer instruction in subject matter designated as "sex education," provided such instruction and subject matter is integrated into an existing course of study such as biology, science, physical hygiene, or physical education. When offered, such instruction shall be available also to nongraded special education students at age-appropriate levels. Except as otherwise required to comply with the provisions of Subparagraph (b) of this Paragraph, whether or not instruction in such matter is offered and at what grade level it is to be offered shall be at the option of each public local or parish school board, provided that no such instruction shall be offered in kindergarten or in grades one through six. Such instruction may be offered at times other than during the regular school day, at such times to be determined by each school board. All instruction in "sex education" shall be identified and designated "sex education."

(b) Effective beginning with the spring semester of the 1992–1993 school year and thereafter, whenever instruction in sex education is offered by any school, such instruction shall be available also to any student in such school, regardless of the student's grade level, who is pregnant or who is a mother or father.

(2) It is the intent of the legislature that, for the purposes of this Section, "sex education" shall mean the dissemination of factual biological or pathological information that is related to the human reproduction system and may include the study of sexually transmitted disease, pregnancy, childbirth, puberty, menstruation, and menopause, as well as the dissemination of factual information about parental responsibilities under the child support laws of the state. It is the intent of the legislature that "sex education" shall not include religious beliefs, practices in human sexuality, nor the subjective moral and ethical judgments of the instructor or other persons. **Students shall not be tested, quizzed, or surveyed about their personal or family beliefs or practices in sex, morality, or religion.**

(3) No contraceptive or abortifacient drug, device, or other similar product shall be distributed at any public school. No sex education course offered in the public schools of the state shall utilize any sexually explicit materials depicting male or female homosexual activity.

(4) The major emphasis of any sex education instruction offered in the public schools of this state shall be to encourage sexual abstinence between unmarried persons and any such instruction shall:

(a) Emphasize abstinence from sexual activity outside of marriage as the expected standard for all school-age children.

(b) Emphasize that abstinence from sexual activity is a way to avoid unwanted pregnancy, sexually transmitted diseases, including acquired immune deficiency syndrome, and other associated health problems.

(c) Emphasize that each student has the power to control personal behavior and to encourage students to base action on reasoning, self-esteem, and respect for others.

B. Notwithstanding any other provisions of law, the qualifications for all teachers or instructors in "sex education" shall be established and the selection of all such teachers or instructors shall be made solely and exclusively by the public local or parish school board.

C. All books, films, and other materials to be used in instruction in "sex education" shall be submitted to and approved by the local or parish school board and by a parental review committee, whose membership shall be determined by such board.

D. Any child may be excused from receiving instruction in "sex education" at the option and discretion of his parent or guardian. The local or parish school board shall provide procedures for the administration of this Subsection.

E. In the event of any violation of the provisions of this Section, the public local or parish school board in charge of administering and supervising the school where said violation has occurred, after proper investigation and hearing, shall correct the violation and take appropriate action to punish the offending party or parties responsible for said violation.

F. No program offering sex education instruction shall in any way counsel or advocate abortion.

G. A city or parish school system may accept federal funds for programs offering sex education only when the use of such funds does not violate the provisions of this Section and only upon approval by the local school board. The acceptance and use of federal funds for sex education shall in no way be construed to permit the use of any federally supplied materials that violate Louisiana law regulating sex education.

H. Notwithstanding any other provision of law, the Orleans Parish School Board may offer instruction in sex education at the third grade level or higher.

"valuable insights for future improvement in abstinence-only programs" (p. 329). For example, they were able to learn that all respondents indicated that the program should be taught in lower grades (the program had been implemented in grades seven through nine) and that responses to the program were mixed: some felt it was of no value and some felt it provided needed information and skills (Yoo and others, 2004). It should be noted, however, that although this inquiry provided participants' opinions toward the program, it still does not provide a behavioral indication of program effectiveness.

As health promotion practitioners and researchers, we must always work within laws and follow policy guidelines as they pertain to program content and the research. Thus, in these instances when certain content cannot be measured or surveyed, a qualitative approach can provide an alternative to quantitative approaches and yield valuable information that would have otherwise been omitted.

Qualitative Research Strategies for Health Promotion Research

Up to this point, we have discussed the features of qualitative research and the instances in health promotion in which qualitative research is warranted; however, we haven't provided a clear discussion of the different types of qualitative research. Essentially, unlike quantitative research, qualitative research does not have specific designs per se; rather, qualitative research has varying strategies that can be thought of as different philosophical orientations providing a general direction for implementing the research. The research strategy can also be thought of as the "tool" for accomplishing a particular research task. These various orientations have historical roots in different disciplines such as anthropology, philosophy, education, zoology, and sociology. The strategy selected is dictated largely by "the purpose of the study, nature of the research question, and the skills and resources available to the investigator" (Morse, 1994, p. 223).

◆ ◆ ◆

In a Nutshell

Qualitative research does not have specific designs per se; rather, qualitative research has varying strategies that can be thought of as different philosophical orientations providing a general direction for implementing the research.

◆ ◆ ◆

Because qualitative strategies are too numerous to describe in great detail, we cover five basic strategies that can be useful for conducting qualitative research in health promotion. Morse (1994) has outlined these five basic qualitative strategies: phenomenology, ethnography, grounded theory, ethnoscience, and qualitative ethology. Each of these qualitative strategies offers "a particular and unique perspective that illuminates certain aspects of reality more easily than others and produces a type of results more suited for some applications than others" (Morse, 1994, p. 223). To illustrate the differences among these strategies, Morse used a hypothetical research scenario involving travelers arriving and departing at an airport. Her conceptualization of each strategy is presented in Table 7.3.

Note the highlighted differences among the five strategies in the nature of the research question, recommended sample sizes, the types of results that could be gleaned, and the types of qualitative methods appropriate for the research question. As we go through each of the strategies in more detail, it may be helpful to apply another hypothetical research example derived from health promotion. For example, a phenomenon that has been highlighted in the literature and

TABLE 7.3. A COMPARISON OF STRATEGIES IN THE CONDUCT OF A HYPOTHETICAL PROJECT: "ARRIVALS AND DEPARTURES: PATTERNS OF HUMAN ATTACHMENT."

Strategy	Research Question or Focus	Participants/ Informants[a]	Sample Size[b]	Date Collection Methods	Type of Results
Phenomenology	What is the meaning of arriving home?	Travelers arriving home; phenomological literature; art, poetry, and other descriptions	≈ six participants	In-depth conversations	In-depth reflective description of the experience of "what it feels like to come home"
Ethnography	What is the arrival gate like when an international plane arrives?	Travelers, families, others who observe the setting, such as skycaps, rental car personnel, cleaning staff, security guards, and so forth	≈ thirty to fifty interviews	Interviews; participant observation; other records, such as airport statistics	Description of the day-to-day events at the arrival gate of the airport
Grounded theory	Coming home: Reuniting the family	Travelers, family members	≈ thirty to fifty	In-depth interviews; Observations	Description of the social psychological process in the experience of returning home
Ethnoscience	What are types of travelers?	Those who observe the setting daily—skycaps, rental car personnel, cleaning staff, security guards, and so forth	≈ thirty to fifty	Interviews to elicit similarities and differences of travelers, card sorts	Taxonomy and description of types and characteristics of travelers
Qualitative ethology	What are the greeting behaviors of travelers and their families?	Travelers and their families	Units—numbers of greetings—one hundred to two hundred	Photography, video, coded	Descriptions of the patterns of greeting behaviors

[a]Examples only.
[b]Number depends on saturation.

Source: From J. Morse (1994), "Designing Funded Qualitative Research," in N. K. Denzin and Y. S. Lincoln (Eds.), *Handbook of Qualitative Research,* Thousand Oaks, CA, Sage, p. 225. Copyright 1994 by Sage Publications, Inc. Reprinted with permission.

sensationalized in the media is the notion of living on the "down low." *Down low* is a term that has been applied mostly to African American men and refers to their living a heterosexual lifestyle (that is, married to a woman) while engaging in sexual intercourse with other men surreptitiously. Of course, this is not a new phenomenon. Many men in the past have lived double lives or remained in "the closet" for fear of social ostracism. However, there is some evidence to suggest that engaging in sexual intercourse with other men place men at risk for HIV infection, which in turn may place their female partners at risk. Given that blacks compose only 12 percent of the total U.S. population but 40 percent of all cumulative AIDS cases (Centers for Disease Control and Prevention, 2005), conducting qualitative research on the phenomenon of living on the down low may help researchers to understand better men's perspectives of this lifestyle and perhaps devise programs that can lead to a reduction in both types of exposure: heterosexual contact and male-to-male contact.

Phenomenology. Within an interpretivist paradigm, phenomenology refers to an analysis made by phenomenological investigation rather than the typological classification of a class of phenomena. Stemming from the discipline of philosophy, phenomenological investigations focus on interpreting "the meaning of events and interactions to ordinary people in particular situations" (Bogdan and Biklen, 1998, p. 23). The emphasis is on understanding the ways in which people construct their realities; that is, an attempt is made to reveal what perspective they hold and how they interpret events that happen. As a research strategy, it is subjective and relies heavily on trying to understand the participants' point of view. You may be wondering at this point, how can a research approach that is subjective also be considered as scientific research? As we have stated previously, quantitative modes of inquiry attempt to be objective and it is that objectivity that serves as a gauge of methodological rigor. Conversely, in the phenomenological interpretivist approach, subjectivity is treated as "a topic for investigation in its own right, not as a methodological taboo" (Holstein and Gubrium, 1994, p. 264). Thus, within this approach, subjectivity is the underlying mode and is embraced.

The method to accomplish phenomenological inquiries may be in-depth conversations and interviews with participants. For researchers using this strategy, however, gaining access to another person's point of view implies that in doing so the researcher may have some influence on the participant's perspective. Nonetheless, there is great utility in this approach, as it involves the collection of data that can provide an in-depth understanding of a phenomenon. Consequently, we may learn something which in turn may be useful for improving some aspect of the human condition. For example, Moore (2000) conducted a phenomenological study to understand the meaning of severe visual impairment to older women diagnosed with macular degeneration. The research question was "What is the lived experience of severe visual impairment in older women diagnosed with macular degeneration?" Interviews with eight women revealed that severe visual impairment meant "persisting toward unfolding ways of being in the world sparked by personal discoveries amidst enveloping losses" (Moore, 2000).

Applying phenomenology to our example of men living on the down low would be very useful for gaining insight into the lives of these men. Our research question could be "What is the meaning of living on the down low?" and could be approached by engaging men in conversations (if you could find them) about sexual orientation, homosexuality, being an African American man in our society, how they view their lifestyle, and how they make sense of their lifestyle. Our emphasis would be on describing the structures (their opinions, values, beliefs, attitudes) of participants' reality that help to explain and interpret the meaning they have attached to their reality. In this example, one hypothetical result could be the following: "For African American men living on the down low, their secretive behavior means keeping their families intact while fulfilling a sexual fantasy that makes them happy and ultimately a better husband or partner."

Ethnography. Ethnography is a qualitative strategy that has its origins in cultural anthropology, the study of human beings in relation to their social interactions and culture. Derived from the Greek term *ethnos*, meaning a people, a race, or a cultural group, and the term *graphic*, meaning descriptive, ethnography is a social scientific description of a people and the cultural basis of their peoplehood (Peacock, 1986). In this context, culture refers to the "acquired knowledge that people use to interpret experience and generate social behavior" (Spradley, 1979, p. 4). Culture is therefore relative and can be interpreted from more than one perspective, such as an outsider's or an insider's point of view. As a qualitative research strategy, ethnography focuses on providing a detailed and accurate *description* of values, behaviors, practices, and beliefs of a given group of people rather than explanation; however, the description should be in terms of the native's point of view rather than from the researcher's. Yet doing ethnography does not entail only studying people and observing their behavior; rather, the ethnographer must go beyond the gathering of observations and facts and learn what they mean. This experience requires the researcher to immerse herself or himself in the culture under study and not only observe the behavior, artifacts, and emotions but also try to understand the meaning attached to them from an insider's perspective. Thus, because ethnography is also concerned with meaning, it is similar to phenomenology, but differs in that its purpose has a much greater scope and culture is the guiding framework used to interpret and attach meaning to the experiences.

◆ ◆ ◆

In a Nutshell

Because ethnography is also concerned with meaning, it is similar to phenomenology, but differs in that its purpose has a much greater scope and culture is the guiding framework used to interpret and attach meaning to the experiences.

◆ ◆ ◆

To conduct ethnography, researchers should use multiple data collection methods such as naturalistic observation, interviews with natives, gathering of artifacts, and examination of archival data. In this way, they can capture a full description of those aspects of culture that shape people's experiences, behavior, beliefs, and emotions. For example, Reisinger (2004) conducted an ethnographic study of an outpatient adolescent drug treatment program. The purpose of the ethnography was to "understand better the treatment experience from the perspective of the adolescent clients" (Reisinger, 2004, p. 244). She conducted four in-depth interviews with each of twenty-five adolescents who presented for treatment. Researchers also observed seventy group sessions and conducted both formal and informal interviews with clinic staff. Moreover, extensive field notes were compiled.

Getting back to our hypothetical example, if we were to apply ethnography to the study of men living on the down low, we would be interested in describing what life is like for men who live this way. In this situation, we might have to enlist the assistance of an *informant,* someone who could be a source of information to help communicate knowledge regarding the experience and serve as a teacher to the researcher. We could conduct interviews with men and perhaps hang out at a bar where they may go to meet other men while observing and taking notes. We would also want to consider interviewing other relevant participants such as a wife or girlfriend, or other members of the community that may play a cultural role in this lifestyle. We would attempt to describe their lives in a way that is in relation to the culture in which they are embedded. This attempt at description involves a *translation process,* which entails "discovering the meanings of one culture and communicating these meanings to people in another culture" (Spradley, 1979, p. 205). In this example, one hypothetical result could be something like the following:

> African American men, who live on the down low, view being gay as religiously immoral and also as detrimental to a person's standing in the community—as many people in the African American community support the view that

homosexuality is taboo, and gay men are viewed as being less than men. They do not describe themselves as gay, as this would contradict their notion of male identity and upset their lives and their family's lives. Instead, personal and social self-preservation requires that they adhere to the cultural norm of heterosexuality. Thus, they fulfill their need for male sexual contact in secret. They justify this behavior by saying it is only an indulgence in male fantasy; it is not a betrayal nor is it hurtful to their wives because they are not sleeping with other women.

Grounded Theory. Essentially, grounded theory is a general methodology for deriving a theory or theories from data systematically gathered and analyzed (Strauss and Corbin, 1994). Grounded theory has been described as a marriage between positivism and interpretivism. First conceptualized as a strategy by two sociologists, Glaser and Strauss (1967), grounded theory is best used for understanding phenomenal processes (Morse, 1994). By processes, we mean that what is being studied or understood is dynamic and may entail stages or phases but may also involve "reciprocal changes in patterns of action-interaction and in relationship with changes of conditions either internal or external to the process itself" (Strauss and Corbin, 1994, p. 278). Because theory development is the main focus of this qualitative strategy, it differs in its central purpose from other qualitative strategies in which meaning and describing are the core purposes. The brilliance of this qualitative approach lies in its logic: explicitly link empirical data to the creation and elaboration of a theory. As you may recall from Chapter Two, we stated that intuition, previous knowledge, or Baconian inductivism were ways in which theory can be developed. Similar in concept to Baconian inductivism, however, the grounded theory approach is a unique and superior way in which theory development should be approached—through research. "A theory is not the formulation of some discovered aspect of a preexisting reality 'out there' . . . rather theories are interpretations made from given perspectives as adopted or researched by researchers" (Strauss and Corbin, 1994, p. 279).

To use grounded theory as your approach you must gather and analyze data in a systematic way, hence grounded theory possesses some features of positivism. The system entails an iterative process sometimes referred to as *constant comparative analysis,* in which data are used first to generate a theory, and then subsequent data are compared against the initial theory. At the beginning of the process, an assumption is made that the initial theory will be provisional; thus, changes and modifications, if necessary, can be made as new data are generated and analyzed, and new patterns and themes emerge. Key to this process is the use of multiple perspectives when gathering and analyzing the data. If you refer back to Table 7.2, note that approximately thirty to fifty participants are recommended when undertaking this approach. Moreover, a distinction should be made when using this approach as to the type of theory that is trying to be developed. *Substantive theory*, which is theory derived from research in one substantive area (for example, short-term and ongoing psychosocial reactions to herpes diagnosis), and *formal theory*, which is a more general theory with broader applications (such as social cognitive theory), are the two overarching categories of theories. The former typically serves as a springboard to the development of the latter. Both types of theories can be developed using grounded theory; however, the approach is better suited to the development of substantive theory. For example, Canales and Geller (2004) conducted a grounded theory study in which they examined mammography decision making across the breast cancer screening continuum: women who consistently got yearly mammograms, women who were inconsistent or failed to get a mammogram, and breast cancer survivors. They were able to develop a theory titled "Moving in Between Mammography," which described the decision-making process and identified several factors that influenced their behavior (Canales and Geller, 2004). Applying a grounded theory strategy to our hypothetical example, we could use this strategy to develop a psychosocial theory that attempted to explain the psychological, psychosocial, and sociocultural factors that influenced the behavior of men on the down low. Using Canales and Geller's theory as inspiration, we could title our theory, "Between Straight and Gay," and potential influencers could be impulsivity, risk-taking, social anxiety, cultural norms, social support, and religiosity.

Ethnoscience. Ethnoscience is a branch of cognitive anthropology, which focuses on the relation between human culture and human thought. Cognitive anthropology strives to understand how people understand and organize their own reality. This branch of anthropology goes beyond studying the behavior of a particular culture by attempting to identify the culturally derived classification systems people use to make sense of their reality. Each person's classification system comprises cognitive categories that provide some order and understanding to life experiences. The main objective of an ethnoscience inquiry is to reliably represent these cognitive categories; that is, reveal a cogent classification system used by people to process and understand behavior, events, emotions, and things—a taxonomy of sorts. Each culture has its own indigenous classification system. Consequently, people from different cultures will have markedly different perceptions of any given set of behavior, events, emotions, or things. Bottorff and others (1998) conducted a qualitative ethnoscience study to examine breast health practices of South Asian women living in Canada. They conducted in-depth interviews with fifty women, which were analyzed and used to develop a taxonomy that represented relationships among emerging cultural themes and domains.

They found that women held four central beliefs regarding breast health practices that ranged from beliefs about taking care of your breasts to beliefs about accessing services.

In our hypothetical example, an ethnoscience study would focus on developing a reliable classification system that the men use to explain their lifestyle. A taxonomy could be developed that would classify men according to their underlying cultural beliefs. An example of this taxonomy could be several domains of beliefs that represented the explanations of their lifestyle choice, such as "cultural taboos against being gay," "homophobia," and "endorsement of the sexual double standard for men that permits promiscuity and adultery."

Qualitative Ethology. Qualitative ethology has its roots in zoology, which is the study of natural animal behavior and falls under the discipline of biology. Typically, ethology involves naturalistic observation designed to ascertain the significance of some naturally occurring behavior and its relationship to the environment. Applying this strategy to humans entails observing them in their natural environment with goals of revealing the cause(s) of the behavior, seeing how the behavior develops, identifying the biological function of the behavior, or determining whether the behavior has evolved. Thus, the ethologist is not interested in the participant's perspective per se. This strategy contrasts with the other qualitative strategies, in which participants' perceptions of events, beliefs, or practices along with their respective meaning are the focus of the inquiry. In qualitative ethology this is not the main emphasis (Blurton Jones and Woodson, 1979, p. 99). This strategy is most useful when the specific behavior of interest can be readily observed in as unobtrusive a way as possible, and also when the behavior is not well-suited to using other self-report methods (such as interviewing).

If we refer to Table 7.3, qualitative ethology is the strategy used to describe patterns of a naturally occurring behavior (in this case, the greeting behaviors of travelers and their families). Instead of in-depth interviews, video and photography of the travelers are the two data-collection modalities used to capture the behavior. In health promotion research, qualitative ethology could be used in clinical settings to characterize interactions between health care providers and their patients (for example, Bottorff and Varcoe, 1995; Solberg and Morse, 1991), to document the interactions between health educators and intervention participants, or to capture certain health-risk behaviors in a field setting (such as drug use or needle sharing). Behaviors of interest to analyze could be communication patterns, both verbal and nonverbal, with an emphasis on how the participant interacts with the particular environment. For example, Morse and Pooler (2002) used qualitative ethology to examine the interactions of patients' family members with the patients and nurses in the trauma room of an emergency department of a hospital. Video was used to film these interactions. Analyzing 192 videotapes, the authors coded the verbal and nonverbal behaviors and were able to categorize these interactions as "families learning to endure, patients failing to endure, family emotionally suffering and patient enduring, patient and family enduring, and resolution of enduring" (Morse and Pooler, 2002, p. 240).

Applying qualitative ethology to men who live on the down low may not be a viable option. Men on the down low are engaging in sexual behavior with other men in secret. Clearly, their behavior would not be open to observation let alone videotaping. Furthermore, it would be difficult to identify a specific setting in which the behavior would naturally occur. Thus, qualitative ethology may not be the best strategy for investigating this type of behavior.

Qualitative Data-Collection Methods for Health Promotion Research

As we have described five main qualitative strategies of inquiry, you may have noted that each strategy was associated with certain data-collection method(s). Primary data-collection methods can include observations and in-depth interviews as well as personal and official documents, photographs, recordings, drawings, e-mails, and informal conversations. For example, in Table 7.2, phenomenology was associated with in-depth conversations, whereas grounded theory used in-depth interviews and observations. Qualitative ethology used video and photography. Thus, the strategy selected by the investigator is connected to a specific method for data collection (Sterk and Elifson, 2004). In this section, we describe and discuss two data-collection methods widely used to conduct qualitative inquiries: interviewing and participant observation.

Interviewing. In general, interviewing can take several different forms that range from unstructured to structured, and may involve interviewing an individual, a dyad, or a group (that is, a focus group). The first form of interviewing we will discuss is considered the least structured and can be thought of more as an informal conversation than a formal interview. When using this method, there are no specific questions asked; rather, topics emerge and flow from the conversation. Of course, the interviewer must prepare a plan to discuss certain general topics related to the research; however, the process is provisional in that certain topics may not get discussed and there is no set order to the discussion (Babbie, 2004). This form of interview is used frequently in phenomenological investigations or other inquiries in which the investigator is interested in understanding the meaning behind participants' experiences, events, practices, or behavior. Thus, it would be difficult to construct specific questions a priori.

The goal of this type of interview is to explore and to probe the interviewee's responses so that an in-depth understanding of the phenomena can be reached. This process places a major emphasis on the details of the interviewee's life experiences and social behavior. The interviewer attempts to engage the interviewee in conversation about the interviewees' attitudes, interests, feelings, concerns, and values as these relate to the research topic. Because this interview is an interaction, meaning is jointly constructed by the interviewer and the interviewee; meaning is rarely revealed as an epiphany by the interviewee, although it may happen! A skilled interviewer allows participants to describe their experiences and explore their thoughts and opinions about the research topic. Because of this dynamic, it is critical that the interviewer try to establish a rapport with the participant and create a sense of trust; however, building trust and establishing a respectful relationship in which the interviewee feels comfortable may be affected by other issues such as gender and race, which may play a role in this process (Fontana and Frey, 1994).

In conducting this type of interview, interviewees should be given a considerable amount of latitude to expand upon the topics because it is they who are "knowledgeable, have a meaningful perspective to offer, and are able to make this explicit in their own words" (Sterk and Elifson, 2004, p. 137). It truly is a conversation taking place between the interviewer, who is an active participant, and the interviewee. Thus, although there is a predetermined topic of interest, the conversation or interview should be viewed as spontaneous and unstructured. A caveat must be stated, however. Even though the interview should be viewed as a conversation, the interviewer must focus on listening to the interviewee. Rather than trying to appear to *be interesting*, the interviewer should *appear interested in* what the interviewee has to say (Babbie, 2004). In fact, Lofland and Lofland (1995) recommend adopting the role of the "socially acceptable incompetent" when interviewing (p. 56).

It is prudent to begin the conversation with less sensitive, benign topics and then gradually ease the conversation toward more sensitive and complex issues. For example, if a researcher were to have a "conversation" with a man who lives on the down low, he or she would want to start the conversation with a discussion of what it is like to be an African American man in today's society, what his experiences were growing up, and what life is like for him in the present. Because this is a highly personal and sensitive topic, it might be best to consider matching the interviewer's gender and race with those of the interviewee (for example, male and African American). This matching may facilitate the establishment of rapport. Then, once trust has been established (this could take from several hours to perhaps several interview sessions over the course of several days), the conversation could be steered toward more sensitive topics such as sexual behavior. During the interview or the conversation, it is also beneficial if the interviewer is cognizant of any responses that would allow for more in-depth probing. Probing takes many forms, but basically entails an effort either verbally or nonverbally on the part of the interviewer to elicit more details, to guide the dialogue, to iterate the meaning of something said by the interviewee, or to allow the interviewee to feel comfortable in preparing his or her response. Probes perform these functions while also allowing the interviewer to establish a relationship with the interviewee and indicate the desire to understand what the interviewee is saying (Fontana and Frey, 1994). For example, the interviewer could ask a directive question such as "Could you tell me more about your thinking on that?" The interviewer could also use the echo probe, in which he or she repeats what the interviewee has just said. This indicates to the interviewee that the interviewer is listening to what they say. The interviewer could also simply use comments such as "uh huh," "I see," "Yes," or "Mm." Nonverbal probes are also effective and include nods of the head or simply remaining silent to give the interviewee time to reflect or prepare their next thought. In any event, the function of the probes is to motivate the participants to communicate more fully and to help them focus on the general topics while keeping the communication flowing.

◆ ◆ ◆

In a Nutshell

Probing takes many forms, but basically entails an effort either verbally or nonverbally on the part of the interviewer to elicit more details, to guide the dialogue, to iterate the meaning of something said by the interviewee, or to allow the interviewee to feel comfortable in preparing his or her response.

◆ ◆ ◆

A more structured type of interview than the unstructured interview is the semistructured interview. This form of interviewing uses a series of open-ended questions that are typically asked of all participants in a predetermined order. The questions are considered directive and are used to ascertain specific topics related to the research. The interviewer should read the question exactly as it is worded to avoid changing the intent of the question in addition to asking all of the questions that apply. Although the interviewer is encouraged to use probes, the probes should be as neutral as possible to avoid introducing bias into the process. For example, if the interviewer asks a question and the participant says, "I don't know," or "I am not sure," one type of neutral probe, called a "clarification probe," that could be used in this instance is, "There are no right or wrong answers to these questions, we are only interested in finding out how you feel about this."

Although there is more structure to this form of interview, the open-ended questions still allow the participant to elaborate and provide significant details on his or her experiences. Thus, this type of interview is well-suited for grounded theory, ethnography, and ethnoscience strategies, when little is known about a certain issue but the research question has a definite direction. For instance, semi-structured interviews were used in a study of fourteen Mexican and Mexican American women staying at a battered women's shelter. The study sought to describe the barriers to the women negotiating condom use with their abusive partners. Themes of physical, psychological, and sexual abuse of the women who requested condom use emerged, as did the influence of power and control exerted over their public, private, and sexual interactions (Davila and Brackley, 1999). The semistructured interview guide used in the study is presented in Box 7.5.

When the interviewer interviews a small group of people at the same time, it is termed a focus group. Focus groups typically involve between six and twelve individuals who are a homogeneous group, but who do not usually know each other. Participants should be chosen specifically on the basis of the research topic. For example, if were we to conduct a qualitative inquiry as formative research to designing an HPP to prevent teen alcohol and drug use, we would choose participants for the focus group that were similar in age, gender, and ethnicity to the targeted intervention population. Focus groups involve a small sample that is usually generated using nonprobability techniques such as convenience sampling (see Chapter Eleven). Although the results may not be generalizable, they can still provide very useful information. In contrast to the one-on-one interview, the emphasis of the focus group is not necessarily on each participant's individual experiences, beliefs, and attitudes; rather it is the interaction between participants that is of interest to the investigator.

Focus groups have been used for a very long time in advertising and marketing research, in which researchers have gathered information about new product ideas, name changes to existing products, or customer's opinions about existing products (Brilhart and Galanes, 1998). In health promotion, focus groups are used quite frequently to provide information about interventions, salient health issues, or health care needs; to identify interests, topics, or concerns of the targeted population; or to develop new scale measures. Focus groups can be unstructured, with the moderator—the person facilitating and conducting the focus group—announcing the topic to be discussed and allowing the participants to respond freely. This should entail participants presenting their own views and then also responding to the views expressed by the other group members. Focus groups can

Box 7.5. English and Spanish Semistructured Interview Guide from a Study of Mexican and Mexican American Women

English

1. Tell me what you know about HIV/AIDS?
   A. How do women and men get it?
   B. What does it do to the body?
   C. Is there a vaccine or cure for HIV/AIDS?
2. What can a person do to keep from getting HIV/AIDS?
   A. What do you do to keep from getting HIV/AIDS?
3. In the past three months, what would you say your chance of being infected with HIV/AIDS has been?
4. In the past three months, how have you protected yourself against HIV/AIDS?
   A. For what reasons have you protected yourself?
   B. For what reasons have you not protected yourself?
5. What do you know about condoms?
6. Tell me what you think or know that is good about condoms?
7. Tell me what you think or know that is bad about condoms?
8. Tell me about your first experience with a condom.
9. Tell me about your last experience with a condom.
10. Tell me about your best experience with a condom.
11. Tell me about your worst experience with a condom.
12. Have you ever asked a male partner to use a condom?
    A. When?
    B. Under what circumstances?
    C. How did you ask him?
13. How does your partner respond when you ask him to use a condom?
14. What additional information would you like to discuss or share related to condom use?

Spanish

1. Dígame lo que usted sabe sobre de VIH/Sida?
   A. ¿Cómo las mujeres y los hombres lo cogen?
   B. ¿Qué le hace al cuerpo?
   C. ¿Hay una vacuna o una cura por el?
2. ¿Qué puede hacer una persona para evitar infección de VIH/Sida?
   A. ¿Qué hace usted para evitar infección de VIH/Sida?
3. ¿En los últimos tres meses, qué piensa ira su peligro de ser infectada con VIH/SIDA?
4. ¿En los últimos tres meses, cómo se ha protegido en contra del VIH/Sida?
   A. ¿Cuál son las razones porque se ha protegido?
   B. ¿Cuál son las razones porque no se ha protegido?

5. ¿Dígame lo qué sabe usted de condones?
6. Dígame que piensa o sabe usted de porque condones son buenos.
7. Dígame que piensa o sabe usted de porque condones son malos.
8. Dígame de su primera experiencia con condones.
9. Dígame de su última experiencia con condones.
10. Dígame de su mejor experiencia con condones.
11. Dígame de su peor experiencia con condones.
12. ¿Usted ha preguntado a su compañero que use condones?
    A. ¿Cuándo?
    B. ¿En qué circumstancias?
    C. ¿Cómo le preguntó?
13. ¿Cómo responde su compañero cuando usted le pregunta que use condones?
14. ¿Qué otra información gustara usted discutir con relacio al uso de condones?

Source: Copyright © 1999 from *Issues in Mental Health Nursing* by Davila and Brackley. Reproduced by permission of Taylor & Francis Group, LLC, www.taylorandfrancis.com.

---

also be semistructured, with the moderator using a guide to cover questions and specific topics presented in some order.

Depending on the topic, there are instances in which the group should be stratified by gender, age, or some other relevant characteristic. For example, Cameron and others (2005) conducted four on-line focus groups (similar in structure to a regular focus group, however, on-line focus groups are conducted in a chat room via the Internet) with Internet-using teens to discover their experiences with, exposure to, and perceptions of sexually oriented Websites and sexually explicit Websites. Because of the sensitive nature of the topic, the researchers stratified each group by gender and age to ensure that participants felt comfortable responding to sexually related content, and to ensure that the topics presented were developmentally appropriate.

One advantage of using a group interview as opposed to conducting individual interviews is the group dynamics. People reacting to each other tend to create a synergy that is much greater than what could be created on an individual basis. Thus, the method is synergistic and holds the potential for generating additional topics and information that might otherwise have been missed. Other advantages include its flexibility, low cost, and speedy results (Krueger, 1988). Yet, there are some disadvantages. At times, there may be one group member who tends to dominate the conversation or who may intimidate other group members. This is a difficult situation that must be addressed skillfully by a trained moderator. Clearly, because there is the group dynamic, the moderator has less control of the situation as compared with individual interviews. There is also the issue of confidentiality. The moderator can assure the participants that whatever is discussed "within the group stays within the group," but the same cannot be said for the participants. If the topic is sensitive, then precautions should be taken such as having participants agree to maintain confidentiality in the informed consent form and also agree to explicit protocol guidelines prior to when the focus group begins (Sterk and Elifson, 2004).

Whether the interviews are semistructured or unstructured, or conducted with an individual or with a group, there are some basic issues for the qualitative researcher to consider. For example, how many participants or focus groups should be conducted? Table 7.2 provides some general guidelines for sample size depending on the research question and the strategy; however, most qualitative researchers agree that these are meant as guidelines and should not be used in the same manner as sample size estimation performed in power analyses. Essentially, the number of participants or the number of focus groups is sufficient when the selected participants represent the range of potential participants in the setting, and at the point at which the data gathered begins to be redundant, that is, when consistent themes are repeated. This latter point of data redundancy and repetition is also referred to as data saturation. It is at this point that the investigator should feel confident in knowing that an adequate sample size has been reached or a sufficient number of focus groups has been conducted.

All interviews and focus groups conducted should be audiotaped with the permission of the interviewee(s). Of course, taping, or in some instances, videotaping, interviews does not preclude the interviewer from taking notes during the interview or writing notes after the interview. Once the interview or focus group is completed, the audiotapes can be transcribed "verbatim" to begin the process of data analysis.

Observation. To emphasize the importance of observation as a research method to the overall research enterprise, one need mention only one name—Charles Darwin. His meticulous attention to detail, copious notes, and commitment to extended and lengthy periods of observation resulted in his formalization of a biological theory of evolution with his assertion that natural selection was the main underlying mechanism. Needless to say, the impact of his research on science, society, religion, education, and politics is immeasurable, and his work is considered by many as scientifically revolutionary. Yet interestingly, rather than study his subjects under controlled settings using manipulation and randomization, Darwin's research method was naturalistic observation. Thus, observation as a scientific method has great utility. In addition to generating new theories, observation can be used to supplement other data-collection methods, such as interviews, to provide an expanded understanding of some phenomenon or to provide "insight into the social context in which people operate" (Sterk and Elifson, 2004, p. 142).

Participant observation is a specific type of naturalistic observation in which the researcher enters the world of the people he or she wants to study. In order to do this, however, the investigator must first identify an appropriate setting and then gain access to that setting. Whether the setting is public or private, there typically is some *gatekeeper,* a person who has the power and authority to control access, with whom the investigator should negotiate to gain access. For public settings, identifying a gatekeeper may be more difficult, or one may not exist. The investigator must also consider the ethics of observing people who are in the public realm without their informed consent. For example, how would you feel if you were out at a coffee shop or at a bar with your friends and you happen to notice a person sitting off in the corner taking notes and watching what you and your friends did? We are not contending that observing people in a public setting is unethical or wrong. In fact, many sociological and anthropological studies of public settings have been conducted in this way (for example, Lofland, 1973; McCoy and others, 1996; Monaghan, 2002; Tewksbury, 2002); however, there are other important issues to consider, and these issues must be weighed against the importance of the research and the balance of ethics and methodological rigor. For example, the investigator must decide what role he or she will adopt when making observations and whether or not to be covert or overt. Gold (1958) outlined four potential roles moving from the more involved and covert to complete detachment and overt.

The first role is that of *the complete participant,* with the researcher allowing the people under study to see him or her as a participant, not as a researcher. Thus, it is considered covert because participants in the setting do not realize this person is researching them. Acting in the role of a participant may also raise methodological problems because the investigator interacts with the participants, which may have an effect on the dynamics of the setting, the participants' behavior, or both. Because of these considerations (ethical and scientific), the decision to adopt the role of the complete participant should be well-justified. In other instances, it may be practical to adopt the second role, that of the *participant as observer.* In the participant-as-observer role, the investigator is overt, in that he or she identifies as a researcher while interacting with the participants in the social process. Thus, this role avoids some of the ethical issues in the complete participant role, but some of the methodological issues remain (for instance, observer effects). The advantage of both roles is they provide a unique insider's perspective that assists in the interpretation of what is being observed.

The third role is that of the *observer as participant,* in which the investigator's main role is that of the observer. She or he identifies as a researcher, but enters

MINCUS AND DINCUS AS "COMPLETE PARTICIPANTS" FOR THEIR CHICKEN STUDY.

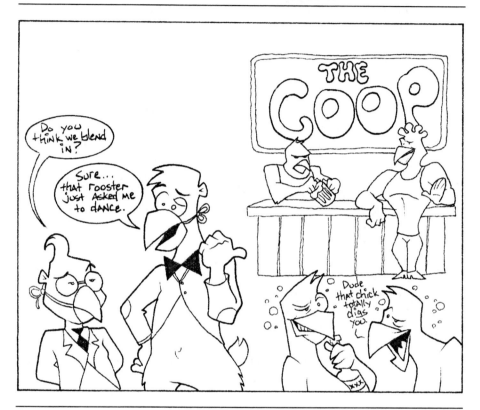

Copyright 2005 by Justin Wagner; reprinted with permission.

the setting periodically and for brief periods of time to conduct the observations. In this role, the ethical issues are rectified; however, because of the higher level of detachment than the first two roles and the lack of involvement in the setting and with the participants, it may be more difficult to garner the perspective of the participants and provide accurate interpretation to the observations. Finally, the fourth role is that of the *complete observer*, in which the researcher observes the social process without ever becoming a part of it. Within this role, there is some variation in the level of detachment. Observations can be made directly by researchers as they passively observe the setting, or there are some instances when researchers may remain completely outside of the setting. In this instance, they may opt to use equipment such as video recorders to make the observations. This role is more along the lines of an "objective" researcher, with ethical issues and observer effects minimized; however, the researcher does not have the benefit of understanding what is going on from the perspective of an insider. Thus, he or she may not interpret the findings in a way that captures accurately the participants' perspectives. Thus, the complete-observer role is more suited to qualitative ethology, in which the participants' perspectives are not the main focus of the inquiry.

Once the researcher has identified the setting, gained access, and worked through the issues of what role to adopt, it is now time to begin observing. How, what, and when you record your observations depend on the nature of the study, whether or not there is freedom to take notes as the observations are being made, and the stage of the research process. Note taking is generally the mode used to record observations. The process of note taking can require some level of expertise and may be approached systematically. In the initial stage of the research process, observations should be more broad and descriptive. These initial observations serve as a guide to identify the key aspects of the setting, people, and behaviors that are of interest. This may involve unstructured note taking in a free form, with the researcher trying to hone in on the most relevant aspects of what is going on and record not only the actual observation but also his or her interpretation of the observation (Babbie, 2004). As the research progresses, the investigator may begin to narrow the focus and record observations of fewer people, interactions, events, times, or processes, but with more detail and elaboration (Adler and Adler, 1994). You may want to try and create a list of key words and participants based on your initial observations, and then use this list to organize and outline your subsequent observations. At this point, field notes should be descriptive as well as reflective about what one has seen, heard, experienced, and thought about during an observation session. You may want to leave wide margins on the page for interpretations or for noting your personal impressions of the event. We cannot emphasize enough the importance of detail when generating field notes. Notes should include at a minimum the date, site, time, and topic. Notes can also include diagrams of setting layout in addition to other pertinent context. To facilitate the process, some researchers create a more structured guide. For example, you could create a form beforehand that allows the recording of essential information regarding participants' characteristics, and their roles, appearances, and interactions.

In addition to knowing how and what to record, the qualitative researcher should be aware of *when* to record. In his study of gay men attending bathhouses, Tewksbury (2002) adopted the role of complete participant. He "entered and spent several hours in the bathhouse, circulated with and among patrons, and carefully observed others, their activities, movements, interactions and the use of the physical features of the environment. Field notes were written during periodic re-treats (usually every 10 to 15 minutes) to one of the private rooms available for rent to patrons" (pp. 84–85). Although it is recommended to take field notes while observing, in this instance because of his covert role, Tewksbury was not at liberty to take field notes while he was observing. Moreover, even if it is possible to take notes while the events are occurring, it may not be feasible to observe everything let alone record everything. To solve this problem, Spradley (1979) recommends using an approach that entails first making a condensed account of what occurs while it is occurring, followed-up with an expanded account in which the researcher fills in the details that were not recorded on the spot. This approach ensures that relevant observations are not missed because of note taking. In addition, Spradley asserted that his "ability to recall events and conversations increased rapidly through the discipline of creating expanded accounts from condensed ones" (p. 75).

Many qualitative researchers also suggest maintaining a fieldwork journal that records feelings, reactions, ideas, fears, and problems that arose during the course of the study. This journal will assist later on in the data analysis and may become an important data source (Spradley, 1979). This process for recording thoughts and ideas is sometimes referred to as "memoing" and can provide a picture of how the study evolved.

Similar to conducting interviews, field notes should be transcribed verbatim on a regular basis. Transcribing the field notes allows the researcher to begin the process of identifying preliminary themes and helps pinpoint the right time to end the study. As was the case with interview data, ending the study should occur at the point of data saturation, when later themes and patterns are consistent with earlier findings and no new themes have emerged.

Qualitative Data Analysis

It is beyond the scope of this chapter to provide an in-depth discussion of qual-itative data analysis. Many texts have been written on the subject and should be consulted (for example, Lofland and Lofland, 1995; Miles and Huberman, 1984, 1994). Yet in this section we thought it would be beneficial to provide a cur-sory overview of the process because the best way to learn how to do qualita-tive data analysis is to actually do it. We realize that the first time it may seem like a formidable task because the data are voluminous and initially unorganized. Therefore, we provide some basic steps for data management and analysis which the novice investigator can draw upon to perform a reasonable qualitative data analysis.

Before data analysis can begin, the data must be processed. This entails revising, deciphering, and editing field notes, and then transcribing notes and audiotaped interviews. Hopefully, this process has been ongoing during the data-collection period. Once all the data have been processed, the first step in analysis is to try to sort the data and impose some type of organization. This process should also be ongoing. You would not want to wait until all data have been collected to begin the process of organization; rather, it should occur parallel to data collection. Some researchers organize their data first by type (for example, interviews, field notes, archival records) and then within each type, an additional sort is done by question, date, people, or places.

Once a system has been created, the next step is to become familiar with the data by reading through it and, if available, reading memos or research journal entries. This will help to identify main concepts or themes and to assist in providing detailed descriptions of the setting, participants, and other activities relevant to the research methods. In addition, researchers may want to continue the method of memoing to record their analytical decisions made and insights into the analysis.

The next step is to create a basic coding scheme. Coding especially in the context of using the grounded theory approach is a multifaceted process. We will consider for the sake of space only three of the main processes: *open coding, axial coding,* and *selective coding* (Strauss and Corbin, 1990). Initially one does open coding, in which the data are considered in detail while developing some initial categories. This is the process whereby qualitative data are first categorized. Codes can be descriptive words or short phrases that are attached to units of data (such as a word, a sentence, or a paragraph) and that represent a core concept, central category, or theme. For example, in their study of gay men's acceptance of a hypothetical AIDS vaccine, one of the codes in the researchers' codebook was "sides," and it signified the side effects from taking the vaccine (Salazar, Holtgrave, Crosby, Frew, and Peterson, 2005). A codebook is a complete description of every code used. For each code you must define what the code means and how it relates to your research.

Coding the data is a relatively simple task. As you read through the data, you systematically code with respect to the core concepts in your codebook. You can underline or highlight the units of data that apply to a particular code while placing the assigned code in the margin (Sandelowski, 1995). This is coding by hand. It is important to note that there are myriad qualitative software packages available to facilitate the entire data-analysis process if desired (for example, QSR NUD*IST, Atlas/Ti, or Ethnograph). Keep in mind that as you develop your codebook and code your data, this is an iterative process in which you may add new codes the deeper you delve into the data, while old codes may be removed.

Later, if using the grounded theory strategy, the next process is axial coding, in which data are put together in new ways. The basic premise is to develop a system of coding that seeks to identify causal relationships *between* categories and reveal connections between categories and subcategories. Thus, axial coding serves to begin the process of developing the theoretical framework underpinning your analysis. Finally, selective coding involves the process of selecting and identifying the core category and systematically relating it to other categories. These relationships eventually are integrated and form the basic theoretical structure. This process is about synthesis and interpretation of the meanings. To aid in this process, it is recommended that data displays be used. Displays of the data entail diagrams, any graphics that are useful, concept maps, or simple cartoons that can act as summarizing devices.

The last step in this process is writing your results. This involves describing in detail the central or core categories using direct quotes from the data to illustrate and support. The challenge is to create an engaging narrative that reveals the underlying meaning to the phenomena under study and tells a story. You should also consider using tables and figures. The ultimate objective is to allow the reader to draw similar conclusions based on what has been presented.

◆ ◆ ◆

In a Nutshell

The challenge is to create an engaging narrative that reveals the underlying meaning to the phenomena under study and tells a story.

◆ ◆ ◆

Integration with the Research Process

Ostensibly, qualitative research does not seem to fit with the overall research process as presented in Figure 1.2; however, with some modification to the existing steps, we can propose a process that illustrates a qualitative mode of inquiry. For example, for step 1, imagine the priority population of low-income rural Americans at risk of diabetes. For step 2, imagine that you want to know what having diabetes means to this population or what the psychological and sociocultural processes associated with developing diabetes are. You would then determine that the research would be observational (step 3) and, in fact, naturalistic, as you would want to interview and observe people in their rural setting. Instead of selecting the most parsimonious research design (step 4) as described in Chapter Four, you would want to consider which qualitative strategy (such as phenomenology, grounded theory, and so on) would best serve the research goals. As you approach step 5, you will note that there is not a selection of variables per se; rather, you select the data-collection method, such as observing or interviewing, that can best capture the phenomena under study. To identify and recruit participants into your study (step 6), your sampling techniques are typically limited to nonprobability sampling, such as purposive, snowball, and convenience. The final steps (7 through 9) are similar except that steps 8 and 9 are iterative rather than occurring sequentially.

Summary

This chapter is unique because it is the only chapter in this book that adopts the interpretivist perspective, which should be viewed with great importance and relevance to health promotion research and practice. Qualitative research can address research questions that cannot be addressed by quantitative approaches. Because it is contextual it provides a more thorough understanding of the phenomena that may be missed with a quantitative strategy. Furthermore, one of qualitative research's greatest strengths is that it can be used to generate testable hypotheses, theories, or both. Qualitative research encompasses varying strategies, uses multiple methods (in other words, triangulation), and involves data-collection methods that are integrated with the setting and the researcher. Qualitative data are descriptive and comprise text and images; thus, data analysis cannot be performed using standardized procedures and techniques; rather, the analysis is iterative, subjective, and subject to the researchers' professional intuition and views. Like quantitative research, although there is no manipulation, the nature of qualitative research may still necessitate attention to certain ethical issues. Contrary to what some may believe (qualitative research is "easier" than quantitative research), qualitative research involves a personal commitment and voluminous amounts of data; thus, qualitative research may not be for the faint of heart. Nevertheless, qualitative research has contributed to the overall research enterprise in substantive ways and will continue to do so. Therefore, we recommend highly that you take your next trip by train and see for yourself!

Issues to Consider

1. One of the roles qualitative researchers can adopt when doing field research is that of the complete participant. This role requires that the researcher's goals remain covert. Thus, people involved are not aware that they are being

studied. What if the goal of the research is to reveal, for example, the heterosexual practices of men who frequent nightclubs and bars. What are the ethics involved when a researcher who in the course of the study has sex with female patrons?

2. For the most part, in addition to the relatively small sample sizes, qualitative research uses nonprobability sampling techniques such as snowball sampling, convenience sampling, and so on to recruit participants. Thus, qualitative research is not generalizable; however, there are many quantitative studies that employ nonprobability sampling techniques. Because these studies use data that are quantitative and perform statistical analyses, are they considered more generalizable than qualitative research?

3. As indicated in this chapter, qualitative research is very useful as a formative research to the development and implementation of HPPs, and as a follow-up or adjunct to program evaluations; however, there is a paucity of these types of published studies. Why might this be true? If the HPP showed no significant effects quantitatively, should this be the end of the road research-wise for this program?

For Practice and Discussion

1. Working with a colleague, formulate a research question that lends itself to a qualitative approach. Next, you and your colleague find another pair of colleagues that can perform the same exercise. Then give this other pair of colleagues your research question and ask them to select the most appropriate qualitative strategy conducive to answering the question, and identify the best data-collection technique(s). Have them provide a rationale for why they chose the particular strategy and methods. In turn, you and your colleague should do the same for their research question. Compare and discuss the outcomes.

2. Ask five other students if they would participate in a phenomenological investigation. You could ask them what health promotion *means* to them. Try to take notes of the conversations you have with them and identify any main themes that emerge from these conversations.

3. Visit several venues in your community, such as a local coffee shop, a public health clinic, a courtroom, or a nightclub, and observe for a couple of hours. Your goal is to conduct a qualitative ethology. If possible, record notes while you observe. Try to determine whether people in the venue are exhibiting a pattern of behavior. You may want to create a form beforehand to assist with your observations.

References

Adler, P. A., and Adler, P. (1994). Observational techniques. In N. K. Denzin and J. S. Lincoln (Eds.), *Handbook of qualitative research* (pp. 377–392). Thousand Oaks, CA: Sage.

Babbie, E. R. (2004). *The practice of social research* (10th ed.). Belmont, CA: Wadsworth.

Barofsky, I., and Sugarbaker, P. H. (1979). Determinants of patient nonparticipation in randomized clinical trials for the treatment of sarcomas. *Cancer Clinical Trials, 2,* 237–246.

Blurton Jones, N. G., and Woodson, R. H. (1979). Describing behavior: The ethologist's perspective. In L. Lamb, S. Suomi, and G. Stephenson (Eds.), *The study of social interaction: Methodological issues* (pp. 97–118). Madison, WI: University of Wisconsin Press.

Bogdan, R. C., and Biklen, S. K. (1998). *Qualitative research in education: An introduction to theory and methods* (3rd ed.). Boston: Allyn and Bacon.

Bottorff, J. L., and Varcoe, C. (1995). Transitions in nurse-patient interactions: A qualitative ethology. *Qualitative Health Research, 5*(3), 315–331.

Bottorff, J. L., and others. (1998). Beliefs related to breast health practices: The perceptions of South Asian women living in Canada. *Social Science & Medicine, 47*(12), 2075–2085.

Brilhart, J. K., and Galanes, G. J. (1998). *Effective group discussion* (9th ed.). Boston: McGraw-Hill.

Cameron, K. A., and others. (2005). Adolescents' experience with sex on the Web: Results from online focus groups. *Journal of Adolescence, 28,* 535–540.

Canales, M. K., and Geller, B. M. (2004). Moving in between mammography: Screening decisions of American Indian women in Vermont. *Qualitative Health Research, 14*(6), 836–857.

Centers for Disease Control and Prevention. (2005). *HIV/AIDS among African Americans.* CDC fact sheet. Retrieved March 30, 2005, from www.cdc.gov/hiv/pubs/facts/afam.htm.

Colangelo, L., Domel, R., Kelly, L., Peirce, L., and Sullivan, C. (1999). *Positivist and interpretivist schools: A comparison and contrast.* Retrieved February 16, 2005, from www.edb.utexas.edu/faculty/scheurich/proj2/index.htm

Davila, Y. R., and Brackley, M. H. (1999). Mexican and Mexican American women in a battered women's shelter: Barriers to condom negotiation for HIV/AIDS prevention. *Issues in Mental Health Nursing, 20*(4), 333–355.

Denzin, N. K. (1978). *The research act: A theoretical introduction to sociological methods* (2nd ed.). New York: McGraw-Hill.

Featherstone, K., and Donovan, L. (1998). Random allocation or allocation at random? Patients' perspectives of participation in a randomized controlled trial. *British Medical Journal, 317,* 1177–1180.

Ferguson, P. R. (2002). Patients' perceptions of information provided in clinical trials. *Journal of Medical Ethics, 28,* 45–48.

Fontana, A., and Frey, J. H. (1994). Interviewing: The art of science. In N. K. Denzin and J. S. Lincoln (Eds.), *Handbook of qualitative research* (pp. 361–376). Thousand Oaks, CA: Sage.

Fraser, J. (1997). Methadone clinic culture: The everyday realities of female methadone clients. *Qualitative Health Research, 7*(1), 121–139.

Glaser, B. G., and Strauss, A. L. (1967). *The discovery of grounded theory: Strategies for qualitative research.* Chicago: Aldine.

Glesne, C., and Peshkin, A. (1992). *Becoming qualitative researchers: An introduction.* White Plains, NY: Longman.

Gold, R. L. (1958). Roles in sociological field observations. *Social Forces, 36*, 217–223.

Grant, C.H.I., Cissna, K. N., and Rosenfeld, L. B. (2000). Patients' perceptions of physicians communication and outcomes of the accrual to trial process. *Health Communication, 12*(1), 23–29.

Holstein, J. A., and Gubrium, J. F. (1994). Phenomenology, ethnomethodology, and interpretive practice. In N. K. Denzin and J. S. Lincoln (Eds.), *Handbook of qualitative research* (pp. 262–272). Thousand Oaks, CA: Sage.

Johnson, J. L., Kalaw, C., Lovato, C. Y., Baillie, L., and Chambers, N. A. (2004). Crossing the line: Adolescents' experiences of controlling their tobacco use. *Qualitative Health Research, 14*(9), 1276–1291.

Krueger, R. A. (1988). *Focus groups: A practical guide for applied research.* Newbury Park, CA: Sage.

Kuhn, T. (1970). *The structure of scientific revolutions* (2nd ed.). Chicago: University of Chicago Press.

Lofland, J., and Lofland, L. (1995). *Analyzing social settings* (3rd ed.). Belmont, CA: Wadsworth.

Lofland, L. (1973). *A world of strangers.* New York: Basic Books.

McCoy, C. B., and others. (1996). Sex, drugs, and the spread of HIV/AIDS in Belle Glade, Florida. *Medical Anthropology Quarterly (New Series), 10*(1), 83–93.

Melville, J., and others. (2003). Psychosocial impact of serological diagnosis of herpes simplex virus type 2: A qualitative assessment. *Sexually Transmitted Infections, 79*, 280–285.

Miles, M. B., and Huberman, A. M. (1984). *Qualitative data analysis: A sourcebook of new methods.* Thousand Oaks, CA: Sage.

Miles, M. B., and Huberman, A. M. (1994). *Qualitative data analysis: An expanded source book* (2nd ed.). Thousand Oaks, CA: Sage.

Miller-García, T. D. (2004). *Gender, power, and the meaning of condom use: A qualitative assessment of condom use among Latino couples.* Unpublished master's thesis, Rollins School of Public Health, Emory University, Atlanta.

Monaghan, L. F. (2002). Opportunity, pleasure, and risk: An ethnography of urban males heterosexualities. *Journal of Contemporary Ethnography, 31*(4), 440–477.

Moore, L. W. (2000). Severe visual impairment in older women. *Western Journal of Nursing Research, 22*(5), 571–595.

Morse, J. (1994). Designing funded qualitative research. In N. K. Denzin and J. S. Lincoln (Eds.), *Handbook of qualitative research* (pp. 220–235). Thousand Oaks, CA: Sage.

Morse, J. M., and Pooler, C. (2002). Patient-family-nurse interactions in the trauma-resuscitation room. *American Journal of Critical Care, 11*(3), 240–249.

Nakkash, R., and others. (2003). The development of a feasible community-specific cardiovascular disease prevention program: Triangulation of methods and sources. *Health Education and Behavior, 30*(6), 723–739.

Peacock, J. L. (1986). *The anthropological lens: Harsh light, soft focus.* New York: Cambridge University Press.

Reisinger, H. S. (2004). Counting apples as oranges: Epidemiology and ethnography in adolescent substance abuse treatment. *Qualitative Health Research, 14*(2), 241–258.

Richardson, M. A., Post-White, J., Singletary, S. E., and Justice, B. (1998). Recruitment for complementary/alternative medicine trials: Who participates after breast cancer. *Annals of Behavioral Medicine, 20*(3), 190–198.

Roberts, F. (2002). Qualitative differences among cancer clinical trial explanations. *Social Science and Medicine, 55*, 1947–1955.

Salazar, L. F., Holtgrave, D., Crosby, R. A. Frew, P., and Peterson, J. L. (2005). Issues related to gay and bisexual men's acceptance of a future AIDS vaccine. *International Journal of STDs and HIV, 16*(8), 546–548.

Sandelowski, M. (1995). Qualitative analysis: What it is and how to begin. *Research in Nursing and Health, 18*, 371–375.

Solberg, S., and Morse, J. M. (1991). The comforting behaviors of caregivers toward distressed postoperative neonates. *Issues in Comprehensive Pediatric Nursing, 14*(2), 77–92.

Spradley, J. P. (1979). *The ethnographic interview.* Orlando: Harcourt Brace Jovanovich.

Steckler, A., and Linnan, L. (Eds). (2002). *Process evaluation for public health interventions and research.* San Francisco: Jossey-Bass.

Sterk, C., and Elifson, K. (2004). Qualitative methods in community-based research. In D. Blumenthal and R. DiClemente (Eds.), *Community-based research: Issues and methods* (pp.133–151). New York: Springer.

Strauss, A. L., and Corbin, J. (1990). *Basics of qualitative research: Grounded theory procedures and techniques.* Thousand Oaks, CA: Sage.

Strauss, A., and Corbin, J. (1994). Grounded theory methodology: An overview. In N. K. Denzin and J. S. Lincoln (Eds.), *Handbook of qualitative research* (pp. 273–285). Thousand Oaks, CA: Sage.

Tewksbury, R. (2002). Bathhouse intercourse: Structural and behavioral aspects of an erotic oasis. *Deviant Behavior, 23*(1), 75–112.

Yoo, S., Johnson, C. C., Rice, J., and Manuel, P. (2004). A qualitative evaluation of the Students of Service (SOS) program for sexual abstinence in Louisiana. *Journal of School Health, 74*(8), 329–334.

Yu-Jen, C., Yiing-Mei, L., Shuh-Jen, S., and Mei-Yen, C. (2004). Unbearable weight: Young adult women's experiences of being overweight. *Journal of Nursing Research: JNR, 12*(2), 153–160.

CHAPTER EIGHT

PROGRAM EVALUATION

Nancy Thompson, Michelle C. Kegler,
and David R. Holtgrave

Evaluation uses social science research methods to determine whether programs or parts of programs are sufficient, appropriate, effective, and efficient. Evaluation also generates information about how to improve programs that do not meet these criteria. If a program has unexpected benefits or creates unforeseen problems, evaluation will let us know about this as well (Deniston and Rosenstock, 1970; Thompson and McClintock, 1998). In short, evaluation provides information to serve a variety of purposes:

- Finding out whether proposed program materials are suitable for the people who are to receive them
- Learning whether program plans are feasible before they are put into effect
- Ensuring that a program is conducted as it was designed

- Serving as an early warning system for problems that could become serious if unattended
- Monitoring whether a program or activity is producing the desired results
- Demonstrating whether a program has any unexpected benefits or problems
- Providing program managers with the information needed to improve service
- Monitoring progress toward the program's goals
- Producing data on which to base future programs
- Demonstrating the effectiveness of the program to the target population, the public, those who want to conduct similar programs, and those who are providing the funding [adapted from Tobacco Technical Assistance Consortium, 2005]

There are also indirect benefits that may result from formally evaluating a program. One is that program staff have the opportunity to hear from the people they are trying to serve. In turn, this lets the program participants know that they have a voice in the running of the program, and that the program personnel respect what they have to say. It conveys the message that the program is not being imposed upon them. Evaluation can also improve staff morale by providing evidence either that their efforts have been fruitful, or that leadership is aware of problems and taking appropriate steps. Staff also get to hear the good news about the program in the words of the people served. A third indirect benefit is that the results can demonstrate such an effect that the media may develop an interest, further promoting the program (Thompson and McClintock, 1998).

Evaluation differs from research in that its primary purpose is to provide information to decision makers to help them make judgments about the effectiveness of a program and to help them make improvements to a program. Evaluations are typically guided by the needs of key stakeholder groups and designed in a way that is sensitive to the dynamic and political organizational settings in which programs exist. More so than with pure research, evaluation methods must balance scientific rigor with the need to produce meaningful findings in a timely manner in a way that is minimally disruptive to program operations.

Illustration of Key Concepts

Numerous texts have been written on evaluation (for example, Rossi, Lipsey, and Freeman, 2004; Patton, 1997; Weiss, 1997). This section draws from these foundational sources, as well as from commonly accepted wisdom in the field, to highlight some of the major concepts and issues in evaluation. Topics covered in this section include planning for evaluation, stakeholders, target population, description of the program, logic models, formative evaluation, process evaluation, outcome evaluation, economic evaluation, and evaluation reports.

Evaluation Planning

A frequent error made in developing a program is to add an evaluation after the fact. Evaluation should begin while the program is being created, in fact, as soon as someone has the idea for a program. Once begun, it should continue through the duration of the program, only ending once a final assessment has measured the extent to which the program met its intended goals. The following scenario describes why it is important to start the evaluation process so early. Suppose a health promotion practitioner created a program to provide free bicycle helmets to youths from low-income neighborhoods. To initiate the program, program staff placed posters in grocery stores and flyers in mailboxes throughout the neighborhoods they hoped to reach. The posters invited youths to come to the program location for a free bicycle helmet. Some youths responded but not as many as had been expected. So, to determine why the numbers were low, the health promotion practitioner decided to evaluate. The staff may learn that youths in the area are in after-school programs during the hours the program is open. They may learn that it is the parents who are most interested in seeing that their children obtained a helmet, but that their messages targeted the youths. They may learn that the location is too far for the youths to travel alone. So the staff now need to rewrite the posters and flyers, change the hours, or move the location. Had the health practitioner assessed interest and access to the location before the program began, it would have saved time, money, and the disappointment and frustration of the program staff.

During the course of running the program, any public health program should produce most of the information needed to evaluate its effectiveness in achieving its goals and objectives. Thus, evaluation activities can and should be integrated into the design and operation of the program. If this happens, then evaluation may require little more than analyzing the information collected throughout the operation of the program.

◆ ◆ ◆

In a Nutshell

Evaluation activities can and should be integrated into the design and operation of the program.

◆ ◆ ◆

Failure to evaluate a public health program can be considered irresponsible, and perhaps unethical. Why? It is evaluation that allows us to determine whether a program benefits or harms the people it is designed to serve. We do not use medications that are untested, and we should not use educational, behavioral, or social interventions that have not been tested either. Ineffective programs can discourage people from behavior change, and insensitive programs can build public resentment, causing people to resist future, more effective, interventions (Thompson and McClintock, 1998).

Let's look at another example. Suppose the staff of an injury prevention program invited a fifty-five-year-old with an automobile-acquired spinal cord injury to talk to students about the hazards of driving above the speed limit. The staff hoped that this person's story about speeding at age sixteen, and the subsequent adverse health effects he suffered, would discourage the students from driving above the speed limit. Evaluation might show, however, that many teenagers do not relate to the problems of people over age thirty and are not influenced by what they have to say. Evaluation could also show what type of people the students would listen to—perhaps sports stars or other young people (their peers) who have had difficulty finding a job because of their driving history. It can be nonproductive, and even counterproductive when the wrong person delivers a message, no matter how good the message is.

Budgeting for evaluation is an important part of the planning. The cost of evaluation varies. Operating a program with a design that includes a comparison group or multiple repeated assessments over time is more expensive than operating a service program only, but evaluation should be built into the program design and included in the cost of the program (Thompson and McClintock, 1998). What is more, programs with comparison groups or repeated measures (see Chapter Four for more detail) are better able to demonstrate whether the program is producing the intended result. Typically, programs with good evaluation components have the greatest likelihood of receiving funding. Figure 8.1 presents a listing of some costs that are commonly encountered when conducting an evaluation.

FIGURE 8.1.   COMMON EVALUATION-RELATED COSTS.

Some costs commonly encountered in an evaluation:

- Flyers, press releases, or other recruitment materials
- Meeting or interview space
- Telephone costs for scheduling or conducting interviews or focus groups
- Purchasing, copying, or printing of data collection instruments or questionnaires
- Recording devices
- Audiotapes or videotapes
- Participant or interviewer transportation
- Mailing
- Incentives for participants
- Transcriptionists for taped material
- Computer(s)
- Data entry personnel
- Statistical consultant
- Printing or copying of final report

Source: Adapted from Tobacco Technical Assistance Consortium, 2005.

Stakeholders

One of the first steps in conducting an evaluation is to identify and engage stakeholders in the planning process. Stakeholders include all persons who have an interest in the program being evaluated, the conduct of the evaluation, and the evaluation findings. Stakeholders include program participants; program staff and volunteers; those providing funding to the program or the evaluation; those providing other resources, such as space, for the program; and evaluation personnel. Depending on the program, the stakeholders may also include parents or family members of participants, or all community members, whether or not they participated in the program. Involving major stakeholders in the process of evaluation planning, execution, and analysis ensures that the evaluation results will have value. It also helps to ensure that the results of the evaluation will be used to improve the program.

◆ ◆ ◆

In a Nutshell

Involving major stakeholders in the process of evaluation planning, execution, and analysis ensures that the evaluation results will have value.

◆ ◆ ◆

Describing the Program

Another early step in the evaluation process is to develop a thorough understanding of the program to be evaluated. Key elements include the target population, need for the program, goals and objectives, program components and activities, underlying logic, resources, stage of development, and program context (Centers for Disease Control and Prevention, 1999).

Target Population. The target population is the group the program is intended to serve. The more clearly this population has been defined, the easier it will be to determine whether the population has been reached and whether the program was effective for these people. As a part of evaluation planning, it is important to determine whether the program intended to reach all people in the county, for example, or only those persons who currently use the services of the county health department, or only males between the ages of eighteen and fifty who use the services of the county health department. How you can best reach each of these groups will vary.

Logic Models. An important part of describing a program is to understand the logic underlying it. The evaluation should identify the program's ultimate goal(s) and enumerate clearly the program's activities and how they are expected to lead to the goal. Putting this information together with sufficient detail to be of value can be a difficult task. A logic model is a tool that is designed to help you with this process. A logic model provides a graphic representation of the relationships among three aspects of the program: the resources put into the program, the program activities, and the results.

The five parts of a logic model are

- Inputs
- Activities
- Outputs
- Outcomes
- Impact (Goals)

Figure 8.2 depicts what a logic model should look like. Inputs are the resources that the program must have in order to conduct the program's activities. These include funding, personnel (staff as well as volunteers), equipment, supplies, and space. They also include collaborations with other organizations and people whose interests are consistent with those of the program. Planning, too, is an input that is required in order to conduct program activities.

Activities are the actual events that take place when the program is occurring (Tobacco Technical Assistance Consortium, 2005), or constitute the program itself. Some activities include the educational program, distributing condoms or smoke alarms, or holding support groups. But activities can also include inviting collaborators to a meeting, sending letters to supporters, building relationships with communities to be served, gathering materials for a resource center, maintaining an inventory of resources, responding to telephone inquiries, and disseminating information to interested parties.

Outputs are measures that can be used to demonstrate that the program was conducted as planned, and reveal the *process* the program goes through to achieve its outcomes. These include indicators such as the number of training sessions

FIGURE 8.2.   BASIC LOGIC MODEL COMPONENTS.

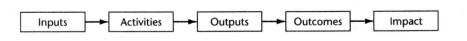

FIGURE 8.3. ABBREVIATED PROGRAM LOGIC MODEL.

| Inputs | Activities | Outputs | Outcomes | | Impact |
			Short-term	Long-term	
Staff	Coalition meetings	Groups attending			Decrease in tobacco-related cancer
Volunteers	Meetings with legislators	Meetings attended	Policies adopted	Decrease in smoking	
Computers		Legislators met with			

held or the number of collaborators in attendance at a meeting. In contrast, outcomes are measures that can be used to demonstrate that program participants *received* what you put out there. Outcomes would include indicators such as an increase in knowledge or changes in attitudes or behavior. In the case of tobacco use prevention programs, outcomes could include an increase in the belief that smoking is dangerous, and a decrease in the rate of smoking.

The impact of a program is the measure of whether or not the overall program goal was achieved and is usually long-term in nature. For health programs, this is usually a measure of decreases in morbidity and mortality. In our smoking example, the program's impact could be a decrease in new cases of lung cancer or deaths from this disease. It could also be a decrease in overall smoking-related mortality, including both cancer and heart disease.

A logic model can be developed for an entire program or for one of its parts, such as a particular activity. Figure 8.3 presents an example of an abbreviated logic model for a program to reduce tobacco-related cancer. Figure 8.4 presents an example of a more detailed logic model for the process portion of a cardiovascular disease prevention program designed to reduce disparities in exercise behavior.

Types of Evaluation

Several typologies exist for the different kinds of evaluations. A common distinction is that between summative and formative. Rossi and colleagues (2004) define summative evaluation as "evaluation activities undertaken to render a summary judgment on certain critical aspects of the program's performance, for instance, to determine if specific goals and objectives were met" (p. 65). They define formative evaluation as "evaluative activities undertaken to furnish information

FIGURE 8.4.   LOGIC MODEL WITH DETAILED INPUTS, ACTIVITIES, AND OUTPUTS.

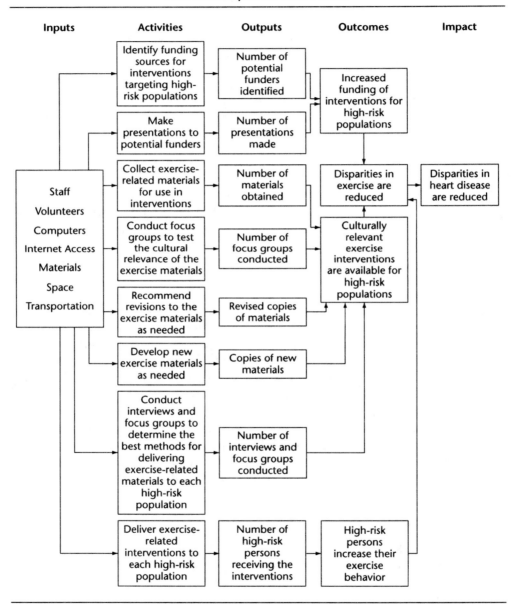

that will guide program improvement" (p. 63). In public health and health promotion, four types of evaluation are widely recognized: formative, process, outcome, and economic. Each of these is described here.

Formative Evaluation. The purpose of formative evaluation is to determine that an element of the program (for example, materials, message, and location) is feasible, appropriate, meaningful, and acceptable to the program's target population (Tobacco Technical Assistance Consortium, 2005). In other words, it tends to focus on the inputs and activities of the program. When we discuss program plans, messages, materials, or strategies with members of the target population before they are put into use, we are conducting formative evaluation. Formative evaluation should be conducted when program materials, messages, and procedures are being developed, before the program begins. It should also be conducted when changes are made, such as revising the materials, adapting the program to a new population or setting, or attempting to resolve problems that occurred with prior materials or procedures.

The methods used in formative evaluation can be qualitative or quantitative. For example, suppose you were working with a program designed to provide diet counseling to citizens of your state in order to reduce deaths from heart attack and stroke. If you needed to find out whether or not it was working to provide the counseling through county health departments, you might use in-depth interviews in a number of ways. For example, you might interview those who have received counseling and those who have not and ask questions such as

- What led you to attend (or not attend) the counseling?
- Was the health department a factor in your decision? If yes, what was its role?
- What do you like about having the counseling through the health department?
- What do you dislike about having the counseling through the health department?

You might also interview the providers of the diet counseling and ask them questions such as

- What works well about the program?
- What does not work well?
- What are the benefits of providing the counseling through the health department?
- What are the problems with providing the counseling through the health department?
- What are some better ways to provide the counseling?

You might interview program administrators and ask

- Why was the health department chosen as the means of providing the counseling?
- What were the perceived benefits of using the health department? Have these benefits been realized?
- What were the perceived drawbacks of using the health department?

You might also interview administrators of the health department and ask

- What do you know about the diet counseling program?
- What are the benefits to the health department associated with this program?
- What are the costs to the health department associated with this program?

Many of these same questions could also be addressed by conducting focus groups with each of these types of program affiliates.

Observation is another qualitative method that can be used for formative evaluation. Suppose you are working with a program designed to provide hypertension screening in rural areas of your state through churches and civic groups and you want to determine whether the civic group screenings were working. An observer at the screening locations could note

- How the facilities are laid out and whether the physical setup works
- What problems participants appear to encounter
- Whether participants appear to know where to go
- How much participants and program personnel interact
- Whether there is any grumbling as people leave

In observing program personnel, the observer could note

- How they set up for the screening
- Who is responsible for what tasks
- How they approach participants
- What steps they take to ensure privacy
- Whether they take time to explain each step
- What feedback they provide to those who were screened

In observing participants, the observer could note

- Do they tend to be of similar ages or social backgrounds?
- Do any people approach and choose not to participate? If so, are their characteristics similar to those of the people who choose to participate?

- How do people respond when approached by program personnel?
- Do they ask questions? What kind of questions do they ask?

Quantitative methods, such as cross-sectional surveys, can also be used to conduct formative evaluation. Suppose, for example, you wanted to assess the effectiveness of your advertising for a screening program such as the one described above. You could query people who did and did not participate in the screening by using a survey similar to that shown in Figure 8.5. Combined with demographic information, the responses to surveys like these could be used to determine for whom the advertising is and is not appropriate and effective.

Process Evaluation. Process evaluation assesses the way the program is being delivered, rather than the program's effectiveness. It documents what is actually being provided by the program and compares that to what was supposed to be provided to determine whether there are any gaps. In other words, process evaluation functions as a form of quality control. It also serves many other purposes, such as providing managers with feedback on the quality of delivery, documenting the fidelity and variability in program delivery across sites and personnel, providing information to assess exactly what components of the program are responsible for particular outcomes, and providing data that can be used to demonstrate how the program affects funders, sponsors, participants, and the public. To serve these purposes, process evaluation focuses on the activities and outputs

FIGURE 8.5.   SAMPLE SURVEY.

Please indicate the extent to which you agree or disagree with each of the following statements	Strongly Agree	Agree	Neither Agree nor Disagree	Disagree	Strongly Disagree
There was enough advertising.	SA	A	N	D	SD
The location of the advertising was good.	SA	A	N	D	SD
The ads were easy to understand.	SA	A	N	D	SD
Overall, I liked the ads.	SA	A	N	D	SD

of the program, for example, what was done in each screening, and how many screenings were held. Program context, reach of the program, dose delivered and received, fidelity to the original program plan, implementation, and recruitment are some of the typical components of process evaluation (Linnan and Steckler, 2002).

Common process evaluation questions (adapted from Patton, 1997) include

- What are the program's main characteristics as perceived by major stakeholder groups?
- Who participates in the program, and how do they compare to the intended target population for the program?
- Which components of the program are working as expected? What is not working well? What challenges and barriers have been encountered?
- What do participants and staff like and dislike?
- What has changed from the original implementation design and why?
- What are the startup costs of the program? What are the ongoing costs of implementation?
- What has been learned about the program that might inform efforts elsewhere?

As in formative evaluation, the methods used in process evaluation can be qualitative or quantitative. For example, suppose you were working with a program designed to provide child safety-seat checks and education to caregivers who transport children under the age of seven years in their vehicles. If you wanted to find out how the checks were being conducted, you could use observation. The observer could note whether or not the program technician checked both the installation of the seat and the placement of the child within the seat. The observer could also note whether the technician involved the caregiver in the seat check, whether or not she or he discussed with the caregiver any problems that were identified, and whether or not she or he provided instruction to the caregiver about how to correct the problem.

Quantitative methods can also be used for process evaluation. For example, counts of number of vehicles checked, number of seats checked, and number of caregivers educated could be used to verify the program's output. If the program was advertised through a radio campaign, counts of radio spots developed and taped, stations contacted and stations accepting spots, number of spots aired, frequency of airing per spot, and minutes of airtime would also be elements of process evaluation. Other common data-collection methods in process evaluation include diaries or logs, document review, record abstraction, and monitoring or tracking systems.

Outcome Evaluation. Outcome evaluation is linked to the outcomes in the program's logic model, and often uses experimental or quasi-experimental study designs, along with quantitative methods. Short-term outcome evaluation can measure the short-term effects of the program on a participant immediately after he or she participates. Consequently, it measures outcomes that can change rapidly as a result of an intervention, such as knowledge, attitudes, and intended behavior. Changes in these outcomes are typically assessed with pretest-posttest designs—that is, administering the measures before and after participants take part in the program. Short-term outcome evaluation provides evidence of the degree to which a program is meeting its short-term or intermediate goals, such as increasing participants' awareness of the hazards of secondhand smoke or changing their knowledge, attitudes, and beliefs about secondhand smoke. Surveys, interviews, and observation are common data-collection methods in these kinds of evaluations.

Changes in outcomes such as actual behavior, for example, quitting smoking indoors, usually take longer to manifest themselves. As a consequence, they are usually assessed over longer periods of time, when a follow-up assessment is administered in addition to the standard pretest-posttest assessment. Control or comparison groups are often used to aid in attributing the observed effects to the program. See Chapters Four and Six for more detailed discussion of experimental and quasi-experimental research designs.

The value of outcome evaluation is that it provides an indicator of both program effectiveness and the extent to which a program's objectives are being met. When combined with process evaluation, outcome evaluation can indicate which activities and outputs appear to have the greatest influence, and allow program managers to shift resources from less effective to more effective elements of the program. Demonstrating a program's ultimate impact upon morbidity and mortality, however, can be challenging due to the long-term nature of these outcomes and the multiple influences on them. Program evaluations in public health and health promotion, therefore, often focus on intermediate outcomes rather than on morbidity and mortality.

Economic Evaluation. Part of evaluating a program is determining whether or not the effects it produces are worth the program's costs. Economic evaluation methods are a family of techniques that can answer questions about the affordability of the program, the efficiency of the program, and the standards the program must achieve to be considered cost-saving or cost-effective. Five cost-related evaluation issues are of real interest to decision makers: (1) affordability; (2) assessing costs of unmet needs; (3) performance standard setting; (4) comparing programs within one disease area to each other; and (5) comparing programs in one area to health-related services in other disease areas.

Cost Analysis (Determining Affordability). Consider the following question. "There is a highly effective risk-reduction program that was developed in another state—can we afford to offer the service in my hometown?" To answer this "affordability" question, we need to know the cost of delivering the program activities. This might mean knowing the dollar cost of conducting each activity per participant served, or it might mean simply knowing, in detail, what types of human resources and materials are needed to conduct the activity.

The economic evaluation technique of cost analysis is well-suited to answering the affordability question (Gold, Siegel, Russell, and Weinstein, 1996; Trentacoste, Holtgrave, Collins, and Abdul-Quader, 2004). In a cost analysis of a prevention program, a table is constructed with the categories of resources consumed by the program as the rows (for example, staff time, incentives given to participants, materials distributed, staff travel time) and inputs as the columns of the table. These inputs include (1) a definition of each resource category; (2) a definition of the unit of each resource category; (3) the number of units of each resource category consumed; (4) the dollar value of each resource category; and (5) the product of the number of resource units consumed and the dollar value of each unit for each resource category. Summing these products across all resource categories gives the total cost of the program. Dividing the total cost by the number of clients yields the per-client cost of the program.

Overall, there are seven basic steps in a cost analysis (Gold, Siegel, Russell, and Weinstein, 1996; Gorsky, 1996):

- Choose a time period for the cost-analysis
- Count the clients served during this time period
- Inventory the resources, in specific units, required for all program activities
- Calculate the cost per unit of each resource used
- Count the number of units of each resource used in the time period specified
- Calculate the total costs of the program
- Calculate the expected cost per client served

If a decision maker is interested in questions of the affordability of particular programs, the economic evaluation technique of cost analysis is well-suited to providing answers. Cost analysis can determine the price of delivering a program, and it can provide detailed information about the exact types (and quantities) of resources consumed by the program.

Cost of Unmet Needs Analysis (Assessing Costs of Unmet Needs). Consider yet another question that might be posed by a health professional in a given community. "How much would it cost to run a program that addresses the unmet prevention service delivery needs

DINCUS FORGETS TO DO A COST-UTILITY ANALYSIS BEFORE IMPLEMENTATION.

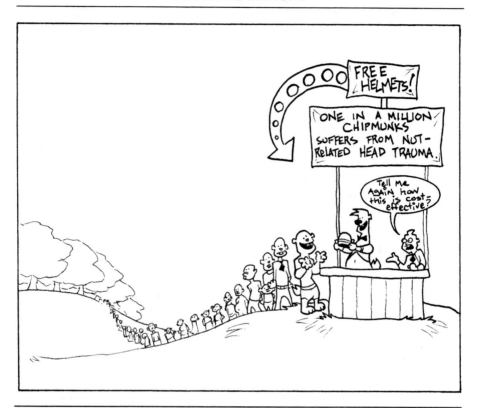

Copyright 2005 by Justin Wagner; reprinted with permission.

of a population?" From time to time, decision makers may need to know how much it would cost to address the unmet needs of any particular population or populations. Cost of unmet needs analysis can answer this question (Holtgrave, Pinkerton and Merson, 2002). A cost of unmet needs analysis has just a few basic steps:

- The number of people in need of a particular activity or service is estimated (for example, using epidemiologic and behavioral information).
- The most effective activities or services for this population are identified (for example, using the published literature or local evaluation information).
- The per-client cost of these activities or services for this population is identified (for example, using the published literature or local cost analyses).

The per-client costs of the programs are multiplied by the number of people needing the programs; this yields the cost of unmet needs for this particular population. Cost of unmet needs analysis can answer cost of unmet needs questions for decision makers, *and* it can also equip decision makers to answer questions from media, state legislators, federal agencies, and others interested in the real cost of unmet needs in a particular locale.

Threshold Analysis (Performance Standard Setting). Another important question might be, "The State Legislature wants to know if it is saving money by preventing disease and averting medical costs. How much disease would this program have to prevent in order to be cost-saving?" In a threshold analysis, we start by taking the cost of a particular program (Holtgrave and others, 1997). Then we divide it by the present value of the lifetime medical care cost of treating one case of the disease the program is designed to prevent. (*Present value* is a technical term meaning, roughly, that we use a 3 percent annual discount rate to bring future health care costs into present value.) The result tells us how many cases of disease would have to be permanently prevented by this program for it to be considered cost-saving. Note that we do not have to know anything about how much disease is actually prevented by this program in order to calculate the cost-saving threshold.

These simple calculations constitute a threshold analysis in its entirety. However, we can go one step further and ask whether the approximate number of cases of disease that might be prevented by a particular program is likely to be above or below the threshold. For instance, if a state does a threshold analysis on its HIV counseling and testing program and finds that only five HIV infections would have to be prevented for the program to be cost-saving, it can try to identify whether there is evidence to suggest that the actual number of infections prevented is above or below five (even if the precise number is unknown). Oftentimes there will be sufficient evidence to determine whether or not it is likely that a threshold is being met, even when the exact level of effectiveness is not known. Identifying whether the number of infections prevented is above or below a threshold can be a much more practical evaluation question to answer, rather than trying to estimate the exact number of infections prevented.

Here, we mention an analysis designed to determine a "cost-saving" threshold. Other, related techniques can be used to determine if an intervention is cost-effective even if not cost-saving.

Cost-Effectiveness Analysis (Comparing Programs Within One Disease Area to Each Other). Again, please consider the following question. "We would like to prevent as many cases of a particular disease as possible given the level of resources that our state has available—how can we do this?" People working in one particular area of disease prevention (for instance, HIV prevention) all desire to avert as many cases of that illness as possible—indeed, that is the very nature of their work. Consequently, they want to give priority to prevention programs that will prevent as many cases of that disease as possible. Of course, a real limitation is the amount of resources available, so, public health personnel have to maximize the cases of disease prevented within those resource constraints.

The technique of cost-effectiveness can help with this decision (Pinkerton, Johnson-Masotti, Holtgrave, and Farnham, 2001). As applied here for illustration, cost-effectiveness analysis estimates the cost-per-case-of-disease-prevented by a given program. Different types of services to prevent that one type of disease could then be compared on a cost-effectiveness basis. For instance, if there were five different types of services to avoid lung cancer, they could be compared on the basis of cost-per-case-of-lung-cancer-prevented.

Cost-Utility Analysis (Comparing Programs in One Area to Health-Related Services in Other Disease Areas). Here, please consider a question posed at the national level. "The Office of Management and Budget in the White House is wondering whether investment in HIV prevention is better than investments in diabetes, cancer, or heart disease. How can we even begin to answer a question like that?" Many public health policymakers must set priorities across disease areas. For instance, appropriations committees in the U.S. Congress must work to make funding decisions across many areas of expenditure, including making health service funding decisions that pit cancer programs versus heart disease programs versus HIV prevention programs versus diabetes control programs (and so on). The Office of Management and Budget in the White House has endorsed cost-benefit and cost-utility analysis as important forms of input into such decision making. (We'll focus here on the more broadly useful cost-utility analysis rather than cost-benefit analysis.)

Cost-utility analysis evaluates a program in terms of the cost-per-quality-adjusted-life-year-saved (or cost per QALY saved, for short) (Gold, Siegel, Russell, and Weinstein, 1996; Pinkerton and Holtgrave, 1998). Note that in the cost-effectiveness analysis discussed earlier, the cost-effectiveness outcomes were in the form of cost per case of a particular disease prevented (for example, case of lung cancer prevented); that outcome form is useful for comparing prevention programs that target the same disease to each other, but is not of use for comparing prevention programs for one disease to those in other disease areas. The cost-utility analysis outcome of cost per QALY saved can be used across disease areas since a quality-adjusted life year saved in one area is (at least theoretically) the same as a QALY saved in another disease area.

Simply put, a cost-utility analysis can show that a program is cost-saving, cost-effective, or not cost-effective. If a cost-utility analysis shows that the costs prevented (usually health care costs prevented) by a program are greater than the cost of delivering the program itself, then the program is said to be cost-saving. Clearly, if a program saves more money than it costs to deliver, it can justifiably be labeled "cost saving."

However, a program may cost more to deliver than it saves but still be quite worthwhile. For instance, kidney dialysis, many forms of surgery, and many medical screening programs cost more than they save, but as a society we readily accept them and invest in them. Although there is no magic cutoff value, very commonly it is cited that programs that are not cost-saving but cost less than $50,000 per QALY saved should be labeled as cost-effective. (Note that some researchers would place the cutoff at $80,000, $100,000, or even $120,000 rather than $50,000.) Programs that cost more than the cutoff value (say, $50,000 per QALY saved) cannot be justifiably labeled as cost-effective.

The Evaluation Report

No matter what type of evaluation is conducted, the results have to be shared with major stakeholders. Generally, the main function of an evaluation report is to provide answers to the questions posed at the beginning of the evaluation and discuss what these answers mean. In evaluation, meaning is often derived through some form of comparison. Patton (1997) discusses comparing program outcomes to outcomes from a similar program, to stated program objectives, to outcomes from the same program in a prior time period, or to external standards of desirability. Other objectives of an evaluation report include providing management with a basis for decisions regarding program changes, soliciting continued funding, providing staff with feedback, making others aware of the program and its contributions, and making recommendations for future action.

The reporting of results is especially important in evaluation, as it becomes the basis for future action. Without an adequate report of the findings, the evaluation is largely worthless. In formulating the report, consider each of the categories of stakeholders, their needs, and their interests. Also consider what actions they might want to take as a result of the report. This will ensure that you provide them with sufficient information to inform their action as fully as possible.

◆ ◆ ◆

In a Nutshell

Without an adequate report of the findings, the evaluation is largely worthless.

◆ ◆ ◆

There are numerous additional issues to consider in reporting evaluation findings. For example, should the report be written or oral? If it is written, options include an executive summary followed by a full report, an executive summary only, press releases, newsletters, or a traditional academic research monograph (Patton, 1997). Other issues to consider include authorship and contributors to the report, as well as whose perspectives are represented. Options range from including only the evaluator's perspective to the evaluator writing the report on behalf of a particular stakeholder group.

Applied Example

Pool Cool is a sun-safety program initially implemented in Hawaii and Massachusetts and currently being disseminated nationwide. Because of its comprehensive evaluation, the Pool Cool program is used here to illustrate many of the key concepts covered in this chapter. Designed as an intervention research study, the project included formative, process, and outcome evaluation. (For a more detailed description of the program and related evaluation findings, please see Glanz, Geller, Shigaki, Maddock, and Isnec, 2002; and Glanz, Isnec, Geller, and Spangler, 2002.)

Stakeholders

Stakeholders are those who have a stake or a vested interest in evaluation findings. This includes individuals who make decisions about a program or simply desire information about the program or its evaluation. For Pool Cool, major stakeholders included the Pool Cool staff (behavioral scientists, health educators, research assistants, and data managers), the aquatics and recreation staff, parents of young children, and children taking swimming lessons at the participating pools. Stakeholders also included those who would ultimately pay medical care expenses for any cases of cancer that might arise in the future. The funding agency is also considered a stakeholder, and for Pool Cool this was the Centers for Disease Control and Prevention (CDC). Patton (1997) advises evaluators to go beyond identification of stakeholders and to develop a strong relationship with at least one primary intended user. This requires evaluators to find strategically located people who are enthusiastic about an evaluation and committed to using the results. For Pool Cool, the project team both designed and evaluated the program. This integration facilitated use of the evaluation findings in making decisions about the program.

Defining the Program

A critical step in designing an evaluation is to develop a thorough understanding of the program to be evaluated. The Pool Cool program uses both behavioral and environmental strategies to prevent skin cancer by improving sun protection behaviors, reducing sunburns, and promoting sun-safety policies and environments at swimming pools (Glanz, Geller, Shigaki, Maddock, and Isnec, 2002). The *target audience* for the Pool Cool program was children who took swimming lessons and their parents, as well as aquatics instructors at the participating pools (Glanz, Isnec, Geller, and Spangler, 2002; Glanz, Geller, Shigaki, Maddock, and Isnec, 2002). Educational strategies included lifeguard and aquatic instructor training, sun-safety lessons to be implemented as part of swimming lessons, a series of interactive activities, and incentives. Environmental strategies included informal consultation on policy change and provision of sunscreen pump bottles, a shade structure (such as a tent, a canvas or tarp cover, or an umbrella), and signage with sun-safe messages.

The Pool Cool program was based on the social cognitive theory, which asserts that behaviors are influenced by the social and physical environment and that people, their behaviors, and the environment have a reciprocal relationship with each influencing the other (Glanz, Geller, Shigaki, Maddock, and Isnec, 2002; Bandura, 1986). The logic underlying the Pool Cool program was relatively straightforward. If knowledge, skills, health beliefs, and social and physical environments can be altered to support sun safety, the prevalence of preventive behaviors will increase among children taking swimming lessons, their parents, and aquatics instructors. An increase in these behaviors will lead to reductions in sun exposure and sunburns among program participants, and in the long-term, reductions in skin cancer. Thus, short-term outcomes included changes in knowledge and skills, health beliefs, social norms, social acceptability, and physical environments. Specific environmental and policy-related outcomes included existence of shade structures and sun-safety signage, and availability of sunscreen at the participating swimming pools. Intermediate behavioral outcomes included use of sunscreen, wearing protective clothing, seeking shade during peak sun hours, and wearing sunglasses. The longer-term outcomes that would, in theory, result from an increase in these preventive behaviors included reduced sun exposure, reduced sunburns, and, ultimately, a lower incidence of skin cancer.

Types of Evaluation

Formative evaluation is usually conducted in the developmental phase of a program to provide input that can be used to modify a program and document the feasibility of program implementation. Data from formative evaluations are useful in crafting and tailoring intervention strategies and messages that effectively reach the target population, resonate with selected audiences, and are culturally appropriate. Planning a successful program requires a solid understanding of the knowledge, attitudes, behaviors, and culture of the target audience (Green and Kreuter, 1999). In Pool Cool, this required learning the culture of the swimming pool environment, and learning about the sun-safety practices and views of lifeguards, aquatics instructors, and pool managers. It also required developing an understanding of sun-safety beliefs and practices of parents and children.

The Pool Cool formative evaluation used multiple data-collection methods (Glanz, Carbone, and Song, 1999; Glanz, Isnec, Geller, and Spangler, 2002). Qualitative evaluation methods included focus groups, discussion groups, and interviews with children, parents, recreation staff, pool managers, aquatics instructors, and lifeguards. Site visits to swimming pools were also completed. Quantitative data were collected through self-administered written surveys. Several issues affecting program design emerged from the formative component of the evaluation.

The process evaluation component of Pool Cool was multifaceted and served several purposes (Glanz, Isnec, Geller, and Spangler, 2002). For example, it assessed the extent of implementation of the educational and environmental program components, how much time was spent delivering the program, exposure to program components, program reach, and how the target audience—lifeguards and children—rated the various aspects of the program. It also was designed to catch any unintended consequences or unexpected circumstances that might influence either program implementation or outcomes.

Three types of data collection were employed in the process evaluation: monitoring forms, observation records, and select items from posttest surveys. The monitoring forms were completed by lifeguards and aquatics instructors and were designed to assess delivery of the eight sun-safety lessons. They were also used to assess the presence of parents at the pools, how well lessons were received, and which components were taught.

Staff logs were used for quality assurance purposes and were completed on site visits to the participating pools. Staff logs helped to document that participation and implementation were affected by the weather. Relevant survey items asked parents about participation, their reactions to the program, and incentives they had received. Overall, the process evaluation findings enabled the project team to feel comfortable that the program was being implemented as planned. Good documentation of the implementation process also shed light on how the program outcomes were achieved. For a more detailed description of the process evaluation, see Glanz, Isnec, Geller, and Spangler (2002).

The outcome evaluation design for the Pool Cool Program was a randomized controlled trial (see Chapter Six for more details on RCTs) with swimming pools as the unit of randomization and analysis (Glanz, Geller, Shigaki, Maddock, and Isnec, 2002). Pools were randomized into either the intervention arm ($n = 15$) or the control arm ($n = 13$), with the latter receiving an attention-matched injury-prevention program. Primary outcome data were collected through self-administered written surveys completed by two cross-sectional samples of parents at the beginning of the summer and eight weeks later. These were parents of children ages five to ten who were taking swimming lessons. Major measures included demographic factors, knowledge about skin cancer and sun protection guidelines, attitudes, policies for sun protection at the pool, parent and child's sun-protection practices, and child's sunburn experiences for the previous summer and the summer when the program took place. Environmental outcomes were assessed through observation at three points in time: the beginning, middle, and end of the summer. Two independent observers completed observations forms to assess availability of sunscreen, shaded areas, sun-safety signage, and lifeguard sun-safety practices.

Results showed significant intervention effects in children's use of sunscreen, staying in shade, and sun-protection habits. Use of sunscreen, wearing a hat, and sun-protection habits also increased among parents. Furthermore, pool sun-protection policies increased in the intervention pools. Environmental results documented greater improvements in availability of sunscreen, posting of sun-safety signs, and lifeguard shirt use in intervention pools relative to control pools. Overall, outcome evaluation results showed a modest, but significant program effect. Evaluation results have been disseminated through publication in peer-reviewed journals. The program is currently being disseminated nationwide. This second phase of the project also included process and outcome evaluations. For a more detailed description of the outcome evaluation, see Glanz, Geller, Shigaki, Maddock, and Isnec (2002).

Integration with the Research Process

Numerous similarities exist between applied research and program evaluation. Both use social science research methods, for example. Both involve developing study questions, selecting a study design, determining what should be measured and how, and sampling decisions. Furthermore, both require attention to reliability and validity of measures, qualitative or quantitative data collection, protection of human participants, data analysis, interpretation of findings, and dissemination of results.

The nine-step model presented in Chapter One can be compared with the framework for program evaluation in public health developed by the Centers for Disease Control and Prevention (1999). The latter model specifies six steps in the evaluation process: engage stakeholders, describe the program, focus the evaluation design, gather credible evidence, justify conclusions, and ensure that evaluation findings are used. Differences in the two models stem largely from the purposes of the two endeavors. In evaluation, the purpose is to provide information to make decisions about a specific program. Common guiding questions include, Is the program meeting its objectives? Is the program effective? Is the program implemented as planned? How can the program be improved? Not surprisingly, the evaluation framework emphasizes attention to stakeholders and the program description, as well as concern with the use of the evaluation findings. These concepts are largely absent in the research model, which makes sense, since the primary purpose of research is to create or discover generalizable knowledge.

◆ ◆ ◆

In a Nutshell

The evaluation framework emphasizes attention to stakeholders and the program description, as well as concern with the use of the evaluation findings.

◆ ◆ ◆

Other, more subtle, differences also exist. Whereas the research process begins with identifying a priority population, identification of a priority population, assessment of needs and assets, and selection of intervention strategies are typically driven by the program planning process in evaluation. Ideally, of course, evaluation planning is fully integrated into program planning, but that is not always the case in practice. The middle steps in the research and evaluation processes are similar, with selecting the design, determining measures, and sampling subsumed under the "focus the evaluation design" and "gather credible evidence" steps of the evaluation framework.

Summary

Evaluation involves the systematic collection of information to answer questions about a program. These questions can be classified into four types of evaluation: formative, process, outcome, and economic (outcome evaluation as a broad category also includes impact evaluation). Formative evaluation is conducted during the developmental phase of a program to determine whether specific components such as materials, message, and learning activities are feasible and acceptable to the program's target population. Both qualitative and quantitative methods are common in formative evaluation. Process evaluation focuses on the internal operations of a program and attempts to provide information that can lead to program improvement. It also uses both qualitative and quantitative methods. In contrast, outcome evaluations usually employ quantitative methods to determine the effectiveness of a program. In other words, Is the program achieving the desired outcomes? As described in this chapter, numerous types of economic analysis can be conducted under the rubric of program evaluation. These include cost analysis, cost of unmet needs analysis, cost-effectiveness, threshold analysis, and cost-utility analysis.

Evaluation is similar to applied research and draws heavily upon social science research methods. It differs from research in its emphasis on stakeholder involvement and its focus on providing information to decision makers to aid them in making judgments about a particular program. Typical steps in the process include engaging stakeholders; describing the program along with its underlying logic; focusing the evaluation design; collecting, analyzing, and interpreting data; and reporting study results. Program evaluation exemplifies how research methods can be applied to real-world situations to make a difference both in how we approach social and public health problems and in people's day-to-day lives.

Issues to Consider

1. An important decision that must be made early on in an evaluation is whether the evaluator should be someone internal to the program or organization being evaluated, or whether he or she should be external to the program or organization (Patton, 1997). External evaluators are typically private consultants, or associated with a university or research organization. They usually conduct evaluations through contracts with the funder or the organizational sponsor of the program. They do not have a long-term relationship with the program and are thus often viewed as more objective and independent than an evaluator who is employed by the program or its organization. Inside evaluators are believed to be more susceptible to organizational pressures to report findings that support a particular point of view. External evaluators, although possibly more objective, often do not understand the program or its context as well as an inside evaluator. Furthermore, the knowledge they gain about the program may not remain with the program once the contract is over. When internal evaluators are used, their knowledge and insights about the program remain

accessible to the organization. Given the pros and cons of internal and external evaluators, which would you generally recommend? Why?

2. In the course of conducting an evaluation, even an external evaluator will develop relationships with program personnel. For an internal evaluator, these relationships can be even stronger. Especially in the case of service programs such as those conducted in public health, evaluators can learn about staff members' motivations and dedication to the program. When volunteers are involved, an evaluator may hear about how these people have given generously of their time for program activities with no compensation. When it comes time to report negative results, it is incumbent upon the evaluator to balance respect for the efforts of program personnel with a clear and truthful accounting of the findings. How would you go about doing that?

For Practice and Discussion

1. You are an evaluator in the State Health Department, and your supervisor approaches you about a new project. It seems that a coalition in one of the cities of your state has received some new funding for its two-year-old program to increase exercise among people with arthritis. The pain associated with arthritis can cause arthritis sufferers not to use their muscles and, as a result, their muscles can atrophy. The goal of the arthritis exercise program has been to increase participants' joint flexibility and aerobic fitness while preventing the loss of their muscle condition. So far, they have served 225 people with arthritis.

   The program planners are excited about the additional funding and the potential to reach more people. The staff has just learned, however, that before the funds will be released, the program must submit a complete evaluation plan to their funder. You are assigned to develop their evaluation plan. How would you begin? Since the program has already been running for two years, what problems might that create in developing the plan? What parts of the plan might be easier to write for an existing program?

2. You have been asked by the director of a local hospital's cardiac rehabilitation department to evaluate a program conducted through the department. In this program, women with a history of myocardial infarction or of coronary artery bypass surgery who exercise regularly are asked to make telephone calls to other women with a similar history who do not regularly exercise. The purpose of the calls is to encourage the nonexercisers to participate in group exercise as a means of providing social support, since studies have found that women who persist in exercising after cardiac rehabilitation are more likely to have social support (Moore, Dolansky, Ruland, Pashkow, and Blackburn, 2003).

Although program evaluations can produce positive findings as well as negative findings, the personnel in charge of the program are not enthusiastic about the evaluation. Specifically, they express fear that it will not show all the good things their program is doing. As the evaluator, what can you do to help the program personnel become invested in your evaluation plan?

3. You have been conducting an evaluation of a state program designed to encourage African Americans to consider becoming organ donors. As a part of the evaluation, television stations in the state aired television spots about the need for organs in the African American community. African Americans in the state were later surveyed, and their knowledge and attitudes about organ donation were compared to those of African Americans in a neighboring state.

After completing the evaluation, you are invited to present your findings at a national meeting. A hepatologist (liver doctor) in the audience complains about your results, saying that you did not randomly assign people to receive the program or not. How would you respond to this person?

References

Bandura, A. (1986). *Social foundations of thought and action: A social cognitive theory.* Upper Saddle River, NJ: Prentice-Hall.

Centers for Disease Control and Prevention. (1999). Framework for program evaluation in public health. *Morbidity and Mortality Weekly Report, 48*(RR-11), 1–40.

Deniston, O. L., and Rosenstock, I. M. (1970). Evaluating health programs. *Public Health Reports, 85*(9), 835–840.

Glanz, K., Carbone, E., and Song, V. (1999). Formative research for developing targeted skin cancer prevention programs for children in multiethnic Hawaii. *Health Education Research, 14*(2), 155–166.

Glanz, K., Geller, A., Shigaki, D., Maddock, J., and Isnec, M. (2002). A randomized trial or skin cancer prevention in aquatics settings: The Pool Cool program. *Health Psychology, 21*(6), 579–587.

Glanz, K., Isnec, M., Geller, A., and Spangler, K. (2002). Process evaluation of implementation and dissemination of a sun safety program at swimming pools. In A. Steckler, and L. Linnan (Eds.), *Process evaluation for public health interventions and research* (pp. 58–82). San Francisco: Jossey-Bass.

Gold, M. R., Siegel, J. E., Russell, L. B., and Weinstein, M. C. (Eds.). (1996). *Cost-effectiveness in health and medicine.* New York: Oxford University Press.

Gorsky, R. D. (1996). A method to measure the costs of counseling for HIV prevention. *Public Health Reports, 111*(supplement 1), 115–122.

Green, L., and Kreuter, M. (1999). *Health promotion planning: An educational and ecological approach* (3rd ed.). Mountain View, CA: Mayfield.

Holtgrave, D. R., Pinkerton, S. D., and Merson, M. (2002). Estimating the cost of unmet HIV prevention needs in the United States. *American Journal of Preventive Medicine, 23*, 7–12.

Holtgrave, D. R., and others. (1997). Setting standards for the Wisconsin HIV counseling and testing program: An application of threshold analysis. *Journal of Public Health Management and Practice, 3*, 42–49.

Linnan, L., and Steckler, A. (2002). *Process evaluation for public health interventions and research.* San Francisco: Jossey-Bass.

Moore, S. M., Dolansky, M. A., Ruland, C. M., Pashkow, F. J., and Blackburn, G. G. (2003). Predictors of women's exercise maintenance after cardiac rehabilitation. *Journal of Cardiopulmonary Rehabilitation, 23*(1), 40–49.

Patton, M. Q. (1997). *Utilization-focused evaluation.* Thousand Oaks, CA: Sage.

Pinkerton, S. D., and Holtgrave, D. R. (1998). Assessing the cost-effectiveness of HIV prevention interventions: A primer. In D. R. Holtgrave (Ed.), *Handbook of economic evaluation of HIV prevention programs* (pp. 33–43). New York: Plenum Press.

Pinkerton, S. D., Johnson-Masotti, A. P., Holtgrave, D. R., and Farnham, P. G. (2001). Using cost-effectiveness league tables to compare interventions to prevent sexual transmission of HIV. *AIDS, 15*, 917–928.

Rossi, P. H., Lipsey, M. W., and Freeman, H. E. (2004). *Evaluation: A systematic approach* (7th ed.). Thousand Oaks, CA: Sage.

Thompson, N. J., and McClintock, H. O. (1998). *Demonstrating your program's worth: A primer on evaluation for programs to prevent unintentional injury.* Atlanta: Centers for Disease Control and Prevention, National Center for Injury Prevention and Control.

Tobacco Technical Assistance Consortium. (2005, January). *The power of proof: An evaluation primer.* Retrieved February 6, 2005, from www.ttac.org/power-of-proof/index.html.

Trentacoste, N. D., Holtgrave, D. R., Collins, C., and Abdul-Quader, A. (2004). Disseminating effective interventions for HIV prevention: A cost analysis of a risk reduction intervention for drug users. *Journal of Public Health Management and Practice, 10*, 130–139.

Weiss, C. (1997). *Evaluation: Methods for studying programs and policies.* Upper Saddle River, NJ: Prentice-Hall.

PART THREE

MEASUREMENT, SAMPLING, AND ANALYSIS

CHAPTER NINE

MEASUREMENT IN HEALTH PROMOTION

Richard R. Clayton and Richard A. Crosby

Measurement is everywhere. It is woven in, on, over, around, and through everything we do. As soon as a baby is born the medical personnel determine "vital statistics"— the height, weight, and Apgar score for the newborn—and record the month, day, year, and time of birth. The time lapsed since birth is used to determine when visits to the pediatrician are scheduled and when certain immunizations are administered. At each postnatal visit, medical staff determine and record the baby's weight and height in order to measure "change," and may take the baby's temperature. Temperature is measured in degrees. Throughout an individual's life, his or her birthday is celebrated and used to mark important developmental transitions such as reaching the ages to drive, to vote, and to drink. Over time, while the specific measures taken may change somewhat, virtually everything in an individual's life is measured. For example, when individuals enter school their attendance or absence will be recorded in a student record database as will their test and achievement scores.

Each of the measures taken and recorded has a metric. Temperature is measured in degrees Fahrenheit or Celsius, weight is measured in pounds or grams and kilograms, test scores are measured in actual numbers (as in SAT and GRE scores) or in percentiles. As you may already know, some metrics are more sophisticated than others. For example, metrics for measures range from a nominal scale to an ordinal to an interval to a ratio scale.

If measurement is everywhere and in everything, then measurement should be viewed as an essential element of health promotion strategies, campaigns, and programs. Measurement is central, critical, and absolutely vital to our understanding of health promotion research. In this chapter, the emphasis will be on *who* and *what* is measured in public health, *when, how,* and *where* the measurements occur, and, most important, *why* public health phenomena are measured. We have chosen to use one behavior, tobacco use, and its role in public health to illustrate the key concepts presented in this chapter. We will also address contextual-level influences on health by using the family unit as an example of a key variable, which may pose several challenges to measurement. Specifically, this chapter will focus on step 5 in the nine-step model described in Chapter One. However, because health promotion research is frequently based on the use of self-reported measures, this chapter precedes a chapter (Chapter Ten) that will provide an in-depth analysis of issues relevant to increasing the validity of self-reported measures. Both chapters are dedicated to providing you with up-to-date techniques for assessment in health promotion research.

◆ ◆ ◆

In a Nutshell

Measurement is central, critical, and absolutely vital to our understanding of health promotion research.

◆ ◆ ◆

Illustration of Key Concepts

Perhaps one of the most fundamental aspects of measurement is determining the metric used for variables. A variable is a single measure that, by definition, can take on more than one value. If only one value is possible, then the measure cannot vary and therefore must be a constant. Distinctions between four metrics used to categorize or quantify variables are commonly made. As will be shown in Chapters Twelve and Thirteen, the metric associated with a variable will determine the type of statistical analysis performed.

Metrics

Nominal data are especially common in health promotion research. A nominal metric simply categorizes or groups according to some *attribute*. Attributes constitute the mutually exclusive and exhaustive response categories for a variable and are qualitative in nature versus quantitative. Before you were born, your mother went through carefully and strategically scheduled measurements. One of those measures determined whether she was pregnant. The answer to the pregnancy test had only two categories—Yes or No. Either you are pregnant or you are not pregnant; thus, this metric does not include a more or less dimension. Something that is measured "Yes or No," "zero or one," or "present or not present," is a dichotomy and is a specific form of a nominal scale. Nominal measures may also extend beyond a dichotomy. Race, for example, is a nominal variable that may have many different attributes. Some attributes of a nominal variable for religion may include Christian, Jewish, Muslim, Buddhist, Hindu. Nominal attributes cannot be ranked in any fashion. Sex is another example of a nominal variable (male or female).

The next metric is *ordinal*. As your mother endured labor, the physician, nurse, and perhaps your father or some other family member might have asked your mother to tell them how bad the labor pains were—say on a scale from low to medium to high. This is called an ordinal level of measurement. It is characterized by transitivity, in which it is clear that high is more than medium which is more than low. Thus, the attributes are ranked along a continuum. However, it is worth noting that the distance between ranks is *not* known to be equal. For example, presenting a statement to people and then asking them to indicate their level of agreement on a scale with five responses that range from "strongly disagree" to "strongly agree" is something that is measured on an ordinal scale. From this example you can see how you *cannot* determine with certainty whether the difference between "strongly agree" and "somewhat agree" is exactly the same as the difference between "somewhat agree" and "neither agree nor disagree."

The next metric is *interval*. Like ordinal measures, an interval scale has transitivity; however, the distance between ranks is equal. Moreover, a score of "zero" does not equate with a complete absence of the variable that is being measured; rather, it is arbitrary. One example of a measure that uses this type of metric is temperature measured by the Fahrenheit or Celsius scales.

The final metric is *ratio*. As your mother went through labor the physician, nurse, or midwife used what is called a ratio scale of measurement—the number of centimeters that her cervix had dilated so that you could be born. A ratio scale has not only transitivity and equal distance between ranks, but also an absolute zero point. Common measures in health promotion such as "knowledge of heart disease prevention practices" are measured on a ratio metric. Other examples include number of cigarettes smoked per day, number of times a person attended a smoking cessation class, and the amount of money a person spends on cigarettes in one week. The advantage of having a measure that is a ratio scale of measurement is that it allows for statements about proportions. In other words, thirty cigarettes smoked per day as compared to ten cigarettes smoked per day represents a ratio of 3:1. You are unable to make these ratio statements with the other three types of metrics.

Measuring Constructs

Measuring physical properties such as weight, height, and age is a relatively straightforward process. In essence, it is easy to measure things that are tangible. If all measurement in health promotion research were this easy, then this chapter would be extremely short. Because health promotion research is intertwined with health behaviors and their underlying psychological and psychosocial influences, research questions are frequently centered upon intangibles such as self-esteem, depression, self-efficacy, attitudes, perceptions, and beliefs. Thus, while weight exists as a physical entity, self-esteem does not. Indeed, a concept such as self-esteem is not directly observable or measurable, but rather is hypothetical and may be linked to a particular theoretical orientation. For example, scholars theorize that people develop a sense of their own value and that this overall evaluation of their worth or value is influential in shaping some behaviors. Thus, self-esteem can be viewed as a concept versus an object. The question becomes, how do we measure something that is not tangible? The answer begins with the brief schematic shown below.

Concept → Operational Definition → Construct → Indicators

Because the epistemology of scientific inquiry is built on objectivity, the first step in measuring a *concept* such as self-esteem is to create a formalized definition. In a sense, this *operational definition* will become "the" definition of self-esteem for the purpose of the study being conducted. The definition does not need to be universally accepted, it simply needs to be provided so that consumers of your research can know, without question, what you mean when you use the term *self-esteem*. Once you have operationalized the concept it becomes a *construct*. The construct now requires measurement. It stands to reason that complex constructs such as self-esteem must be measured with multiple questions or items. The questions or items should be designed to be distinct *effect indicators* of the construct. Effect indicators signify that each question or item relating to the construct infers some "effect" or influence on an observable behavior and "taps into" the construct (Streiner, 2003). Rarely will a single-item indicator provide a complete assessment of a construct. Therefore, it is quite common to use multiple indicators to assess one construct.

◆ ◆ ◆

In a Nutshell

Once you have operationalized the concept it becomes a construct.

◆ ◆ ◆

Self-esteem represents a unitary construct for which multiple effect indicators can be used to measure it. In this instance, the measure of self-esteem would be called a *scale*. Specifically, a scale is a measure that is composed of "theoretically correlated items" (Streiner, 2003, p. 217) that are measuring the same construct. Examples of scales include the Rosenberg Self-Esteem Scale (Rosenberg, 1989) and the Beck Depression Inventory (Beck, Ward, Mendelson, Mock, and Erbaugh, 1961). Each of these scales has multiple effect indicators that theoretically relate to how self-esteem and depression would manifest. For example, one item from the Rosenberg Scale is "I am able to do things as well as most other people."

Although you may encounter instances when other terms are used interchangeably in the literature or in other texts to describe a collection of items or questions such as scale, test, questionnaire, index, or inventory, it is important to note that there are specific distinctions between a scale and an *index*. Thus, these two terms should not be used interchangeably, as they mean different things. An index refers to a measure in which the items are considered *causal indicators* because they themselves define the construct and influence the value of the construct (Streiner, 2003). The items in an index typically are heterogeneous and may not necessarily be correlated with each other. The Apgar Scale, mentioned previously in this chapter, specifically rates newborns on several characteristics such as heart rate, respiration, muscle tone, reflex response, and skin color and is an excellent example of an index. As you may be able to extrapolate, items composing indexes are not tapping into a unitary construct. In health promotion research, other examples of indexes are quality-of-life questionnaires, tests that assess levels of physical functionality, and knowledge tests. To illustrate these

Box 9.1. Example of a Scale

Below is a list of the ways you might have felt or behaved. Please tell me how often you have felt this way during the past week.

Rarely or None of the Time (< than 1 day)	Some or a Little of the Time (1–2 days)	Occasionally or a Moderate Amount of Time (3–4 days)	Most or All of the Time (5–7 days)

1. I was bothered by things that usually don't bother me.
2. I did not feel like eating; my appetite was poor.
3. I felt that I could not shake off the blues even with help from my family or friends.
4. I felt that I was just as good as other people.
5. I had trouble keeping my mind on what I was doing.
6. I felt depressed.
7. I felt that everything I did was an effort.
8. I felt hopeful about the future.
9. I thought my life had been a failure.
10. I felt fearful.
11. My sleep was restless.
12. I was happy.
13. I talked less than usual.
14. I felt lonely.
15. People were unfriendly.
16. I enjoyed life.
17. I had crying spells.
18. I felt sad.
19. I felt that people dislike me.
20. I could not get "going."

Source: Center for Epidemiologic Studies Depression Scale (CES-D) (Radloff, 1977).

distinctions, an example of a scale is shown in Box 9.1 and an example of an index is shown in Box 9.2.

Two key questions about any scale or index are Is this measure reliable? and Is it valid? *Reliability* means that a measure consistently provides the same answer every time it is used. So if one has a yardstick but it is forty-two inches long, it will still consistently provide the same measurement each time you use it. Unfortunately for the person using this "yard" stick, the consistency is always six inches too long. This brings us to the topic of validity. Although this "yard" stick

---

Box 9.2. Example of an Index

Quality of Life—Modified

I want to find out how you feel about various parts of your life. Please tell me the feelings you have in general according to the following responses.

Very Happy	Happy	Mostly Satisfied	Mixed	Mostly Dissatisfied	Unhappy	Very Unhappy

1. How do you feel about your life overall?
2. In general, how do you feel about yourself?
3. How do you feel about your personal safety?
4. How do you feel about the amount of fun and enjoyment you have?
5. How do you feel about the responsibilities you have for members of your family?
6. How do you feel about what you are accomplishing in your life?
7. How do you feel about your independence or freedom—that is, how free do you feel to live the kind of life you want?
8. How do you feel about your emotional and psychological well-being?
9. How do you feel about the way you spend your spare time?

Source: Andrews and Withey, 1976.

---

may be reliable, it is certainly not valid. Validity refers to whether or not the measure is measuring what it is supposed to measure.

Determining the reliability of a measure could be achieved in several ways. First, reliability could be established by administering the index or the scale to a sample at two points in time and looking for a relatively strong correlation in scores for time 1 and time 2. This is known as *test-retest reliability*. Notice that the underlying assumption here is that the construct is stable; therefore, a reliable measure should produce the same score at time 2 that it did at time 1 for each person in the sample. Thus, a principle in establishing test-retest reliability is that the construct must not be one that undergoes dramatic change over time.

Second, reliability can be established by computing the inter-item correlations between all items comprised in the scale. Note that this technique is appropriate for establishing the reliability of a scale because scale items should be tapping into a unitary construct. Thus, they should be intercorrelated. The same is not true for indexes, however. Computing inter-item correlations is not appropriate

MINCUS REVEALS A VALID MEASURE OF CHIPMUNK I.Q.

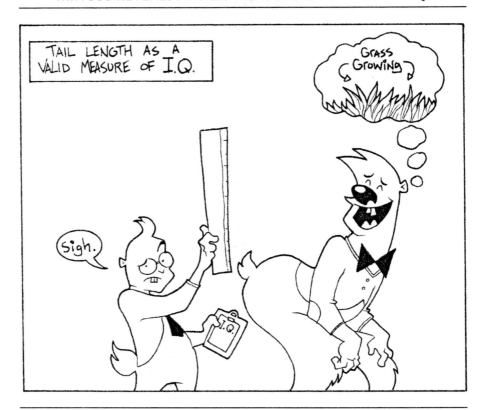

Copyright 2005 by Justin Wagner; reprinted with permission.

for establishing the reliability of an index (Streiner, 2003). Calculating the inter-
item correlations is called assessing the *internal reliability* of the scale.

We can determine the intercorrelations between items on a scale by employing a statistical procedure that yields the statistic Cronbach's alpha. Cronbach's
alpha (α) has a range of 0 to 1, with higher scores representing greater inter-
item reliability. Although hard-and-fast rules don't exist, an α of .70 or higher is
considered sufficient evidence of reliability. It is, however, worth noting that
extremely high alphas such as .95 suggest that there may be redundancy among
some of the indicators. In effect, a scale with an alpha close to 1.0 could probably be reduced to fewer indicators. Note that inter-item correlation could be used
in conjunction with the test-retest technique. Conversely, it is also noteworthy that

the inter-item reliability method can be used in a cross-sectional study, whereas the same cannot be said about the test-retest method.

Third, reliability could be established by using the *split-half* method. Like the inter-item reliability method, this test for reliability could be performed in the context of a cross-sectional study. This analytic procedure begins with dividing the scale into two parallel forms of the measure. For example, an eight-item scale would be randomly divided into two four-item measures. These two shortened forms would then be administered to a sample. The correlation between scores for the two halves is calculated and then used in a formula (such as the Spearman Brown) to estimate the reliability of the total measure (Ghiselli, Campbell, and Zedeck, 1981). Similar to inter-item reliability, this method is not appropriate for indexes, as splitting the index into parts would not be meaningful.

As mentioned previously, validity refers to the index or scale measuring exactly what it is supposed to measure. So a yardstick that is forty-two inches long might be reliable, but it is not valid. A valid measure measures what it is supposed to *and* does so consistently. Thus, for a measure to be valid it must also be reliable, whereas a reliable measure is not necessarily valid.

◆ ◆ ◆

In a Nutshell

For a measure to be valid it must also be reliable, whereas a reliable measure is not necessarily valid.

◆ ◆ ◆

Like reliability, validity can be established through the application of several different techniques. Two of the most elementary techniques are *face validity* and *content validity*. Both techniques employ a *jury of experts* (a panel of professionals who possess expertise with respect to the construct(s) under consideration). Face validity is judged by asking the jury, Does the index or scale appear to measure the construct? Content validity, on the other hand, goes a bit further. For scales you would want to ask, Do the items represent the "universe" of all possible indicators relevant for the construct? For indexes, you would want to ask, Do the items represent a census of items underlying the construct? Content validity can be assessed for both scales and indexes, but judgments made regarding the items differ. Scales assume that there is a universe of potential items from which to draw a sample that represents the unitary construct, whereas items composing an index should be viewed more as a census of items and are dependent on the underlying theory of the construct and prior research (Streiner, 2003). Nevertheless, for both types of validity, the support for a measure being valid is a judgment. Because all constructs are measured by self-report, the more sophisticated techniques of establishing validity are an integral part of the next chapter (Chapter Ten), which is devoted to increasing the validity of self-reported measures.

Types of Variables

Variables can be qualitative or quantitative, can have different levels of measurement, and can represent myriad constructs that are not directly observable or measurable. All of these things have an effect on how the variables can be used and analyzed. In addition to knowing these important aspects of variables, it is also important to understand the role variables can adopt given a particular research context. Variables can be classified into several different types based largely on their function in serving the research question. The first level of distinction is whether the research question is descriptive or causal in nature (see Chapter Four for more detail). The second level of distinction is whether the variable is intended as a "causal" element or an outcome.

Variables in Descriptive Research. In health promotion descriptive research, observational designs rather than experimental designs are used, and the variable of interest is typically known as the *outcome measure*. Outcome measures can be physical indicators of morbidity such as lung cancer, atherosclerosis, blood serum cholesterol levels, emphysema, and chronic obstructive pulmonary disease. Outcome measures may also be health-risk behaviors such as smoking cigarettes, using chew tobacco, eating a diet low in cruciferous vegetables, and being exposed to asbestos. An excellent way to gain first-hand knowledge of health promotion outcome variables considered important to the federal government is to review the document *Healthy People 2010* (Department of Health and Human Services, 2000).

In descriptive research, variables presumed to cause or precede specified outcomes are typically known as *predictor variables*. The mark of a good predictor variable is its ability to reduce error when one makes predictions about an outcome. For example, in 1964 the Surgeon General of the United States issued the first report on the relationship between smoking and lung cancer. In essence, knowing whether (and how much) someone has smoked enables a more accurate prediction of the outcome, in this case lung cancer. Does that mean that smoking cigarettes is the only cause of lung cancer? The answer obviously is no. Some individuals who have never smoked get lung cancer. It does mean, however, that smoking behavior can be used as one of many predictors of developing lung cancer. This concept of using predictors to improve the estimate of an outcome is called *proportional reduction in error.*

◆ ◆ ◆

In a Nutshell

The mark of a good predictor variable is its ability to reduce error when one makes predictions about an outcome.

◆ ◆ ◆

One problem in labeling a given variable as a predictor is that there must be a reasonable level of certainty that the predictor is actually preceding the outcome. This certainty is made possible by assessment of the predictor at a point in time before assessment of the outcome occurs. Consider, for instance, a research question that asks whether nonsmoking teens who believe that smoking causes lung cancer are less likely to ever begin smoking. In this study, the predictor variable can be measured before the outcome occurs (as the sample comprised only nonsmokers). Over the next five years or so, many of those nonsmokers are likely to become smokers. If those who believed, during their teen years, that smoking causes lung cancer were statistically less likely to initiate smoking in the next five years, then it is safe to say that the belief preceded the outcome. But what if you don't have the luxury of doing a longitudinal (prospective) study? Instead, imagine that you have funding for only a cross-sectional design. You wisely sample all teens (not just those who are nonsmokers) to ensure variability in your outcome variables: smoking status and belief that smoking causes lung cancer. You are quite satisfied when the results support your research hypothesis. You find that those holding the belief are statistically less likely to smoke than those not holding the belief. The downside of this finding is that you cannot establish a *temporal order* (see Chapter Four). Thus, one could make the reverse argument (that smoking *causes* a person to deny that a connection between tobacco use and lung cancer even exists). Therefore, in a cross-sectional design, the concept of a predictor variable is problematic. Instead, the term *correlate* is used. Within this context, correlate represents a variable hypothesized to precede the outcome.

The discipline of public health is population oriented. Therefore, in public health, correlates and predictor variables are often measured at the macro or population level. One example of a population-level variable is the state excise tax rate for each of the fifty states in the United States. We could obtain the tax rate while also measuring the percentage of the population that reports being a current smoker. The correlate would be the amount of the state excise tax, ordered from the lowest to the highest. The percentage of the population that smokes would be the outcome variable. One hypothesis to consider would be the higher the state excise tax on cigarettes the lower the percentage who report being a current smoker. If there was an association between the correlate (excise tax) and the outcome (smoking behavior), then it would be reasonable to assume that by manipulating the excise tax rate we could influence smoking behavior. Health economists would be very interested in what would happen to the current smoking rate if the excise tax were increased. In such a case, the results might be reported as "a 10 percent increase in the price of cigarettes yielded a 7 percent decrease in the percentage of people who are smokers."

Variables in Causal Research. Causal research in health promotion uses mainly experimental or quasi-experimental designs (see Chapter Four). The *dependent variable* in experimental research designs is the counterpart to the outcome measure in observational research designs. In a randomized controlled trial (RCT) of a health promotion program (HPP) designed to prevent teens from *ever* initiating tobacco use, the dependent variable might be intent to ever smoke. Thus, intent would be assessed at some point after teens complete the program or the equivalent control condition. If the research hypothesis is supported, then those receiving the program will have less intent to smoke than those receiving the control program.

◆ ◆ ◆

In a Nutshell

The dependent variable *in experimental research designs is the counterpart to the outcome measure in observational research designs.*

◆ ◆ ◆

In health promotion research we often are interested in a variety of dependent variables. For example, mass media is used often in health promotion campaigns to influence individual level change. The dependent variables might be (1) awareness of the campaign (yes or no), (2) remembering the central theme or message of the campaign (knowledge beyond mere awareness), (3) a change in knowledge about the content of the campaign, (4) a change in one's attitude about the topic of the campaign, (5) a change in intention to change a behavior pattern that puts one at greater risk for a negative health outcome, or (6) a change in one's behavior thus reducing the risk for a negative health outcome. All of these are desirable outcomes and are related to each other.

Alternatively, in experimental research designs, *independent variables* cannot take on several different forms. Instead, these variables are limited to group assignment in the randomization process. By definition, the independent variable is manipulated by the investigator. Therefore, assignment to condition (the HPP or the control group) is an example of an independent variable.

◆ ◆ ◆

In a Nutshell

By definition, the independent variable is manipulated by the investigator.

◆ ◆ ◆

Mediating Variables. In the smoking–lung cancer relationship example, one might ask, How does smoking actually "cause" lung cancer in some people? This is a question about the mechanisms and processes that occur after the cause and before the effect. These mechanisms are said to *mediate* the observed relationship between smoking and lung cancer. In health promotion, the focus is more often on factors that might, at a population level, cause a reduction in lung cancer. For example, suppose a state embarks on a comprehensive and large-scale campaign to reduce the amount of smoking in that state. The health promotion campaign involves a substantial increase in the state excise tax on cigarettes; a universal prohibition on smoking in restaurants, bars, and other public places; the dissemination of effective prevention programs in schools; and the funding of effective smoking cessation interventions in health insurance plans and in worksites. All of this would be presented as an integrated strategy via a huge public awareness and marketing campaign. On average, it takes about twenty to twenty-five years of chronic smoking for lung cancer to appear, and the ultimate mediating variable for the smoking–lung cancer relationship is gene mutations. However, by reducing the levels of smoking through the use of massive campaigns that involve raising cigarette taxes, reducing environmental tobacco smoke, preventing dependency, and mass media, one might expect the rates of lung cancer and other tobacco-related illnesses and deaths to decline. A targeted outcome of the anti-smoking campaign could be a change in social norms surrounding smoking so that smoking is frowned upon. In this instance, affecting social norms is one mechanism that allows the intent of campaign to be translated into reduced risk for lung cancer. In essence then, mediating variables "come between" the cause (in this case the antismoking campaign) and the effect (in this case the reduction of cigarette use in a population).

Moderating Variables. Moderating variables identify the conditions under which the relationship between two variables might be stronger or weaker. For example, if the relationship between smoking and lung cancer was statistically stronger among whites than among blacks and Hispanics, then race or ethnicity would be considered the moderating variable. If the relation was stronger among those who are from rural rather than suburban and urban areas, then place of residence would be the moderating variable. Social support is a classic example of a moderating variable in the health promotion literature, in which perceptions of high levels of social support serve as a buffer (that is, moderator) against experiencing the negative effects of stress on health outcomes. Furthermore, some variables may moderate the effectiveness of HPPs. One example could be that HPP was effective in reducing smoking, but only for women. For men, it was not effective. Thus, in this example gender serves the moderating variable. It is important to consider what variables may serve as moderators both of significant relationships between correlates and outcomes and of HPP effectiveness.

In a Nutshell

Moderating variables identify the conditions under which the relationship between two variables might be stronger or weaker.

Measuring Behavioral Variables

Think about how to measure a rather simple variable, a behavior, such as smoking cigarettes. All of us have seen individuals smoking so we know what the behavior involves or looks like. Some of us are "experts" on smoking because we may have tried smoking cigarettes in the past, or we may be (hopefully not) a current smoker.

Tobacco use is important from a public health perspective because 430,000 deaths each year in the United States are attributable to smoking. This figure is more than the combined deaths from suicide, homicide, automobile accidents, alcohol, drug abuse, and HIV/AIDS. Second, smoking is a leading cause of cardiovascular disease, the leading cause of death in the United States. Third, 90 percent of lung cancer is attributable to smoking. Simply put, there is no other health-related variable as important as smoking in terms of its consequences for society.

Given the enormous consequences from smoking, it is essential that we understand how to measure this behavior so that valid and useful conclusions can be drawn from our research. Therefore, in this section we will review some of the ways that smoking is measured in both observational and experimental studies. In almost all studies individuals are asked to self-report their behavior on either a self-administered questionnaire or to an interviewer.

Lifetime Experience with Smoking. An example of a question designed to measure lifetime experience with smoking specifies that "ever" smoking includes as little as taking even a puff from a cigarette. Consider the following example.

Have you ever tried cigarette smoking, even a puff? (mark one box)

      ❑ Yes

      ❑ No

There is nothing inherently wrong with this question. One could presume that a "yes" is different from a "no," and that those who have ever smoked may be different from those who have never smoked. One goal of prevention in tobacco use is to increase the number and percentage of the population that has never tried cigarettes. However, this is a very gross measurement. It tells us nothing about when in a person's life they had this experience. Presumably, those who try cigarettes earlier in their life rather than later may be different on a number of dimensions. Presumably, the earlier that people try cigarettes, the more likely they are to continue. These are hypotheses that require more precise measurement than *ever* versus *never*. The ever-never dichotomy (nominal variable) doesn't tell anything about whether smoking was a transitory behavior or something that continued, perhaps increased, and became a chronic behavior pattern. Yes or no response to "ever tried smoking?" doesn't provide much data, certainly not enough information to guide the design of a health promotion program.

Recognizing the need to understand how long smoking has occurred, one could ask two questions, one about age at the onset of smoking and one about current smoking. In fact, the following question about one's first experience with smoking is also a question about lifetime ever smoking. If they provide an age at onset it means that they have smoked. If they answer that they have never smoked even a puff of a cigarette, then they are a no on ever smoking. There is also a subtle difference between the first question and the one that follows. In the ever-never question, the investigator is assuming that the person answering the question never smoked. In the question below, there is an implicit assumption that the person answering the question has smoked. They are then required to deny the behavior.

How old were you the very first time you smoked even a puff of a cigarette?
(mark one box)

❑ I have never smoked even a puff of a cigarette
❑ 8 years old or younger
❑ 9 years old
❑ 10 years old
❑ 11 years old
❑ 12 years old
❑ 13 years old
❑ 14 years old
❑ 15 years old
❑ 16 years old
❑ 17 years old
❑ 18 years old
❑ 19 years or older

The second question that will help one develop at least a preliminary picture of the extent of smoking asks about current smoking. In the tobacco field, "current" is defined as the past thirty days or past month.

During the past thirty days, on how many *days* did you smoke one or more cigarettes? (mark one box)

❑ 0 days
❑ 1 or 2 days
❑ 3 to 5 days
❑ 6 to 9 days
❑ 10 to 19 days
❑ 20 to 29 days
❑ All 30 days

This question is more precise than the previous questions. It does provide some information about current use of cigarettes. The answers to this question provide an investigator with information about the frequency of use (an ordinal variable).

We assume that current cigarette use is related to a host of other variables measured at the same time. So, from a health promotion perspective, current cigarette use could be a predictor variable that is associated with some other variable (for example, use of alcohol and other drugs, recent respiratory illnesses, or dependence on nicotine). It could be an outcome variable that is associated with epidemiological and demographic variables that have public health relevance (nominal variables such as race or ethnicity, sex, or rural urban residence, or ordinal variables such as attitudes toward tobacco use, stress, and so on).

One of the problems with subjects such as the number of days one smoked in the past thirty days is that some people may not organize their memory around thirty days, some of which may have occurred during the current month and some in the previous month. The month is a much more common organizing framework for memory. However, if the question were about the "past month," what month would we be asking about? If it were March 20, would we be asking about the nineteenth days of March or about the entire month of February? Another problem is the categorization of number of days. Ten to nineteen days covers a lot of time. One might assume that someone who has actually smoked ten days (assuming it is possible to remember accurately this number) may be different from someone who has smoked nineteen days (assuming it is possible to remember accurately this number). Therefore, the preceding question is often coupled with the following question to create a two-question measure of current cigarette use. Some of these issues related to recall are discussed in more detail in Chapter Ten.

On the days that you smoke, how many cigarettes do you typically smoke?
(mark one box)

- ❑ I have never smoked even a puff of a cigarette
- ❑ Less than 1 cigarette per day
- ❑ 1 to 2 cigarettes per day
- ❑ 3 to 7 cigarettes per day
- ❑ 8 to 12 cigarettes per day
- ❑ 13 to 17 cigarettes per day
- ❑ 18 to 23 cigarettes per day
- ❑ At least 24 cigarettes per day

This is an interesting way to measure current cigarette use. Think about how cigarettes come packaged. A pack contains twenty cigarettes. Notice that none of the categories are easily translated into one-half a pack or two packs. Regular or heavy smokers may gauge how much they smoke in terms of packs rather than individual cigarettes. Another problem with the question is that it requires the individual answering the question to engage in some mathematical computations. Most of us are not very good at such math. Another major problem with this approach to measuring a simple but evidently complex behavior is the assumption that smokers are consistent from day to day in how much they smoke. This may be true for individuals who have been smoking for some time. For relatively new smokers, however, their pattern from day to day and week to week may be erratic.

These limitations can be seen most clearly in Figure 9.1. Data in the figure come from an adolescent smoker who was asked the two previous questions— number of days smoked and number of cigarettes per day. She reported that she smoked twenty to twenty-nine days and that she smoked eleven cigarettes a day. She was then asked to keep a daily diary of her smoking patterns.

As shown in Figure 9.1, of the thirty days in the month, the subject smoked for nineteen days (thirty minus the eleven days that she didn't smoke at all). So, in terms of the categorization, the appropriate answer would have been that she smoked ten to nineteen days, not twenty to twenty-nine days. She smoked on 63 percent of the days in that thirty-day period. She did accurately report that she smoked eleven cigarettes a day, but for only eight of the thirty days in the month. The average number of cigarettes per day was 4.9.

FIGURE 9.1.   A FEMALE ADOLESCENT'S DAILY SMOKING PATTERN.

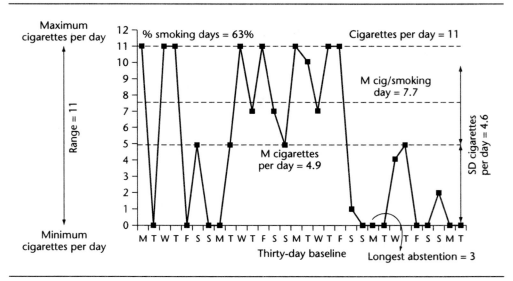

As you can see by now, measurement of a behavior, a behavior with which we are all familiar, a behavior that is based on consumption of a discrete commodity (each cigarette in a pack of twenty cigarettes is not connected to the others in the pack) is not a simple task. From a public health perspective, these examples should make it clear that our traditional approach to measuring this very important health-related behavior is fraught with limitations. In health promotion research it is critical that our measurement be valid. That is, the measures we use should represent the actual behavior as closely as possible. Next, we will attempt to show two less traditional approaches to measurement that may get us closer to understanding this very important behavior. If we are going to be successful in preventing or reducing the consequences of this behavior, it will be necessary for us to do a better job of measuring it.

A Web-Driven Approach. Thirty days is a long time. Smoking occurs in real time—in minutes and hours in a day. The burn time on a cigarette is typically five minutes—three hundred seconds. A smoker typically takes about ten puffs on a cigarette, each of which lasts about three seconds—a total of thirty seconds. This being true, a day is a long time. So, to measure the behavior accurately we have to be more precise.

One of the more modern ways to collect data, and thus measure important variables, is to use a Web-driven approach. Hypothetically, it is possible for individuals involved in a Web-driven study to answer questions at any time of day or night, seven days each week. However, until there is more experience with this approach to measurement, the most common approach is to ask study participants to complete periodic on-line questionnaires.

To illustrate how this approach to measurement works, we will report on a study conducted among 912 members of the freshman class of 2002 at Purdue University. A total of 4,690 in this freshman class completed a short, paper-and-pencil screener questionnaire in the summer during their orientation, when they received their schedule for the fall semester. Of these, 2,001 had some previous experience with cigarettes, somewhere between "just a puff" and much more involvement. These 2,001 were invited to participate in the Web-based study, and 912 agreed to participate.

In addition to completing a forty-five-minute baseline questionnaire, these freshmen participants agreed to provide weekly data (usually on a Sunday) via a secure server once a week for thirty-five weeks. They were asked specifically to report on their use of cigarettes, alcohol, and marijuana for each of the previous seven days. A logical question that you may have is, Why seven days? There are two reasons. The first is that this is a relatively short period of time, less time available for the memory to decay. Second, most people, particularly students,

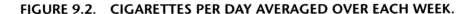

FIGURE 9.2. CIGARETTES PER DAY AVERAGED OVER EACH WEEK.

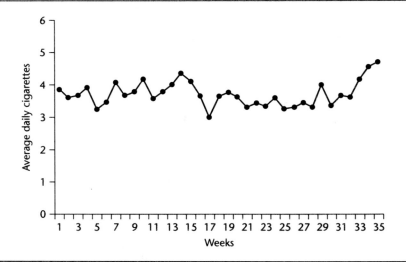

think about their life in terms of weeks. Simply put, the investigators were concerned about the reliability of the data, and a seven-day period of recall seemed reasonable to collect "close to real time" data. Furthermore, because these data were collected on the Web, every response was day and time dated, so it was possible to know when the data were provided and what reference point was being used to report the cigarette use.

> During the past seven days, about how many cigarettes did you smoke each day? If you haven't smoked on a particular day in the last week, enter "0." If you smoked less than a whole cigarette, enter "1."

Figure 9.2 shows the data on cigarettes smoked per day averaged over each of the thirty-five weeks. This is what cigarette use data look like when they reflect a smaller interval. They are still subject to the concerns often raised about self-report data (see Chapter Ten for an in-depth discussion of self-reported data).

The data can be broken down even further to obtain more precision for each week reported. Figure 9.3 indicates the average number of cigarettes per day reported by the sample of 912 freshmen for the period. Every individual in the study who reported smoking had a trajectory of smoking. Therefore, it is possible to show the trajectory for each individual (see Figure 9.1) or, as is the case for Figures 9.2 and 9.3, data are aggregated for the entire sample.

FIGURE 9.3. CIGARETTES: AVERAGE DAILY NUMBER.

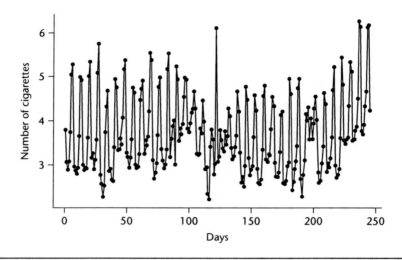

Figure 9.4 breaks the data down even further to show smoking behavior on days when both smoking and drinking occurred. The added dimension of "drinking behavior" provides an interesting context that helps enrich the understanding of smoking. College students will immediately recognize what is happening with these freshmen. Their smoking is mostly low on Sunday, Monday, Tuesday, and Wednesday. However, smoking in this sample is higher on Thursday than on the previous days. The first question that comes to mind is, Is Thursday a weekday or part of the weekend? The second question is, Why the higher rates of use of cigarettes on Friday and Saturday? The answer to this question is simple—this is when students tend to party. As Figure 9.4 indicates, there is a strong connection between smoking and drinking among college freshmen. In fact, a careful examination of the data in Figure 9.4 reveals that over 50 percent of the cigarettes smoked on Friday and Saturday were smoked while students were drinking. Although sophomores, juniors, and seniors were not studied, the data suggest that similar patterns would most likely be found for these students.

In Figure 9.3, the daily smoking data were reviewed for the first thirty-five weeks. Much more precise data allow an investigator to ask a number of questions that are not possible with less precise data. For example, the investigators in the Purdue study asked, What is the highest Thursday with regard to smoking? The answer is Halloween. They also asked about the lowest and highest smoking day for the first semester. You can probably guess the answer. The lowest day was

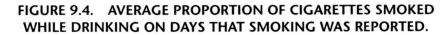

FIGURE 9.4.   AVERAGE PROPORTION OF CIGARETTES SMOKED WHILE DRINKING ON DAYS THAT SMOKING WAS REPORTED.

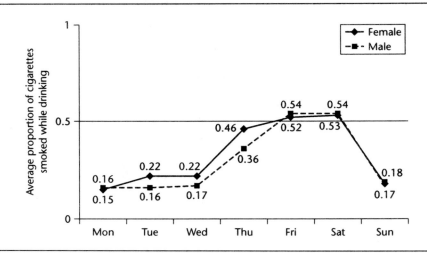

Christmas Day when the students were probably with their parents, who may not know of their smoking. The highest day was seven days later—you guessed it—New Year's Eve.

New Strategies for the Measurement of Behavioral Variables. There is every reason to believe that with improvements in technology there will be a number of new and exciting ways to measure health-related behaviors, which are vitally important to health promotion in particular and to public health in general. One of the more recent developments has been the personal digital assistant (PDA) and the hand-held computer, while there has been a parallel development in observational approaches for data collection known as Ecological Momentary Assessment (EMA). EMA is an outstanding example of an innovative strategy made possible with technological advancements. EMA can greatly improve the reliability and validity of measures pertaining to smoking behavior.

To illustrate the application of EMA to smoking behavior, it is important first to establish several points. The time interval between initially trying cigarettes and becoming a regular user is about two to three years on average. The progression from experimentation to regular use, and often addiction, involves multiple social, psychological, and biological factors, all of which should be measured as reliably and validly as possible. There is evidence that these factors may contribute differentially to stages of transition in smoking. However, this stage categorization may be an artifact of an over-reliance on retrospective questionnaire measures, long periods between observations, and statistical treatment dictums. Only a few studies have examined whether there are differential predictors of stages of smoking. They suggest that stages of transition in smoking may be artificial and that development of dependence on nicotine may be more of a continuum than a switching point. Past research on smoking has usually measured smoking in very gross ways and often on a yearly basis using self-reports of smoking in the past thirty days as "the" measure of smoking. Thus, the lack of precision in some of this research may have contributed to a conceptualization of smoking behavior in "stages" rather than on a continuum.

Although smoking is a behavior exhibited by individuals, smoking among adolescents may occur more frequently within certain contexts. EMA provides a window into the lives of adolescents and serves as a way of examining the influences of specific contexts. EMA is able to capture more accurately than other measurement approaches the frequency, intensity, and tone of social experiences as they occur, as well as the mood associated with those exchanges. EMA data can be collected by PDAs or hand-held computers (Shiffman, 2000). These are used to collect data on adolescents' lives and smoking episodes in real time.

How does EMA work? One study by Mermelstein and her colleagues had the adolescents carry PDAs for seven consecutive days every six months (Mermelstein, Hedegar, and Flay, in press). They were trained to respond to *random prompt interviews* (the PDA or hand-held is programmed to beep randomly, thereby prompting participants to answer questions) and also to self-initiate recordings both of smoking episodes and of no-smoke events (defined as times when the adolescent considers smoking, has an opportunity to smoke, but makes an active decision not to smoke). The interviews took approximately sixty to ninety seconds to complete and asked about mood, activity (what the adolescent was doing), companionship (with whom or alone), presence of other smokers, where they were, and other behaviors (eating, drinking, substance use). At the end of each data-collection week, adolescents underwent an extensive semistructured qualitative interview about their experiences during the week and also reported on their past six-month smoking through a *time-line follow-back interview*. In this type of interview, study participants are asked to recall events as they occurred (that is, in chronological order).

So, do EMAs facilitate adolescents' reporting of their smoking behavior? The average number of random prompts answered during the week of data collection was 33.5. The average number of missed prompts was 5.7. On average, the adolescents answered 85 percent of the random prompt interviews. A total of 89 percent of the prompts were answered within three minutes. There may be times when adolescents can't answer a prompt. In this measurement strategy they can suspend the hand-held computer for up to two hours at a time when it would be difficult to respond. There was, however, some data loss due to damage to the equipment. In follow-up assessments compliance to prompts was about 90 percent.

Compliance with any data-measurement approach is important. Being able to embed the behavioral patterns in situational contexts is also important. We need to know who is doing what with whom, where, how, and of course, why. The *what*, the behavior, can be readily measured in close to real time using EMA, especially if the PDA or hand-held alerts the participant on multiple occasions every day for some specified period. The *who* involves strategic selection of samples that are meaningfully different on important characteristics. The *with whom* and *where* can be measured by simple questions inserted into the computer program. The *why* is also possible by asking specific questions about proximal events and circumstances, such as those that are occurring at the time the PDA or hand-held beeps and asks the participant to provide some answers. For example, Mermelstein and her colleagues were interested in the association of positive and negative mood with smoking (Mermelstein, Hedegar, and Flay, in press). It appears that among adults who smoke, smoking events are more likely to occur in negative-mood situations (depression, anger, anxious). Among adolescents, many of whom are new smokers, the question was whether smoking events were more likely to occur simultaneously with positive rather than negative mood states.

In addition to measuring behaviors and their contextual influences, another application for EMA is with program evaluation. A good example might be the measurement of the influence of certain media events (a health promotion campaign) to see whether people are exposed to the public service announcement by beeping them following the appearance of the PSA on a particular station. By knowing who is watching what programs, it might be possible to more strategically place the health promotion ads and to tailor them for specific types of individuals.

In addition to using EMA with PDAs and hand-helds, consider other new technologies that are either brand new to the health promotion field or close to being tested. For example, in response to the question of *where* certain behavioral events are occurring, it is now possible for the hand-held computer to use a GPS (global positioning system) technology to pinpoint exactly where the person is when he or she is beeped. To determine *with whom* certain behavioral events are occurring, it is now possible to use cameras built into PDAs and hand-helds to get a picture of the space from all four points of the compass. This may create some problems with regard to human subjects' issues, but the limitation is not with the technology. With regard to *why*, there are a host of portable measurement devices that can simultaneously assess heart rate, blood pressure, and a number of other potentially relevant biometric variables.

Finally, think about the fact that every individual is embedded in a variety of contexts. Think about those contexts as if the individual were a pebble dropped in a calm pool or lake. The circles emanating from the pebble (individual) represent the contexts in which he or she is embedded from the most intimate to the most distal. We need better ways of measuring all of the spaces between the various waves coming from the center. This might include, with regard to smoking, the rules and policies present in the home regarding smoking, the rules and policies regarding smoking at school and the programming designed to prevent or treat smoking, laws regarding point of purchase advertising, the rules and policies regarding environmental tobacco smoke, and the laws that vary from state to state about state excise taxes on tobacco products.

Measurement of Contextual Variables

In the previous section we have outlined a host of issues regarding measurement. In addition to understanding how best to measure the behavior of individuals, we also need to measure the contexts within which they are embedded and the influence of certain contextual factors on behavior. This moves us back into the "population"-based world of public health where, in order to change behavior, we have to implement interventions that have broad reach and penetration— interventions that attempt to change behavior through changing the environmental constraints within which individuals live their lives.

In health promotion we are interested in knowing whether and how individuals change their health-related behaviors over time. We also recognize that individuals are embedded in ecological contexts that have a great deal of influence on these health-related behaviors. To understand who and what needs to be changed, it is critical that these contexts be measured reliably and with validity.

There is a plethora of contexts in which individuals may be embedded. This includes families, peer groups, neighborhoods, communities, counties, states, and nations. There is also a variety of organizational contexts such as schools, religious organizations (church-synagogue-mosque), and work organizations (a particular company or a work group within that company) that are potentially important in understanding how and why behaviors change for some and not for other individuals. We will not describe all of the different ways that each of these contexts can be measured. Instead, we will use one of these contexts, the family, to illustrate the difficulties inherent in the measurement of contextual variables.

In studying changes in health behavior it is possible that families exert an influence on the individuals embedded in them to change, or to not change. Think about this for a moment. If we were to treat *family* as a variable to be measured in a health promotion study, how would you measure it? Would you develop a nominal variable? Families have many different dimensions, and as such, it is important to measure these. One of these dimensions is structure. Structure is composed of the different roles that individuals play within families. These roles are mother, father, child, only child, oldest child, second, third, and so on child, youngest child, grandmother, grandfather, aunt, uncle, cousin, and so on. Should we try to create a nominal variable that includes all of the potential structures? If so, then this variable would have too many attributes, rendering the variable impractical for application. In the 1960s Sheppard Kellam and his colleagues began a longitudinal study of first-graders and their families who lived in Woodlawn, a neighborhood in Chicago. Virtually all of the residents of Woodlawn were African American. Kellam asked a rather simple question of these first-graders and their mothers to obtain a measure of family structure. He asked, Who lives with you? The answer was surprising. While many of the first-graders were living in so-called traditional family structures (mother-father-children, mother-children, father-children), overall, there were close to seventy-five different family structures in that one neighborhood. Many of these structures did not have many people in them, but they were nevertheless each a unique family structure (Kellam, Ensminger, and Turner, 1977).

So, how would a public health researcher characterize family context as a variable in this type of situation? Before we decide how to measure family context, perhaps we could use the research hypothesis to guide us. The hypothesis guiding the Kellam research was that children would be more likely to exhibit psychological well-being and social adaptation if they were in an intact family. Intact was defined as living in the presence of both a mother and a father. Family could therefore be a nominal variable—intact or not. However, what could be done to recognize the heterogeneity in the family structure variable? One option is to create *dummy variables* that allow for the comparison of the intact-family category to each of the other seventy-four family categories. Dummy variables are considered nominal variables that distinguish two or more attributes of the variable and can be used to code information concerning group membership into a series of binary distinctions (Bakeman, 1992, p. 205). One category (for example, intact-family) would be used as the referent category, and each of the other categories would be compared to it. The referent category would be coded as zero, and every other category (for example, the other family structures) would be coded as 1. A few examples from the Kellam study, which used a dummy variable coding scheme, follow.

Referent category = mother-father-child   coded as   0
Referent category = Mother-child   coded as   1

Referent category = mother-father-child   coded as   0
Referent category = Father-child   coded as   1

Reference category = mother-father-child   coded as   0
Referent category = Mother-grandmother-child   coded as   1
[Kellam, Ensminger, and Turner, 1977]

As shown, in this approach, every structural combination would be compared to the referent category, and thus the influence of each structure on the outcome variables (psychological well-being and social adaptation) could be assessed.

The importance of this approach is apparent from what Kellam and his colleagues found when these first-graders were studied again in their teen years. As teenagers, children who lived with their mother and had another adult present, regardless of who that other person was, were less likely to be involved in drug use and other forms of delinquent behavior. The conclusion was rather dramatic and counter to common beliefs of society at that time. It was that father absence is less important in predicting psychological well-being and social adaptation in children than mother aloneness. We believe this conclusion is profound because Kellam began his study at about the same time that the federal government claimed that the African American family (notice that the government did not recognize the heterogeneity) was in deep trouble because of the absence of the black male in the family. The larger lesson here is that measurement is important because it establishes boundaries and directions for the analysis, which in turn can have profound effects on the findings, interpretation, and implications of the study.

◆ ◆ ◆

In a Nutshell

Measurement is important because it establishes boundaries and directions for the analysis, which in turn can have profound effects on the findings, interpretation, and implications of the study.

◆ ◆ ◆

Applied Example

To apply some of the issues discussed, we have selected an example that pertains to how the Internet might influence certain health behaviors. The study is ongoing and has several components. One important component of the study assesses the feasibility of recording participants' Web use. One of the major strengths of the proposed research is that it measures the effects of exposure to sexual content on the Web by capturing participants' *actual exposure* to sexual content as opposed to relying entirely on self-reported exposure. This approach is possible because all Web pages visited by participants are stored, processed, and viewed electronically. The process of tracking Web usage and screening Web pages for sexual content is automated. Proprietary technology is used to allow the tracking of all the Web sites visited by individuals by running all household Web activity through a proxy server. This technology allows for capturing the URLs of Web sites visited by the study volunteers. A unique and tailored algorithm is employed. It is based on key words and predesignated categorizations to "bucket" Web sites that are coded as "adult," and to reduce the number of Web pages to be coded. This procedure results in a queue to be viewed and content analyzed for sexually explicit and sexually oriented images and text by human coders. All data are recorded using only a unique study identifier. Data are then encrypted and stored on a secured server.

Integration with the Research Process

Although measurement (step 5 in the nine-step model) appears to be a "middle step," it actually permeates decision making in steps 1 and 2. Implicit in this chapter, the measures selected must be tailored to the needs (literacy and culture) of the selected priority population. An index, for example, might have established reliability and validity for use with African American women. Does this mean that the same index will be reliable and valid for white women, Latinas, or African American men? The answer, of course, is no. The degree to which indicators constitute a construct is a function of the study population.

In a Nutshell

The degree to which indicators constitute a construct is a function of the study population.

The research question should also be selected with a priori attention to the question of measurement. If the research question entails assessment of a behavior such as smoking, then asking, Can I perform a procedure such as EMA? may be wise question before proceeding to set up the research project. As demonstrated in this chapter, a simple retrospective recall assessment of smoking may be far less than rigorous. The point, then, is to ensure that your available resources can match the implied needs of your research question relative to measurement.

This chapter has also shown that measurement decisions potentially can have a dramatic bearing on the research findings. This point should be at the forefront of thought when the findings are being disseminated. Part of disseminating your findings involves listing the limitations of your study (see Chapter Fourteen). Without question, the most common limitations are those related to measurement. This is particularly true with respect to the issue of validity (again, this is also why Chapter Ten addresses the validity of self-reported measures in greater detail).

Summary

Achieving rigor in measurement can be a vast undertaking. Once the level of measurement (nominal, ordinal, interval, or ratio) for any given variable is determined, the task is to decide how the variable will be used. Essentially, the research team must determine what variables will be designated as predictor variables (or correlates if a cross-sectional design has been used), mediating variables, moderating variables, and outcome variables. If the design is experimental, the same question applies, except the terms *independent variable* and *dependent variable* replace *predictor* and *outcome*, respectively. Once all the necessary variables have been identified, the task becomes one of determining how each will be measured. For variables that represent constructs, the additional task is to create an operational definition of the concept being measured. Although variables such as age, gender, income, and education level are relatively easy to measure, the assessment of variables such as smoking frequency or self-esteem may pose tremendous challenges to the research team. This challenge brings several issues to the table. Among these issues are the length of the recall period, the wording of the question(s), the response alternatives, and the technique that will be employed to actually collect the data. Although long-standing techniques such as paper-and-pencil questionnaires may serve the research question well, advances in technology have created a host of new options that may add to the validity of the measure. Moreover, these innovations may be very useful for assessing the context of behavior rather than simply the behavior in isolation.

Issues to Consider

1. Given that *how* a variable is measured can greatly influence the obtained value, it may be critically important to consider how findings from any given study may have been much different based on the use of a different measurement protocol. For example, a descriptive study may conclude that "49 percent of American teens report they have ever smoked a cigarette." Such a finding would result from the use of a question that simply asked teens, Have you

ever smoked a cigarette? The issue to consider is, What value does this type of information have for health promotion research and public health?

2. Suppose that you read a journal article which concludes, "Our findings support the hypothesis that women who have low self-esteem are less likely to eat a balanced diet than women who do not have low self-esteem." The finding is intriguing. But, upon reflection, you remember reading that the inter-item reliability alpha for the measure of self-esteem was .59. You also find no evidence in the article that the measure of self-esteem was validated. Unfortunately, this type of scenario is all too common in health promotion research. The issue, then, is, How can this type of potentially misleading dissemination be avoided?

For Practice and Discussion

1. Please refer back to the first Issue to Consider. You may have answered that the value is quite small because the measure does not capture habitual use. More specifically, the question that is not addressed is, What percentage of American teens smoke cigarettes habitually? Given this research question, how would you proceed to measure "habitual use"?

2. Please return for a moment to the second Issue to Consider. Imagine that you have decided to replicate this study. How would you go about achieving each of the following tasks?
   - Operationalize isolation
   - Identify indicators of isolation
   - Establish reliability of the index
   - Establish face and content validity of the index
   - Collect data from women without recall periods of more than forty-eight hours

3. Please return for a moment to the portion of this chapter that describes EMA. In particular, the data shown in Figure 9.3 are quite striking. These data suggest the possibility that the finely tuned measures may produce results that have previously been masked by the use of less precise measures. While EMA has been applied to the outcome variables of smoking behaviors and sexual behaviors, it is nonetheless a relatively new technology as applied to health promotion research. Please identify at least three other outcome variables (or dependent variables) that you believe would have a much different complexion if they were assessed by EMA rather than traditional retrospective recall methods.

References

Andrews, F. M., and Withey, S. B. (1976). *Social indicators of well-being: Americans' perceptions of life quality.* New York: Plenum.

Bakeman, R. (1992). *Understanding social science statistics: A spreadsheet approach.* Hillsdale, NJ: Erlbaum.

Beck, A. T., Ward, C. H., Mendelson, M., Mock, J., and Erbaugh, J. (1961). An inventory for measuring depression. *Archives of General Psychiatry, 4,* 561–571.

Department of Health and Human Services. (2000). Healthy people 2010. Retrieved March 10, 2005, from www.health.gov/healthypeople.

Ghiselli, E. E., Campbell, J. P., and Zedeck, S. (1982). *Measurement theory for the behavioral sciences.* New York: W. H. Freeman.

Kellam, S. G., Ensminger, M. E., and Turner, R. J. (1977). Family structure and the mental health of children. *Archives of General Psychiatry, 34,* 1012–1022.

Mermelstein, R., Hedegar, D., & Flay, B. (in press). Real-time capture and adolescent cigarette smoking: Moods and smoking. In A. Stone, S. Shiffman, and A. Atienza (Eds.), *The science of real-time data capture: Self-report health research.* New York: Oxford University Press.

Radloff, L. S. (1977). The CES-D scale: A self-report depression scale for research in the general population. *Applied Psychological Measurement, 1*(3), 385–401.

Rosenberg, M. (1989). *Society and the adolescent self-image* (Rev. ed.). Middletown, CT: Wesleyan University Press.

Shiffman, S. (2000). Real-time self-report of momentary states in the natural environment: Computerized ecological momentary assessment. In A. A. Stone (Ed.), *The science of self-report: Implications for research and practice.* Mahwah, NJ: Lawrence Erlbaum.

Streiner, D. L. (2003). Being inconsistent about consistency: When coefficient alpha does and doesn't matter. *Journal of Personality Assessment, 80*(3), 217–222.

CHAPTER TEN

IMPROVING VALIDITY OF SELF-REPORTS FOR SENSITIVE BEHAVIORS

Rick S. Zimmerman, Katherine A. Atwood, and Pamela K. Cupp

The important outcomes in health promotion research and interventions are often behaviors, such as smoking, condom use, and breast self-examination. For a variety of reasons, people often feel a bit uncomfortable about telling the truth in reporting health or risk behaviors, lest they feel they have let their educators or instructors down (for example, what foods they have eaten that they weren't supposed to eat or how often (or little) they came to the gym to work out), or they may not feel comfortable talking about other behaviors at all (for example, about marijuana use or having sex without a condom).

◆ ◆ ◆

In a Nutshell

People often feel a bit uncomfortable about telling the truth in reporting health or risk behaviors.

◆ ◆ ◆

V alid and reliable measurements of sensitive risk behaviors, such as drug use and sexual behaviors, are important for a number of reasons. Accurate measurements of sensitive behaviors allow researchers to estimate their prevalence in the population, which is needed for adequate resource allocation and planning. Careful measurement of these behaviors helps researchers assess the characteristics of the person and the environment associated with risk, and aids in the development of theoretical models of behavior change. In addition, valid and reliable measurements of sensitive behaviors allow for more rigorous evaluation of the very programs designed to reduce their prevalence in the population.

This chapter focuses on how to address threats to validity when measuring sensitive behaviors. For the purposes of illustration, we focus on two sensitive behaviors, drug use and sexual activity. We use these examples to demonstrate how biases can emerge when obtaining estimates of self-reported behaviors and what can be done during the design and administration of surveys to reduce these biases.

Illustration of Key Concepts

We will present the chapter in two sections. First, we present issues to consider related to cognitive processes in improving validity of reports of sensitive behaviors. Second, we present issues to consider related to situational factors in improving validity of these self-reports. We conclude by reviewing evidence about the use of objective or unobtrusive measures to provide additional validation of survey responses.

Validity and Reliability

Let's start by defining what we mean when we talk about validity and reliability and then clarify the focus of this chapter. First, validity has two kinds of possible meanings in research: sometimes we talk about the (internal or external) validity of a study or research design, but we can also talk about validity of a measure. The internal validity of a study or research design is the extent to which we are able to derive clear, causal conclusions from our study; the external validity of a study or research design is the extent to which we are able to generalize to a specific population or other populations beyond those involved in our study.

Our focus in this chapter is on the validity of measures used in health promotion interventions and research. Validity is the degree to which a survey item and its response alternatives measure the phenomenon they are suppose to measure (Bainbridge, 1989). Put differently, it is the extent to which our variables in fact measure the constructs we intend for them to measure. For example, it has been reported that some scientists in the early 1900s believed that one's hat size was associated with intelligence. However, we know that this is not true. So asking about someone's hat size is not a valid measure of intelligence (Bainbridge, 1989). There are several different kinds of validity of measures: two types related to the issues to be discussed in this chapter are *construct validity* and *criterion validity.* Construct validity is defined as the extent to which a measure relates to other measures in theoretically predictable ways. Construct validity can be assessed in studies of adolescent sexual behavior by examining how age of initiation of sexual activity is related to age of initiation of alcohol use, cigarette or marijuana smoking, or frequency of delinquent behaviors, as these behaviors often have been found in previous research to be related to early initiation of sexual activity. A measure can be considered to have strong construct validity when it is significantly correlated with these other variables, or these other factors account for a reasonable proportion of the variance in the sexual behavior measure.

◆ ◆ ◆

In a Nutshell

Validity is the degree to which a survey item and its response alternatives measure the phenomenon they are suppose to measure.

◆ ◆ ◆

Criterion validity is the relationship of a measure to an outcome to which, by the very definition of the measure, it should be related. The SAT (scholastic aptitude test) was created to predict college success; the correlations between the SAT and measures of college success are ways to assess the criterion validity of the SAT. If a self-report measure of condom use were to have high criterion validity, it should be related to a measure of condom sales in the community. If, for people treated for any current STDs, it is unrelated to incidence of new STDs over the next six months, it would be said to have low criterion validity. Both of these types of validity are used by researchers in assessing the validity of measures, and will be referred to throughout the chapter.

Besides validity, the other key dimension for assessing the quality of a measure is reliability. *Reliability* is the degree to which a measure produces stable and consistent results (Bainbridge, 1989). It is important to note that a measure cannot be valid without also being reliable. If a measure of condom use yields different responses every time a respondent answers the measure, how could it possibly be a good, that is, valid, measure of condom use? However, an item can be reliable (give consistent results) and not be valid; asking people how many fingers they have will provide consistent results, though it is probably not a valid measure of number of sexual partners in the past twelve months for most respondents. Because of this relationship between reliability and validity, that reliability is a necessary though not sufficient condition for validity, evidence of reliability can yield greater confidence about the validity of the measure, and so some of the data presented in this chapter concerning validity also references evidence about reliability of measures.

In the section that follows, we discuss the sources of validity problems that may emerge when obtaining self-report data on sensitive behavior. To help organize the discussion about threats to validity, we use Brener and colleagues' definitions of two theoretical perspectives, under which most threats to validity can be organized: (1) cognitive processes and (2) situational processes (Brener, Billy, and Grady, 2003). *Cognitive processes* are defined as the "mental processes underlying self-reported data." These processes are responsible for the inaccurate reporting of events that arise from problems with comprehension of the survey question, recalling relevant events, and placing them in the appropriate time frame (Brener, Billy, and Grady, 2003). *Situational processes* are defined as "problems that arise from factors related to social desirability and interviewing conditions" (Brener, Billy, and Grady, 2003).

Threats to Validity of Self-Report Data Due to Cognitive Processes

The cognitive process of retrieving information from one's memory is said to involve four distinct steps, though more detailed models have been developed to describe this process of retrieval (Oksenberg and Cannell, 1977; Cannell, Miller, and Oksenberg, 1981; Means, Habina, Swan, and Jack, 1992). Threats to validity can occur at each of these steps (Brener, Billy, and Grady, 2003).

Step 1: Comprehension of the Question. The first step involves comprehension of the question. Comprehension is the way in which the respondent understands the question. Understanding involves prior knowledge and experience, how the interviewer interacts with the respondent, perceived goals of the research, and implicit messages communicated by previous survey questions (Means, Habina, Swan, and Jack, 1992).

Step 2: Retrieval of Information. The second step involves retrieval of the information. Retrieval of information requires scanning one's memory and rebuilding the event based on what can be retrieved and then "filling in the gaps" to produce a coherent response (Means, Habina, Swan, and Jack, 1992; Loftus, Smith, Johnson, and Fiedler, 1988). The respondent is often unable to distinguish between what comes directly from his or her memory bank and what has been reconstructed. The process of "reconstruction" allows respondents to provide responses to questions, instead of blurred memories, but can also lead to inaccurate reporting (Loftus, Smith, Johnson, and Fiedler, 1988).

Step 3: Judgment Process. The third step is when one assesses whether the information retrieved is sufficient, referred to as the judgment process. If the information is insufficient, additional retrieval attempts are made. Even after repeated retrieval attempts, the information that is retrieved will not necessarily conform to the parameters of the question. The respondent may use his or her own heuristics (which vary from person to person) to arrive at an estimate, based on the information retrieved (Means, Habina, Swan, and Jack, 1992).

Step 4: Response Generation. The last step is response generation. During this step, the retrieval information is reviewed to assess the extent to which the response is reflective of the respondent's belief system (Brener, Billy, and Grady, 2003) and whether the response meets the needs of the interviewer (see Figure 10.1). Situational factors such as the setting and circumstances of survey administration can affect these four steps of cognitive processing. Brener and colleagues (2003) point out that cognitive and situational factors can overlap or act independently to create bias in survey responses.

Now that we have described the cognitive processes involved in information retrieval and response formulation, let us turn our attention to what can be done when designing surveys to reduce inaccurate reporting of sensitive behaviors.

FIGURE 10.1. MODEL OF THE COGNITIVE PROCESS OF INFORMATION RETRIEVAL.

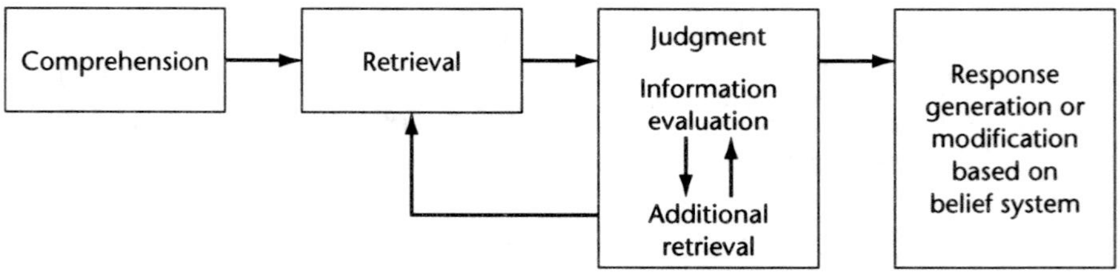

Source: Brener, Billy, and Grady, 2003.

Frequency and Timing. One of the challenges of survey construction is how to word questions about sensitive behaviors to yield accurate responses. The retrieval of information from one's memory is made even more challenging when the behavior involves licit or illicit drug use. A general rule is, the simpler the question, the more accurate the reporting. For example, it is easier to remember whether you have ever engaged in a behavior (such as using a drug or having sexual intercourse) than having to estimate the numbers of times you have engaged in that specific behavior in the past thirty days or in the past year.

◆ ◆ ◆

In a Nutshell

A general rule is, the simpler the question, the more accurate the reporting.

◆ ◆ ◆

When it is necessary to ask more detailed questions about the frequency of a given behavior, estimates are generally more valid when the question asks about the more recent past and shorter time periods (Brener, Billy, and Grady, 2003; Forsyth, Lessler, and Hubbard, 1992). For example, in the substance abuse research, Bachman and O'Malley found that asking high school seniors about the past thirty days of drug use yielded year-long prevalence rates that were approximately three times larger than reports of use in the past year (Bachman and O'Malley, 1981). They reached these estimates by extrapolating twelve months of use from usage over the past thirty days. Their findings were consistent across licit and illicit drugs and different levels of use. In this example it is possible that one of two things were going on: respondents were overreporting their drug use in the shorter time periods, or they were underreporting their use over the past year (Bachman and O'Malley, 1981). It is possible that respondents may overreport behaviors in the past thirty days due to *telescoping*—recollecting events that occur in the past several months and attributing them to the past thirty-day time period. However, researchers tend to concur that as the time from the event increases, the validity of responses deteriorates. This has been found in a wide variety of studies comparing self-report data to external records such as medical records, consumer purchases, and financial statements. For example, in a recent study that examined participants' reports of drug use during sex, fewer inaccuracies were found when the event occurred more recently than when the event occurred in the more distant past (Bell, Montoya, and Atkinson, 2000). In these cases respondents tend not to remember events as well in the distant past as they do in the more recent past.

Although recalling events in the more recent past may improve accuracy, there are some drawbacks to this approach. A thirty-day time period, for example, may not be long enough to capture sufficient numbers of events for meaningful statistical analysis. This is often the case when researching adolescent sexual or drug use behaviors. In these cases, researchers may need to rely on questions that ask about past behaviors over longer time periods.

When surveying substance-using populations, especially treatment populations (in other words, people currently receiving therapy for their addictions), measurement issues can be even more complex. Treatment populations tend to provide more valid estimates of use when the measurement is *more distant* than more recent (Willis, 1997). Substance users are more willing to report past drug use than recent use due to socially desirable responding or fears of reprisal. For example, treatment populations in particular may fear that if they admit to recent drug use certain benefits may be taken away, or others will hold less than favorable opinions about them. Parallel results were found for reports of masturbation, a sensitive sexual behavior which young adult males said they had done as adolescents at much higher rates than they had reported while adolescents (Halpern, Udry, Suchindran, and Campbell, 2000).

Like all elements of designing and implementing research, one must constantly weigh the costs and benefits of certain approaches to survey measurement. For example, in surveys for active drug users, the quality of the information may be compromised when asking about behaviors in the distant past. However, this bias must be weighed against possible invalid reporting of recent drug use if respondents revise their answers to present themselves in a more favorable light.

Retrospective or Longitudinal Assessment of Change.
The way that time is conceptualized and assessed in surveys may affect the validity of self-report data in that respondents are asked to measure their own levels of change. Due to the very nature of cross-sectional surveys (data collection at one time point only), if one is interested in assessing respondents' change in some behaviors or attitudes, one must ask the respondent to *estimate* his or her change over time. However, in longitudinal designs, researchers can assess differences between reports of attitudes or behaviors at two or more time points by calculating differences between those reports given at different times. Which assessment strategy is more valid? Common sense, as well as many studies conducted to assess results of interventions, suggests that people are prone to overreport positive changes when reporting retrospectively, as compared with researchers' calculations of differences between pre- and postintervention change. Some recent research, however, suggests that

under certain circumstances, retrospective reports may be more accurate (Stone, Catania, and Binson, 1999).

Placement and the Sequencing of Questions. Decisions about the order of survey questions involve a series of strategic decisions. In some circumstances, such as in face-to-face interviews, when it is important for the interviewer to develop a relationship with the respondent, the placement of questions within the survey may make a difference (that is, whether toward the beginning, in the middle, or near the end). For example, to increase the likelihood that respondents will answer sensitive questions, the optimal place for them is in the middle of the survey. By this time, rapport has been established and respondents will have successfully answered questions about less emotionally charged topics. Conversely, by the end of the survey participants may be experiencing fatigue, boredom, or annoyance with the survey process (Bachman and O'Malley, 1981).

However, in self-administered surveys of college students and young adults, other researchers have found that the placement of questions near the beginning, middle, or end of the survey has little impact on the validity of responses to questions about sexual behaviors (Catania, McDermott, and Pollack, 1986). It has been proposed that it is not so much the placement but the "sequencing" or context of questions (near, before, or after certain other questions) that may affect validity (Catania, Binson, Van der Straten, and Stone, 1995). For example, asking questions about a person's attitudes about a specific behavior first may affect the "social meaning" (Catania, Binson, Van der Straten, and Stone, 1995) of the behavior and reduce socially desirable responding about the behavior. Johnson found that married couples reported higher levels of extramarital affairs when questions about their attitudes about affairs preceded questions about having an affair, as compared to reported levels of infidelity when attitude questions appeared after behavior questions (Johnson, 1970). It is suggested that attitudinal questions implicitly communicate to the respondent that they will not be judged for having attitudes that support these behaviors or for engaging in these behaviors (Catania, Binson, Van der Straten, and Stone, 1995).

Daily Data Collection. Daily data collection is another approach that is used to increase the accuracy of self-report data and reduce measurement error by reducing errors attributable to retrospective recall. Using this method the respondent completes either a daily diary or a phone interview detailing his or her daily behaviors. Those involved in a diary study make notes about their target behaviors and send the diary back to the research team at scheduled intervals (for example, each day or each week). One advantage of daily diaries over the phone interview method is that the respondent has greater flexibility since he or she doesn't have to schedule phone calls with the research team. However, diaries may not be successfully completed and mailed, particularly among higher-risk populations who tend to lead disruptive lives and experience low literacy rates. Another benefit of daily diaries over telephone interviews is that the data may be less affected by socially desirable responding because the diaries are completed privately. Using the phone interview approach, either the interviewer or the respondent initiates a daily call to obtain or provide information about behaviors that occurred since the last call. Having the respondent initiate contact with the research staff leads to increased flexibility for the participant; however if the respondent forgets to call, entire days of recording can be missed (Morrison, Leigh, and Rogers, 1999). The advantage of having the interviewer initiate contact with the respondent is that missing days may be minimized because the burden is left on the interviewer to reach the respondent; however disconnected phones can become a significant problem for transient populations. In addition, the interviewer may call when others are present, introducing further bias if the participant responds differently because of the presence of a third party.

There are significant drawbacks to either of these methods. In each of these approaches, researchers tend to include both sensitive and nonsensitive behaviors (for example, physical activities levels, care use) and to nest hypotheses into a larger questionnaire about health behaviors to reduce socially desirable responding (Morrison, Leigh, and Rogers, 1999). Unfortunately, this leads to longer questionnaires. A final concern is *reactivity*. Reactivity has been described as changes in behavior that occur due to the frequent recording of the behavior and the implicit message that this behavior is nondesirable or merits changing (Fremouw and Brown, 1980; Gillmore and others, 2001). It is problematic if surveys designed to simply *assess* behaviors implicitly encourage *change* in these behaviors. The research literature is mixed regarding the extent to which reactivity affects the validity of data collected using daily collection strategies (Fremouw and Brown, 1980; Gillmore and others, 2001).

In response to some of these concerns, a more innovative method that has been used is the *experience sampling method*. Using this method a respondent is paged, or beeped, at random times during the day, and he or she provides responses at that moment. This method can reduce recall bias and reactivity because respondents are more likely to remember the event, cannot anticipate when they will be contacted, and will have less opportunity to alter or rehearse responses. This method may *not* be useful for behaviors such as sexual intercourse that do not occur at predictable times, nor appropriate for institutional settings, where beeping the respondent may be considered intrusive (Kubey, Larson, and Csikszentmihalyi, 1996). Table 10.1 summarizes the discussion of the past several pages, presenting

TABLE 10.1.   ADVANTAGES AND DISADVANTAGES OF APPROACHES RELATED TO COGNITIVE FACTORS.

Survey Construction	Advantages	Disadvantages
1. Frequency and timing	Enhances recall	Problematic for sporadic behaviors
Dichotomous questions	Yields higher prevalence	May over-report due to telescoping
More recent reports	Improves accuracy	Reduces number of events for statistical analysis
2. Retrospective versus longitudinal reports of changes	Not well understood	Not well understood
3. Placement and sequencing	Middle of interview best Appropriate context may yield higher prevalence	
4. Daily data collection	Enhances recall	Significant respondent burden May be inappropriate for sporadic behaviors or less stable populations Increased recall bias if diaries completed days later Reactivity possible

advantages and disadvantages of various survey approaches that relate to cognitive factors in the completion of those surveys.

Threats to Validity of Self-Reports Due to Situational Processes

Situational factors are defined as "characteristics of the external environment" (Brener, Billy, and Grady, 2003). Situational factors are factors related to socially desirable responding and interviewing conditions, such as the real or perceived level of privacy and confidentiality, characteristics of the interviewer, and method of survey administration. Social desirability and fear of reprisal are two forms of bias that may be reduced or exacerbated by situational factors such as the setting and method of survey administration; how privacy and confidentiality are explained, perceived, and adhered to; characteristics of the interviewer; and how research is perceived within the broader community. Socially desirable responding takes place when subjects respond to questions in such a way that their responses will leave a more favorable impression on others (DeMaio, 1984). For example,

MINCUS HAS DOUBTS ABOUT SELF-REPORTED BEHAVIOR.

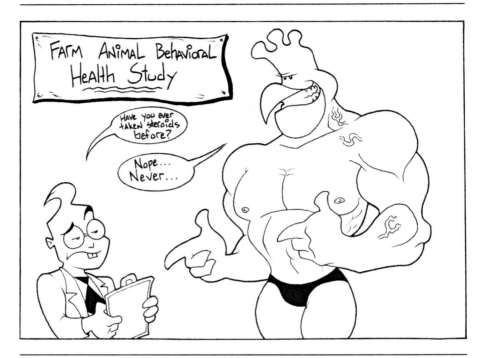

Copyright 2005 by Justin Wagner; reprinted with permission.

respondents may be less inclined to report current drug use if an interviewer administers the survey as opposed to the survey being self-administered.

Fears of reprisal are a second threat to validity that can be affected by situational factors. For example, fear of reprisal may arise when interviewing adolescents or in-treatment populations about illicit drug use; respondents may be concerned that this information could be disclosed to others such as administrators, parents, or teachers. In the following sections we review a variety of situational factors and examine how they may affect the validity of survey responses.

Mode of Survey Administration. Overall, respondents tend to report a higher prevalence of sensitive behaviors when the survey is self-administered—in other words, completed by the subject, rather than by the interviewer. Self-administered questionnaires (SAQ) have been found to yield a higher prevalence for a number of sensitive behaviors including drug and alcohol use, condom use, and number of sexual partners when compared with face-to-face interviews or telephone surveys (Catania, Gibson, Chitwood, and Coates, 1990; Aquilino and LoSciuto, 1990; Gfroerer and Hughes, 1991; Turner and others, 1998; Tourangeau, Jobe, Pratt, and Rasinski, 1997; Boekeloo and others, 1994).

Despite the higher prevalence of sensitive behaviors reported on self-administered questionnaires, there are some advantages to an interviewer-administered survey that should not be overlooked. For example, interviewer-administered questionnaires can significantly reduce the number of missed questions and help to ensure completeness of the interview. If the questionnaire has a more sophisticated design, interviewers also can successfully move the client through the instrument to prevent navigational problems. Many of these former "advantages" of interviews, discussed in reviews and textbooks in the 1960s through the early 1990s, can now be addressed within self-administered surveys using computer-enhanced data-collection techniques.

Computer-Enhanced Data Collection. One of the significant challenges to the validity of self-administered surveys is literacy. Recent developments in computer-assisted and audio-computer-assisted self-interviewing (A-CASI) have helped overcome measurement problems that were due to low literacy levels. These newly emerging technologies have been found to increase perceptions of privacy and reduce social desirability bias, as well as enable respondents to understand both questions and responses and to navigate complex surveys. Computer-assisted software programs have been found to yield higher rates of responding about alcohol, drug use, and sexual-risk behaviors when compared to self-administered paper surveys or interview-administered surveys. In the 1995 National Survey of Adolescent Males, subjects were randomly assigned to an A-CASI ($n = 1,361$) survey condition or self-administered paper survey condition ($n = 368$) (Turner and others, 1998). Males randomized to the A-CASI condition were significantly more likely to report engaging in some type of male-to-male sexual contact (5.5 percent versus 1.5 percent) and in injection drug use (5.2 percent versus 1.4 percent), when compared with those randomized to the paper questionnaire condition (Turner and others, 1998). They were also more likely to report other sensitive behaviors including being drunk or high during sex or having sex with someone who injected drugs. Other researchers have found that while adolescents reported higher rates of drug and alcohol use via computer-assisted assessment, young adults did not (Wright, Aquilino, and Supple, 1998). The observed effects for adolescents varied by level of stigmatization of the drug in question. For example, questions about less sensitive drugs, such as ever smoking a cigarette or ever use of alcohol, were less affected by the mode of survey administration than those about more stigmatized drugs (Wright, Aquilino, and Supple, 1998). The researchers also found that adolescents had fewer concerns about privacy and had more positive attitudes toward computer technology than did older participants (Wright, Aquilino, and Supple, 1998).

While computer-assisted technologies have been heralded as innovative and have allowed for more sophisticated survey design, some classroom-based studies using A-CASI have found no difference in prevalence estimates when compared with self-administered paper surveys (Hallfors, Khatapoush, Kadushin, Watson, and Saxe, 2000). In addition, computer-assisted technologies may be prohibitively expensive and physically cumbersome when surveying large samples. Other considerations include attention to detail in downloading and saving data and, particularly if the research occurs in high-crime areas, issues of safe transport and storage.

Three other computer-enhanced data-collection methods are telephone A-CASI (T-ACASI), touchtone data entry (TTDE), and audio-enhanced personal digital assistant (APDA) technologies. In the T-ACASI methodology, either respondents call in and listen to an interviewing system that asks questions in a standardized, prerecorded way (stopping for responses by use of the touchtone pad), or a human interviewer calls the respondent and then switches over to the recorded interview when the respondent is ready. Unlike typical phone interviews, questions are asked in a standardized way and privacy is provided even if others are in the same room through the use of the telephone touchtone pad. In the TTDE application, human interviewers ask questions over the phone that are responded through use of the touchtone pad. The APDA method involves the use of small, hand-held personal digital assistants (Palm Pilots and similar devices) by students completing surveys in the classroom, with an audio channel via earphones that "reads" the survey to the students. The technology is very similar to A-CASI, but is significantly less expensive, takes up less space, and provides a greater sense of privacy for respondents. Results to date indicate that T-ACASI (Gribble, Miller, Rogers, and Turner, 1999) and TTDE systems (Blumberg, Cynamon, Osborn, and Olson, 2003) yield greater reports of sensitive behaviors than do more traditional telephone interviewing methods, suggesting greater validity of responses. The APDA technology is still in initial testing phases by a small number of researchers, but initial results suggest it can be used effectively, is perceived as providing greater privacy, and yields less missing data than do self-administered questionnaires (Trapl and others, forthcoming). Between the time this chapter was written and the time you are reading it, undoubtedly some of the information about the usefulness of various existing technologies provided here will no longer be accurate, and new technologies not available now will probably be used to improve the validity of self-reported responses of sensitive behaviors.

Internet-Based Data Collection. Increasingly, Internet- (or Web-) based surveys are becoming standard practice. A primary advantage of Web-based surveys involves access to respondents, as researchers clearly have easy access to a variety of populations via the Web that would require more time and resources to recruit elsewhere (from general adolescent and college student populations to marginalized populations such as gay men and transgender individuals). But with that access comes questions about external validity: are those who access and respond to surveys on the Internet different in substantive and meaningful ways from respondents who might have been accessed using more standard or more random sampling procedures? Answers to this question are only beginning to emerge and seem to vary considerably across populations. They are also not directly relevant to the central issue of this chapter, as this chapter is concerned with the validity of measures and not external validity.

More relevant to our concerns here is whether responses to Web-based surveys and surveys completed in other formats (interviews, self-administered paper-and-pencil surveys, or A-CASI surveys) demonstrate comparable validity. The small amount of data available to date suggest that Web-based surveys may produce about the same level of reports of alcohol and illicit substance use as do mail or self-administered questionnaires and yield similar levels of reliability of measures. However, levels of missing data may be greater for respondents to Web-based surveys (Mustanski, 2001; Smith, 2003; McCabe, Boyd, Couper, Crawford, and D'Arch, 2002; Lenert and Skoczen, 2002; and McCabe, 2004).

Interviewer Effects. The effective training of interviewers is a key element in obtaining valid data. Regardless of the shared demographic characteristics or life experiences of the interviewer and the respondent, it is the degree to which the interviewer is able to accomplish the following that is most important: (1) enlist the cooperation of potential research subjects, (2) encourage respondents to answer questions thoughtfully, (3) ask questions in a standardized fashion that does not sway respondents, (4) take his or her time, and (5) be a good listener (Fowler, 1984). For example, if an interviewer rushes through a questionnaire, he or she leaves the impression that the respondent should move quickly, increasing the possibility of error or leaving the impression that the respondent's answers are not important (Fowler, 1984).

Other characteristics that have been assumed to affect validity include the gender, ethnicity, age, or sexual orientation of the interviewer when compared with that of the interviewee. However, it remains an underanswered empirical question as to when and under what circumstances it is necessary to match age, race, sexual orientation, or gender of the respondent and interviewer (Catania, Gibson, Chitwood, and Coates, 1990; Fowler, 1984). Some in the research community believe that both male and female respondents are more likely to report engaging in more stigmatized sexual behaviors to female interviewers than to male interviewers, but these assumptions are based more on anecdotal evidence than recent studies. Recent reviews suggest that the measurement of some sensitive behaviors may in fact yield the most valid responses when interviewers are matched to respondents on demographic characteristics (Catania, 1999).

Setting. The setting where the survey is administered is an additional important situational factor that can affect the validity of self-report data. Some studies suggest that among adolescents there is significant underreporting of sensitive behaviors (including illicit drug use and sexual behaviors) when surveys are completed in the household as compared with school settings (Kann, Brener, Warren, Collins and Giovino, 2002; Gfroerer, Wright, and Kopstein, 1997), although some earlier studies have found no such affects. For example, in an analysis of two national surveys, Kann and colleagues found that of the fourteen behaviors related to alcohol and illicit drug use, students who completed the school-based survey were significantly more likely to report higher levels of alcohol and illicit drug use than were youths responding to the household survey (Kann, Brener, Warren, Collins, and Giovino, 2002). With regard to sexual behaviors, those who completed the school-based survey were significantly more likely to report first intercourse before age thirteen, multiple sex partnerships, and use of alcohol or drugs during their last sexual encounter (Kann, Brener, Warren, Collins, and Giovino, 2002). The comparative analysis did not find differences in prevalence estimates for less stigmatizing behaviors such as physical-activity levels. Kann and colleagues concluded that privacy or perceived privacy is an important element in obtaining valid estimates of stigmatized or illicit behaviors.

When researching substance abuse behaviors among adults in institutional settings, researchers have found that the setting also can have a significant impact on data quality to the extent that respondents perceive that their privacy and confidentiality can or cannot be maintained, with potential fear of reprisal related to significant underreporting in self-report surveys among treatment and incarcerated populations.

Experimental Manipulations to Increase Validity of Self-Reports. A variety of methods to enhance the validity of self-reports have been used by survey researchers using experimental methods, that is, involving significant manipulations beyond such things as word variation and order of questions. Two promising such methods are presented here: the "Bogus Pipeline" procedure and the "Randomized Lists Technique." Information about the first is presented here, and information about the second is presented in Box 10.1.

Box 10.1. The Randomized Lists Technique: A Promising But Experimental Approach to Improving Validity in Surveys

A very interesting, creative, and promising technique to improve the validity of people's self-reports about sensitive behaviors was called by the original author (Miller, 1984) the "Item/Count Paired Lists Technique," and more recently has been called by Zimmerman and Langer (1995) the "randomized lists technique." In this approach the respondent is given a list of behaviors, which includes the sensitive behavior of interest and a set of innocuous (unrelated) items, and is instructed to report the total *number* of activities in the list that he or she has participated in. A second, randomly selected sample of respondents is given a list that is similar in all respects, except that the sensitive behavior has been removed. An estimate of the prevalence of the sensitive behavior is achieved by subtracting the mean count of items reported by respondents who received the list including the sensitive behavior, *minus* the mean count of items reported by respondents who received the list excluding the sensitive behavior. For example, let's say the researcher is interested in how many respondents used marijuana. Half of the sample of respondents then answers how many of the following they have ever done: used marijuana, lied to someone, cheated on a test, kissed someone, or killed someone. The other half indicate how many of the following they have ever done: lied to someone, cheated on a test, kissed someone, or killed someone. If the average number of things done for people responding to the first list is 3.5 and the average number of things done for people responding to the second list is 3.2, the difference of 0.3 (or 30 percent) is then the estimated proportion of people who have used marijuana.

We are aware of six reported studies that have used the technique to assess the prevalence of substance use or sexual behavior. An early test of the technique was promising, but only for young men with less than a higher education who, using this technique, were estimated to have used heroin at a higher rate than when the direct question was asked (Miller and Cisin, 1983); the researchers found little difference between direct and paired lists techniques in prevalence estimates for marijuana and cocaine use in the national household population, however (Miller, Cisin, and Harrell, 1986). Equivocal results were also found in a study conducted by Droitcour and others (1991), which found that prevalence estimates of injecting drug use and receptive anal intercourse were not significantly different from estimates based on direct questions. Some more promising results have been found more recently, however. Wimbush and Dalton (1997) found higher reports for stealing from one's company using the technique than when asking the question directly to respondents. Similarly, Zimmerman and Langer (1995) found higher reports of adolescents having had sex, using marijuana, or having sex with someone of the same gender using this technique than using direct questions, as did LaBrie and Earleywine (2000) when college students were asked about having sex, having had sex without a condom, or having sex without a condom after drinking.

(We think this is a technique that might be used more frequently to assist researchers in obtaining valid prevalence estimates of very sensitive behaviors. We would encourage you to consider using this technique in your own research!)

Researchers, specifically in the smoking-prevention field, have used various forms of the "Bogus Pipeline Procedure" in an effort to increase validity of self-reported use. The Bogus Pipeline Procedure, initially developed by Jones and Sigal (1971), instructs participants that after completion of the survey they will be asked to provide some sort of biologic marker that would presumably verify reported drug use. This procedure is "bogus" because it assures the participant that his or her substance use will be validated by a biologic measure, when it will not. Various "bogus" methods that are used include getting a saliva sample from a cotton swab or having the participant breath into a tube to detect smoking levels. Bogus pipeline procedures must be authentic enough to convince the respondent that the testing procedure can actually verify use (Akers, Massey, Clarke, and Lauer, 1983).

The impact of the Bogus Pipeline Procedure on improving the validity of self-reported data about smoking, alcohol use, and other drug use has been mixed. In many studies, researchers have randomized students either to an intervention condition that includes the Bogus Pipeline Procedure and the completion of a self-reported survey or to a control condition where they complete the self-reported survey only (Campanelli, Dielman, and Shope, 1987). In some cases, students were randomized to a third condition that includes the discussion of the use of the procedure some time in the future but has the students only complete the survey (Werch, Gorman, Marty, Forbess, and Brown, 1987). The purpose of this third condition is to try to answer whether it is the threat of using the procedure or the procedure itself that is associated with increased reporting. Generally, studies have found small or nonsignificant differences in reported levels of drug use, smoking, or alcohol use between these conditions (Werch, Gorman, Marty, Forbess, and Brown, 1987; Akers, Massey, Clarke, and Lauer, 1982). A recent study of the impact of the Bogus Pipeline Procedure on reporting about sexual behaviors found that stereotypical, potentially socially desirable responses reflected in gender differences in reports were smaller in the bogus pipeline condition; this suggests that the Bogus Pipeline Procedure may have yielded more valid responses, in particular involving less overreporting by males and less underreporting by females (Alexander and Fisher, 2003). Table 10.2 summarizes the discussion of the past several pages, presenting the advantages and disadvantages of various survey approaches that relate to situational factors in the completion of those surveys.

TABLE 10.2.   ADVANTAGES AND DISADVANTAGES OF APPROACHES RELATED TO SITUATIONAL FACTORS.

	Advantages	Disadvantages
1. Survey mode: Self	Higher prevalence estimates Reduces socially desirable responding Greater privacy	Cannot ensure completeness Cannot prevent navigational problems
2. Technology-enhanced methods A-CASI T-ACASI TTDE APDA	Reduces socially desirable responding Reduces problems due to low literacy Allows for internal consistency checks Allows for sophisticated branching and skip patterns	May be cumbersome and expensive when surveying large samples Safe storage and transport problematic Risks of losing data if not properly saved
3. Internet-based surveys	Easier access to study samples Access to hidden populations On-line data is collected about survey completion process	Representativeness of sample is unknown or low Concerns about identity and eligibility of respondents
4. Interviewer effects: Training important Matching by demographics to respondent	Reduces social desirable responding Increases comfort level and reports about sensitive topics	May be expensive When and for whom this is important is not well understood
5. Setting: School versus household Treatment facilities Criminal justice systems	Higher prevalence estimates Greater perceived privacy Easier to reach target population Easy to reach hardcore drug users Easier to reach high risk populations	May be problematic for longitudinal studies Underreporting due to socially desirable responding Underreporting posttreatment Underreporting due to fears of reprisal
6. Experimental manipulations Bogus Pipeline Procedure Randomized Lists Technique	Possibly reduces socially desirable responding	Small or nonsignificant impact on reporting Respondent burden

Objective Measures

One of the most persistent criticisms of behavioral research, particularly around sensitive behaviors, is whether self-reports are valid. As discussed so far in this chapter, there is a wide variety of approaches researchers can use within their survey designs and implementations to improve the validity of self-reports. However, even when using a number of these methods, behavioral researchers and medical scientists may still be skeptical of self-reports. Other types of data may be required before a conclusion can be made that relationships among variables or effects of interventions have public health or medical significance. To address this criticism, researchers often compare self-reports to more objective measures that are thought to be less influenced by bias, recall, or socially desirable responding. Thus, while assessments of construct validity and reliability (in other words, correlations to other self-report measures and consistency of the self-report measures themselves, respectively) can contribute to increased confidence in these data, criterion validity (association with outcome data beyond self-reports) may afford an even greater level of confidence about these measures and related results. We will briefly discuss two sorts of these objective measures: biologic measures or markers, and unobtrusive measures.

Biologic Measures or Markers. In the substance abuse literature from the early 1980s, it was generally assumed that self-reports of drug use were valid since validity studies comparing self-reported use with urine testing found similar results. However, at that time urine analysis was less sophisticated than it is now and was less likely to detect drug use; therefore self-reports tended to concur with urine testing (for historical review see Wish, Hoffman, and Nemes, 1997). With the advance of more sophisticated hair and urine testing, the validity of self-reported drug use has been called into question. In addition, with the onslaught of the War on Drugs and stiff prison sentences for possession, reporting of drug use has become a high-risk venture, particularly among treatment and criminal justice populations. A recent meta-analysis of twenty-four validity studies published between 1985 and 1996 compared biochemical measures with self-reported drug use among high-risk populations. Overall, 42 percent of those who tested positive for drug use reported drug use in self-report surveys (Magura and Kang, 1996).

Generally, it has been found that underreporting increases with the severity of the drug, with greater underreporting for cocaine and heroin than for marijuana (Fendrich and Xu, 1994; Mieczkowski, Barzelay, Gropper, and Wish, 1991; Magura and Kang, 1996; Dembo, Williams, Wish, and Schmeidler, 1990). In addition, underreporting seems greatest among criminal justice populations. It is presumed that inmates and arrestees are skeptical of assurances of confidentiality and fear disclosure to those in authority (Magura and Kang, 1996). Other studies have delineated differences in underreporting within incarcerated populations. They found that levels of underreporting were greater among those with more severe criminal offenses (Page, Davies, Ladner, Alfassa, and Tennis, 1977). Among substance abusers, rates of underreporting of drug use are greater after drug treatment than at admission (Magura and Kang, 1996; Hinden and others, 1994), inviting concerns about treatment outcome studies. For example, Hindin and colleagues found that at admission to a residential treatment program, 96 percent of heroin-positive and 89 percent of cocaine-positive clients accurately reported their drug use. At posttreatment, 67 percent of heroin-positive and 51 percent of cocaine-positive users accurately reported their drug use (Hinden and others, 1994). Similarly, Wish and colleagues, in a small study of drug treatment clients, found that 96 percent of clients who tested positive for opiate use at intake reported opiate use. Three months after discharge 46 percent of those who tested positive for opiate use accurately reported their drug use (Wish, Hoffman, and Nemes, 1997), with greater discordance among those who were heavier drug users.

Although self-reported data may be imperfect, biologically assessed measures are not without their drawbacks, including possible contamination, false negatives, limited time windows for detecting the presence of a drug, and considerable expense. There are no extant biologic markers or measures related to sexual behavior that serve as the "gold standard" as urine and hair analysis do for substance use. There are no direct biologic measures to assess whether an individual has had sexual intercourse, has used a condom, or has had a certain number of partners over a given interval of time. However, several measures have been used in preliminary tests.

Udry and Morris (1967) assessed the presence of sperm in women's urine and correlated it to their self-report of recent unprotected intercourse, finding concordance between the two in twelve out of fifteen women. For individuals treated for STDs in a clinic setting, contraction of an incident STD over a period of time can be correlated with self-reported condom use to validate the condom self-report measure; Zenilman and others (1995) found a relatively high, but not perfect, correspondence between the two; 15 percent of men and 23 percent of women who reported always using condoms had new STDs at follow-up. STD testing has increasingly become the "silver standard" for assessment of behavioral effects in interventions related to HIV, pregnancy, or STD prevention. Halpern, Udry, and Suchindran, (1998) report on testosterone as a correlate of levels of sexual activity; this may become useful in validating reports of sexual behavior. More recently, Zenilman, Yuenger, Galai, Turner, and Rogers (2005) have developed a measure to detect the recent presence of sperm in the vaginal cavity of women through assessment of the Y chromosome, indicating recent unprotected sexual intercourse.

Unobtrusive Measures. Unobtrusive measures are those that "do not require the cooperation of a respondent and that do not themselves contaminate the response" (Webb, Campbell, Schwartz, and Sechrest, 1966, p. 2). With respect to measures of substance use or sexual behavior, these may include measures such as alcohol consumption at the community level; use of condom vouchers by study participants; STD or teen birth rates in a community to assess the impact of an intervention; reports of others (partners, close friends, or counselors); or arrest or treatment records. However, these methods also have disadvantages. It is not always possible to interview third parties about a participant's substance abuse, causing possible sampling bias if the study is limited only to those who provide a third-party contact. Some studies have suggested that, in fact, third parties and arrest or treatment records may provide less information about drug use behaviors than the actual respondent (Maisto, McKay, and Connors, 1990). Community-level rates of STDs or teen births require reporting in both cases and exclude spontaneous or voluntary abortions in the latter case.

Concluding Thoughts About Objective Measures. As Webb and colleagues persuasively argued nearly forty years ago, "Over-reliance on questionnaires and interviews is dangerous because it does not give us enough points in conceptual space to triangulate. It is only when we naively place faith in a single measure that the massive problems of social research vitiate (bring into question) the validity of our assumptions" (Webb, Campbell, Schwartz, and Sechrest, 1966, p. 34). Use of objective or unobtrusive measures, alongside self-report data, at a minimum provides stronger evidence for the validity of our measures and results than when they are not used. Indeed, in a review of the literature on self-reports of condom use and STDs over thirty-five years later, Fishbein and Pequegnat (2000, p. 110) arrive at a very similar conclusion: "Both behavioral and biological measures are important outcomes for studying the efficacy and effectiveness of behavior-change interventions. However, one measure cannot substitute for or validate the other, and neither serves as a true surrogate for HIV prevalence or incidence." Use of both self-report and objective measures of sensitive behaviors contributes to our understanding of both the behaviors and their relationship to public health or medical outcomes.

Applied Example

In this section we present an in-depth example for heuristic purposes.

National Survey of Adolescent Males

The primary objectives of the National Survey of Adolescent Males (NSAM) are to "obtain information about patterns of sexual activity and condom use among U.S. teenage males 15–19 years old; to assess their knowledge, attitudes, and risk behaviors relative to AIDS; and to conduct analyses which would identify determinants of condom use" (Pleck, Sonenstein, and Ku, 1993). The first survey was conducted with 1,880 young men in 1988, who were followed up in 1991; a new cohort of 1,741 males were surveyed in 1995. Choices made in developing these surveys and in changes made in administering the 1988 survey and that in 1995 are illustrative of a number of the issues we've discussed here (see Pleck, Sonenstein, and Ku, 1993, and Turner, Miller, and Rogers, 1997, for more details about survey development and methodological issues surrounding the survey).

Three days of training were conducted for the 1988 and 1991 surveys and five days of training for the 1995 surveys. Interviewers were trained in not being judgmental and the sensitive nature of the questions. Interviewers also were allowed to choose other surveys to work on if they felt uncomfortable with these topics, and supervisors screened out interviewers who performed at less than ideal levels. The training was one way of improving the *situation* in which the interview took place to reduce potential respondent bias or perceptions of social desirability.

The researchers also spent considerable resources and time on the mode of survey administration. In the 1988 and 1991 surveys, primarily face-to-face interviews were conducted by trained interviewers. In addition, a self-administered questionnaire was used to assess some of the most sensitive behaviors. In the 1995 survey, the newer A-CASI methodology was used for most respondents, based on successful pilot-testing that showed higher reports of sensitive behaviors using A-CASI compared with self-administered questionnaires. Results for the 1995 survey were again supportive, also showing higher rates of reporting of sensitive behaviors for A-CASI than for self-administered questionnaires (Turner and others, 1998).

The researchers reported various methods for clarifying the wording of questions—for example, those related to whether respondents had had sex. At each time point, they conducted focus groups and pretests of small samples of young men to determine questions or words that were not clear. They also opted for a simpler rather than lengthier definition of intercourse, selecting "Have you ever had sexual intercourse (sometimes this is referred to as 'making love,' 'having sex,' or 'going all the way')?" The researchers also focused on the cognitive processes involved in responding to surveys in their decisions about methods for increasing recall. They asked questions first about the most recent partners, with more limited information being collected about the previous four partners, believing that the most accurate information was likely to be recalled about most recent partners. They also asked about various behaviors, including condom use on a partner by partner basis, rather than overall, expecting it to be remembered better this way. Basing their decision on previous data (indicating most fifteen- to nineteen-year-old males had fewer than six partners in the past twelve months, but many had only episodic sexual experiences during that time interval), they decided to collect information about number of partners using a twelve-month interval because a significantly shorter period might have resulted in loss of data about sexual activity for a substantial portion of the sample.

As a final method for assessing and even improving the quality of their data, the researchers have shown correlations between trends in condom use (from their data) to condom sales nationwide and with pregnancies and births reported by males for their female sex partners in the longitudinal sample between their reports in 1988 and 1991. They have also added the collection of biologic markers, specifically using urine samples from respondents over the age of eighteen in their 1995 testing for chlamydia and gonorrhea to further validate reports of behaviors such as condom use and to add further information to the self-report data.

Integration with the Research Process

The issues discussed in this chapter—how to improve the validity of self-reports of sensitive behaviors by considering cognitive and situational factors as well as biologic and unobtrusive measures—are key elements of the research process. Several key questions pertain to step 5 of the nine-step model shown in Chapter One. What type of survey will be administered? Will it involve interviewers, self-administration using paper and pencil, A-CASI, telephone, Internet, or PDA administration? Should the design be cross-sectional or longitudinal? Will other sorts of validating data, such as biologic markers or unobtrusive measures, be used? How can the research questions be answered while placing the least possible burden on the respondent? In particular, the question of "how" is embedded into this step. How will the questions be worded? What time periods should be used in asking about behaviors? Will questions ask about ever engaging in a behavior or frequency of engaging in that behavior? What will the order of questions be?

Consideration of the sample population (step 6 in the nine-step model) is also important. Clearly, the answers to many of the questions posed in the previous paragraph will be contingent on a thorough knowledge of the people who will be included in the study. Finally, step 7: (implement the study protocol with attention to fidelity) is also connected to the issues discussed here. How will interviewers be trained? Will quality controls or observations be conducted to assess their performance or behavior throughout the study? What checks will be implemented within the survey to reduce missing data, inappropriate skips, inconsistency in reporting, or a respondent completing a Web survey multiple times?

Summary

When asking questions about sensitive behaviors one must be acutely aware of potential threats to the validity and reliability of the survey items that are used and the responses that are provided. In this chapter we reviewed drug use and sexual behaviors as examples of sensitive behaviors for which the validity of self-reports is frequently called into question. We describe validity as being affected by two separate factors (1) cognitive factors and (2) situational factors. Factors that affect cognition, or the remembering of events, include how the question and response items are crafted and the ways that the data are collected to enhance the recollection of past events. Situational factors such as who administers the survey, where the survey takes place, who is present, and how research is perceived are external factors that can affect how likely it is that respondents will provide valid answers to questions about sensitive or stigmatized behaviors. Both cognitive and situation factors affect the overall validity of self-report behaviors.

All of these techniques for improving the validity of self-report data have their strengths and their limitations. Constructing surveys and conducting research is a balancing act. Some cognitive approaches, such as daily diaries, can enhance recall of past events but may be too difficult or too burdensome for some higher-risk populations to use. In other cases, situational factors such as the use of brief close-ended questions about highly stigmatized behaviors may provide the data you are interested in, but if you don't build rapport with the respondent or sequence these questions with other attitudinal questions, respondents may provide invalid answers due to socially desirable responding.

This chapter has also reviewed objective measures that are used to externally validate self-report responses, such as urinalysis and STD testing. While these methods allow you to compare self-reports to an outside criterion measure, biologic testing is labor intensive and expensive, and may provide limited time windows when it is possible to validate the behavior. Creating opportunities for assessing the construct validity of survey items, which is being able to compare responses to behavior questions with other behavior or attitude questions in the survey, is a critical method for assessing validity when more laboratory-based measures are not feasible or appropriate.

Issues to Consider

1. As we move away from open-ended, qualitative methods of data collection and move toward more technologically advanced, quantitative data-collection methods, are we losing richness in exchange for improved validity and reliability?

Under what conditions are technologically based quantitative assessments appropriate, and when are more qualitative, open-ended, or interviewed administered research techniques more appropriate? What about areas of research where we don't know very much?

2. Throughout this chapter we have reviewed some of the available evidence regarding the validity of self-reports of sensitive behaviors, particularly when compared with outside criteria such as drug testing or STD testing. What do you conclude about the overall accuracy of self-report data? Is the cup half full or half empty? If you were presenting to a room full of physicians, could you report that you were confident the survey data you collected were accurate? Or would you prefer to present to a room full of prevention and behavioral scientists and enthusiastically support the use of biologic markers whenever possible to validate self-report data? Defend your argument based on the available evidence for drug use and sexual behaviors.

For Practice and Discussion

1. You are writing a grant to study the frequency of unprotected sexual intercourse among adolescents and want to understand the influence of drugs or alcohol use on your target outcome behavior. You are deciding how you want to design and administer the survey to ensure that you can make a link between drug use and the sexual behavior and to ensure valid reporting of the behaviors. Work in groups to define the following: (1) the population and setting of the study; (2) the mode of survey administration (A-CASI, paper and pencil, daily diaries); (3) whether self-administered or interview administered; (4) specific survey questions to measure frequency of the behavior; (5) survey items or other data-collection methods that will provide construct validity; and, finally, (6) whether you will use biologic measures, unobtrusive measures, or both to validate self-reported behaviors. Discuss the advantages and disadvantages of your approach and defend your design decisions based on how they will improve the validity of responses.

2. Use the information learned in this chapter to describe how the issues clearly related to self-reports of *very sensitive* behaviors such as illegal drug use and stigmatized sexual behavior might relate to self-reports of *less sensitive* behaviors, such as assessing exercise behavior as part of an evaluation of an exercise or wellness program in the workplace. To what extent do you think that mode of administration, use of technology-enhanced data-collection techniques, issues of timing and frequency, longitudinal versus retrospective reports, and use of

biologic or unobtrusive measures might be more or less important in the case of exercise behavior as compared with more sensitive behavioral reports?

References

Akers, R. L., Massey, J., Clarke, W., and Lauer, R. M. (1983). Are self-reports of adolescent deviance valid? Biochemical measures, randomized response and the Bogus Pipeline in smoking behavior. *Social Forces, 62,* 234–251.

Alexander, M. G., and Fisher, T. D. (2003). Truth and consequences: Using the Bogus Pipeline to examine sex differences in self-reported sexuality. *The Journal of Sex Research, 40*(1), 27–35.

Aquilino, W. S., and LoSciuto, L. A. (1990). Effects of interview mode on self-reported drug use. *Public Opinion Quarterly, 54,* 362–395.

Bachman, J. G., and O'Malley, P. M. (1981). When four months equal a year: Inconsistencies in student reports of drug use. *Public Opinion Quarterly, 45,* 536–548.

Bainbridge, W. S. (1989). *Survey research: A computer-assisted introduction.* Belmont, CA: Wadsworth.

Bell, D. C., Montoya, I. D., and Atkinson, J. S. (2000). Partner concordance in reports of joint risk behaviors. *Journal of Acquired Immune Deficiency Syndromes, 25,* 173–181.

Blumberg, S. J., Cynamon, M. L., Osborn, L., and Olson, L. (2003). The impact of touch-tone data entry on reports of HIV and STD risk behaviors in telephone interviews. *The Journal of Sex Research, 40*(2), 121–128.

Boekeloo, B. O., and others. (1994). Self-reports of HIV risk factors at a sexually transmitted disease clinic: Audio vs. written questionnaires. *American Journal of Public Health, 84,* 754–760.

Brener, N. D., Billy, J.O.G., and Grady, W. R. (2003). Assessment of factors affecting the validity of self-reported health risk behavior among adolescents: Evidence from the scientific literature. *Journal of Adolescent Health, 33,* 436–457.

Campanelli, P. C., Dielman, T. E., and Shope, J. T. (1987). Validity of adolescents' self-reports of alcohol use and misuse using a Bogus Pipeline Procedure. *Adolescence, 22*(85), 7–22.

Cannell, C. F., Miller, P. V., and Oskenberg, L. (1981). Research on Interviewing Techniques. In S. Leinhardt (Ed.), *Sociological methodology.* San Francisco: Jossey-Bass.

Catania, J. A. (1999). A framework for conceptualizing reporting bias and its antecedents in interviews assessing human sexuality. *The Journal of Sex Research, 36*(1), 25–38.

Catania, J. A., Binson, D., Van der Straten, A., and Stone, V. (1995). Methodological research on sexual behavior in the AIDS era. *Annual Review of Sex Research, 6,* 77–125.

Catania, J. A., Gibson, D. R., Chitwood, D. D., and Coates, T. J. (1990). Methodological problems in AIDS behavioral research: Influences on measurement error and participation in studies of sexual behavior. *Psychological Bulletin, 108*(3), 339–362.

Catania, J. A., McDermott, L., and Pollack, L. (1986). Questionnaire response bias and face-to-face interview sample bias in sexuality research. *Journal of Sex Research, 22,* 52–72.

DeMaio, T. (1984). Social desirability and survey measurement: A review. In C. Turner and E. Martin (Eds.), *Surveying subjective phenomena* (pp. 257–282). New York: Russel Sage Foundation.

Dembo, R., Williams, L., Wish, E. D., and Schmeidler, J. (1990). Urine testing of detained juveniles to identify high-risk youth. In *National Institute of Justice: Research in Brief.* Washington, DC: National Institute of Justice.

Droitcour, J., and others. (1991). The item count technique as a method of indirect questioning: A review of its development and a case study application. In P. P. Biemer, R. M. Groves, L. E. Lyberg, N. A. Mathiowetz, and S. Sudman (Eds.), *Measurement errors in surveys* (pp. 185–210). New York: Wiley.

Fendrich, M., and Xu, Y. (1994). The validity of drug use reports from juvenile arrestees. *International Journal of the Addictions, 29*(8), 971–985.

Fishbein, M., and Pequegnat, W. (2000). Evaluating AIDS prevention interventions using behavioral and biological outcome measures. *Sexually Transmitted Diseases, 27,* 101–110.

Forsyth, B. H., Lessler, J. T., and Hubbard, M. L. (1992). Cognitive evaluation of the questionnaire. In C. Turner and J. Lessler (Eds.), *Survey measurement of drug use: Methodological studies* (pp. 13–52). Rockville, MD: National Institute of Drug Abuse, Division of Epidemiology and Prevention Research.

Fowler, F. J., Jr. (1984). *Survey research methods.* Thousand Oaks, CA: Sage.

Fremouw, W. J., and Brown, J. P. (1980). The reactivity of addictive behaviors to self-monitoring: A functional analysis. *Addictive Behaviors, 5,* 209–217.

Gfroerer, J. C., and Hughes, A. L. (1991). The feasibility of collecting drug abuse data by telephone. *Public Health Reports, 106*(4), 384–394.

Gfroerer, J., Wright, D., and Kopstein, A. (1997). Prevalence of youth substance use: The impact of methodological differences between two national surveys. *Drug and Alcohol Dependence, 47*(1), 19–30.

Gillmore, M. R., and others. (2001). Daily data collection of sexual and other health-related behaviors. *Journal of Sex Research, 38*(1), 35–43.

Gribble, J. N., Miller, H. G., Rogers, S. M., and Turner, C. F. (1999). Interview mode and measurement of sexual behaviors: Methodological issues. *Journal of Sex Research, 36,* 16–24.

Hallfors, D., Khatapoush, S., Kadushin, C., Watson, K., and Saxe, L. (2000). A comparison of paper vs. computer-assisted self-interview for school, alcohol, tobacco and other drug surveys. *Evaluation and Program Planning, 23*(2), 149–155.

Halpern, C. T., Udry, J. R., and Suchindran, C. (1998). Monthly measures of salivary testosterone predict sexual activity in adolescent males. *Archives of Sexual Behavior, 27*(5), 445–465.

Halpern, C. T., Udry, J. R., Suchindran, C., and Campbell, B. (2000). Adolescent males' willingness to report masturbation. *Journal of Sex Research, 37,* 327–332.

Hays, R. D., and Huba, G. J. (1988). Reliability and validity of drug use items differing in the nature of their reponse options. *Journal of Consulting and Clinical Psychology, 56*(3), 470–472.

Hinden, R., and others. (1994). Radioimmunoassay of hair for determination of cocaine, heroin, and marijuana exposure: Comparison with self-report. *International Journal of Addiction, 29,* 771–798.

Johnson, R. (1970). Extramarital sexual intercourse: A methodological note. *Journal of Marriage and Family, 32,* 279–282.

Jones, E. E., and Sigal, H. (1971). The Bogus Pipeline: A new paradigm for measuring affect and attitude. *Psychological Bulletin, 76,* 349–364.

Kann, L., Brener, N. D., Warren, C. W., Collins, J. L., and Giovino, G. A. (2002). An assessment of the effect of data collection setting on the prevalence of health risk behaviors among adolescents. *Journal of Adolescent Health, 31*(4), 327–335.

Kubey, R., Larson, R., and Csikszentmihalyi, M. (1996). Experience sampling method applications to communication research questions. *Journal of Communication, 46,* 99–118.

LaBrie, J. W., and Earleywine, M. (2000). Sexual risk behaviors and alcohol: Higher base rates revealed using the Unmated-Count Technique. *Journal of Sex Research, 37,* 321–326.

Lenert, L., and Skoczen, S. (2002). The Internet as a research tool: Worth the price of admission? *Annals of Behavioral Medicine, 24,* 251–256.

Loftus, E. F., Smith, K. D., Johnson, D. A., and Fiedler J. (1988). Remembering "when": Errors in the dating of autobiographical memories. In M. Gruneberg, P. Morris, and R. Sykes (Eds.), *Practical aspects of memory* (pp. 234–240). Chichester, UK: John Wiley and Sons.

Magura, S., and Kang, S-Y. (1996). Validity of self-reported drug use in high-risk populations: A meta-analytical review. *Substance Use & Misuse, 31*(9), 1131–1153.

Maisto, S. A., McKay, J. R., and Connors, G. J. (1990). Self-report issues in substance abuse: State of the art and future directions. *Behavioral Assessment, 12,* 117–134.

McCabe, S. E. (2004). Comparison of Web and mail surveys in collecting illicit drug use data: A randomized experiment. *Journal of Drug Education, 34,* 61–72.

McCabe, S. E., Boyd, C. J., Couper, M. P., Crawford, S., and D'Arch, H. (2002). Mode effects for collecting alcohol and other drug use data: Web and U.S. mail. *Journal of Studies on Alcohol, 63,* 755–761.

Means, B., Habina, K., Swan, G. E., and Jack, L. (1992). Cognitive research on response error in survey questions on smoking. *Vital and Health Statistics, 6*(5) (DHHS Pub. No. PHS 89–1076). Washington, DC: Government Printing Office.

Mieczkowski, T., Barzelay, D., Gropper, B., Wish, E. (1991). Concordance of three measures of cocaine use in an arrestee population: Hair, urine, and self-report. *Journal of Psychoactive Drugs, 23*(3), 241–249.

Miller, J. D. (1984, July). *A new survey technique for studying deviant behavior.* Unpublished dissertation. Dissertation Abstract: 1984-56841-001. *Dissertation Abstracts International, 45*(1-A), 319.

Miller, J. D., and Cisin, I. H. (1983). *The item-count/paired lists technique: An indirect method of surveying deviant behavior.* Unpublished manuscript. Washington, DC: George Washington University, Social Research Group.

Miller, J. D., Cisin, I. H., and Harrell, A. V. (1986). A new technique for surveying deviant behavior: Item-count estimates of marijuana, cocaine, and heroin. Paper presented at the annual meeting of the American Association for Public Opinion Research, St. Petersburg, Florida.

Morrison, D. M., Leigh, B. C., and Rogers, G. M. (1999). Daily sata collection: A comparison of three methods. *Journal of Sex Research, 36*(1), 76–82.

Mustanski, B. S. (2001). Getting wired: Exploiting the Internet for the collection of valid sexuality data. *Journal of Sex Research, 38,* 292–301.

Oksenberg, L., and Cannell, C. (1977). Some factors underlying the validity of response in self-report. *Bulletin of the International Statistical Institute, 48,* 325–346.

O'Malley, P. M., Bachman, J. G., and Johnston, L. D. (1983). Reliability and consistency in self-reports of drug use. *International Journal of Addictions, 18*(6), 805–824.

Page, W. F., Davies, J. E., Ladner, R. A., Alfassa, J., and Tennis, H. (1977). Urinalysis screened versus verbally reported drug use: The identification of discrepant groups. *International Journal of the Addictions, 12*(4), 439–450.

Pleck, J. H., Sonenstein, F. L., & Ku, L. (1993). Changes in adolescent males' use of and attitudes toward condoms, 1988–1991. *Family Planning Perspectives, 25,* 106–110.

Smith, T. W. (2003). An experimental comparison of knowledge networks and the GSS. *International Journal of Public Opinion Research, 15,* 167–179.

Stone, V. E., Catania, J. A., and Binson, D. (1999). Measuring change in sexual behavior: Concordance between survey measures. *The Journal of Sex Research, 36*(1), 102–108.

Tourangeau, R., Jobe, J. B., Pratt, W. F., and Rasinski, K. (1997). Design and results of the Women's Health Study. (1997). In L. Harrison and A. Hughes (Eds.), *The validity of self-reported drug use: Improving the accuracy of survey estimates* (NIDA Monograph Series No. 97-4147, pp. 344–365). Rockville, MD: National Institute of Drug Abuse.

Trapl, E. S., and others. (forthcoming). *Use of audio-enhanced personal digital assistants for school-based data collection.* Manuscript under review.

Turner, C. F., Miller, H., and Rogers, S. M. (1997). Survey measurement of sexual behavior: Problems and progress. In J. Bancroft (Ed.), *Research Sexual Behavior* (pp. 37–60). Bloomington, IN: Indiana University Press.

Turner, C. F., and others. (1998). Adolescent sexual behavior, drug use, and violence: Increased reporting with computer survey technology. *Science, 280*(5365), 867–874.

Udry, R. J., and Morris, N. M. (1967). A method for validation of reported sexual data. *Journal of Marriage and the Family, 29,* 442–446.

Webb, E. J., Campbell, D. T., Schwartz, R. D., and Sechrest, L. (1966). *Unobtrusive measures: Nonreactive research in the social sciences.* Chicago: Rand-McNally.

Werch, C. E., Gorman, D. R., Marty, P. J., Forbess, J., and Brown, B. (1987). Effects of the Bogus Pipeline on enhancing validity of self-reported adolescent drug use measures. *Journal of School Health, 57*(6), 232–236.

Willis, G. B. (1997). The use of the psychological laboratory to study sensitive survey topics. In L. Harrison and A. Hughes (Eds.), *The validity of self-reported drug use: Improving the accuracy of survey estimates* (NIDA Research Monograph Series No. 97-4147, pp. 416–438). Rockville, MD: National Institute of Drug Abuse.

Wimbush, J. C., and Dalton, D. R. (1997). Base rate for employee theft: Converge of multiple methods. *Journal of Applied Psychology, 82,* 756–763.

Wish, E. D., Hoffman, J. A., and Nemes, S. (1997). The validity of self-reports of a drug use at treatment admission and at follow-up: Comparisons with urinalysis and hair assays. In L. Harrison and A. Hughes (Eds.), *The validity of self-reported drug use: Improving the accuracy of survey estimates* (NIDA Research Monograph Series No. 97-4147, pp. 344–365). Rockville, MD: National Institute of Drug Abuse.

Wright, D. L., Aquilino, W. S., and Supple, A. J. (1998). A comparison of computer-assisted and paper and pencil self-administered questionnaires in a survey on smoking, alcohol, and drug use. *Public Opinion Quarterly, 62,* 331–353.

Zenilman, J., Yuenger, J., Galai, N., Turner, C. F., and Rogers, S. M. (2005). Polymerase chain reaction detection of Y chromosome sequences in vaginal fluid: Preliminary studies of a potential biomarker for sexual behavior. *Sexually Transmitted Diseases, 32,* 90–94.

Zenilman, J. M., and others. (1995). Condom use to prevent incident STDs: The validity of self-reported condom use. *Sexually Transmitted Diseases, 22*(1), 15–21.

Zimmerman, R. S., and Langer, L. M. (1995). Improving estimates of prevalence rates of sensitive behaviors: The Randomized Lists Technique and consideration of self-reported honesty. *Journal of Sex Research, 32,* 107–117.

CHAPTER ELEVEN

PRINCIPLES OF SAMPLING

Richard A. Crosby, Laura F. Salazar, and Ralph J. DiClemente

Ultimately, the utility of a research project is a function of its generalizability. In turn, generalizability is a function of how well the sample represents the selected priority population. Sampling is a science unto itself; one that is used to predict winners of political elections before the polls even close, and one that may someday be used in place of a "head by head" count for the U.S. census. In health promotion research, sampling methods can be divided into two main categories: (1) methods that are admittedly weak in generalizability (nonprobability sampling methods) and (2) methods that yield high generalizability (probability methods). Despite its limitations, the former category is often very useful in the early stages of the research chain or when the nature of the selected population precludes the application of probability methods. The latter category, although far more rigorous, is often problematic to apply, as it depends on the existence of a sampling frame.

Indeed, asking the question, Does a *sampling frame* (a listing of people in the population) exist? is the most effective way to determine if a nonprobability sample or a probability sample should be used. Because this basic decision about sampling is so critical, this chapter is devoted to an in-depth discussion of the nonprobability and probability sampling techniques that are most often used in health promotion research.

Illustration of Key Concepts

The Sampling Goal

As with most endeavors, the key aspect of successful sampling is a great deal of attention to planning. Planning, in a sense, is the "art" of sampling; it requires creativity and cautious optimism regarding possibilities. At the foundation of this planning, the researcher is formulating an operationally defined goal. Three vital decisions are needed to formulate this goal: (1) What is the sampling element? (2) Is a sampling frame accessible? and (3) What type of sampling technique should be employed?

Sampling Elements. The goal of any sampling technique is to maximize the *generalizability* of the sample to the population. In this sense, the term *population* refers to all possible *elements* of a defined group. An element, in turn, can be people (as is usually the case) or well-defined units (or clusters) that have importance in public health (such as emergency care centers, schools, and homeless shelters). When people are the sampling element, the research questions are centered on the person (for example, Do outpatients from cardiac care centers consume a healthy diet?). Conversely, when elements compose well-defined units the research questions will involve "behavior" of an entire system such as, How effectively do cardiac care centers teach outpatients to consume healthy diets? Thus, an initial step in defining the sampling goal is to determine whether the research questions necessitate investigation of individual-level behavior or the collective behavior of an organized system. Table 11.1 presents several examples of health promotion research questions shown by this essential division in purpose.

◆ ◆ ◆

In a Nutshell

An initial step in defining the sampling goal is to determine whether the research questions necessitate investigation of individual-level behavior or the collective behavior of an organized system.

◆ ◆ ◆

TABLE 11.1.   EXAMPLES OF RESEARCH QUESTIONS DISPLAYED BY LEVEL OF ANALYSIS.

Person-Level Research Questions	System-Level Research Questions
How does condom availability influence teens' use of condoms?	What factors influence school systems to adopt condom distribution programs?
Is religiosity associated with lower rates of domestic violence?	Do churches actively teach couples and families conflict-resolution skills?
Are first-time parents able to properly install infant car seats?	Do hospitals offer first-time parents training in the installation of car seats?
Do women residing in low-income nursing homes consume diets adequate in fiber?	Do low-income nursing homes provide women with diets that are adequate in fiber?
Is affiliation with social organizations associated with decreased substance abuse?	To what extent do urban social organizations provide teens with alternatives to substance abuse?
Do people with adult-onset diabetes practice the consistent and correct use of insulin?	What is the extent of postdiagnostic education provided to adults newly diagnosed with diabetes in state-funded health clinics?

Sampling Frame Accessibility. Once the type of element has been identified, the next question that presents itself is whether a *sampling frame* exists (or can be created). A sampling frame can be loosely defined as an exhaustive list of elements. The word *exhaustive* is critical here because the list must represent every element in the population. For example, imagine that the research question is, Are unemployed men residing in rural counties more likely to be heavy smokers than unemployed men residing in urban counties? At first, the existence of a sampling frame seems intuitive—unemployed men are "listed" by offices that provide government assistance (that is, unemployment benefits). Ignoring for a moment whether such lists would even be made available, the researcher needs to ask the question, Is this frame exhaustive of the population?

An unfortunate reality of sampling is that very few sampling frames are truly exhaustive of the population. For example, do all unemployed men collect government assistance? Even seemingly clear-cut cases of an effective sampling frame can be problematic. A classic example of this is the use of telephone directories as a sampling frame. The directory is not exhaustive because it will not include people who use cell phones exclusively, people who cannot afford phone service, people who pay extra for an unlisted number, or people who have recently moved into the listing area. Thus, the question, Is this frame exhaustive of the population? is answered by degree rather than by a simple "yes" or "no." ("No" would almost always be the answer.) Table 11.2 displays examples of sampling

TABLE 11.2.   SAMPLING FRAMES WITH HIGH AND LOW DEGREES OF GENERALIZABILITY.

Higher Generalizability	Lower Generalizability
Research Question:	Research Question:
Is parental monitoring associated with health risk behavior among boys thirteen to sixteen years of age from low-income homes?	Are cancer patients who remain optimistic likely to survive longer than those who lose hope?
Sampling Frame:	Sampling Frame:
Boys enrolled in reduced-cost lunch programs at public schools	People diagnosed with cancer at publicly funded medical offices.
Note: Findings could be generalized to low-income boys attending public schools, but not to those who have dropped out or been placed in an alternative setting (including juvenile detention)	*Note:* Publicly funded medical offices may represent only a very small portion of the locations where cancer is diagnosed—thus generalizability is quite low.
Research Question:	Research Question:
Are women who receive WIC benefits at risk of rapid repeat pregnancy?	What behavioral factors predict iron-deficiency anemia among pregnant women?
Sampling Frame:	Sampling Frame:
Women enrolled in WIC programs	Women receiving prenatal care
Note: In this scenario, the sampling frame and the research question "line up" perfectly! Thus, generalizability would be optimal.	*Note:* The key question to consider is what portion of pregnant women do not receive prenatal care. To the extent that pregnant women in any given setting may not receive this care, generalizability decreases.
Research Question:	Research Question:
To what extent do hospital-based pediatricians meet guidelines for children's vaccination schedules?	Are low-income elderly women less likely than their male counterparts to exercise on a regular basis?
Sampling Frame:	Sampling Frame:
Hospital registry of pediatricians with privileges	Women and men receiving Medicare benefits
Note: Again, the sampling frame and the research question appear to line up quite nicely. Thus, potential for generalizability is high.	*Note:* Here, it is important to realize that all low-income elderly people may not receive Medicare benefits. Further, not all people receiving Medicare benefits are likely to be low-income and many may not perceive themselves to be "elderly." Thus, generalizability is likely to be quite low.

frames that adequately represent the population (providing a higher degree of generalizability) and those less likely to represent the population (providing a lower degree of generalizability).

Careful scrutiny of Table 11.2 will reveal two important points. First, note that none of the examples involves units as the sampling element. In each example, including the one regarding pediatricians, the research question is about behavior at the individual level. The question here is, Why weren't examples provided for elements defined by well-defined units? The answer is that, with some exceptions, well-defined units typically have a sampling frame that will offer a high degree of exhaustion. As a principle, exhaustion is generally far more likely when the sampling element is defined by a unit rather than by people. The difference is that social structures and law often protect individual identities, whereas group identities are often made public by intention. For example, churches, voluntary health agencies, schools, and neighborhood organizations are units that, by design, can be easily identified. Hospitals, soup kitchens, youth organizations, and drug treatment centers are just a few other examples of potential elements that are amenable to sampling for research questions at the system level.

Second, deeper scrutiny of the left-hand column in Table 11.2 raises an essential question: Can these sampling frames be accessed? Access to lists of pediatricians with hospital privileges may be possible; however, one can easily imagine "lists" that could not be obtained (for example, people receiving psychotherapy, convicted felons, persons living with tuberculosis, people who have survived cancer). This key concern leads to compromise between two competing conditions: (1) the need for the sample to be generalizable to the target population, versus (2) the practical reality of obtaining sampling frames that list people.

This compromise is often inevitable, and it may shape the research question. For example (from Table 11.2), imagine that the initial research question is to investigate the relationship of parental monitoring to health risk behavior among low-income boys attending public schools. That the sampling frame exists is not in question, but whether this list will be provided to a researcher is another question entirely. Thus, compromise occurs by altering the research question to accommodate the sampling frame that is accessible. For example, the question could become, What is the relationship of parental monitoring to health risk behavior among boys attending public schools? Note that the slightly altered research question no longer includes the term *low-income*. Because of privacy regulations, disclosing a comprehensive list of boys who qualify for a reduced or free lunch is problematic, whereas disclosing a comprehensive list of *all* boys may be acceptable. Moreover, the advantage of this inclusive sampling frame is that the original research question could still be evaluated. For example, the study questionnaire could ask all boys, Do you qualify for a free or reduced-price lunch at school? Then the analysis could compare low-income boys (defined by the "lunch" criterion) to remaining boys. In fact, such a comparison could lead to a more elaborate version of the initial research question: What is the relationship of parental monitoring to health risk behavior among low-income boys attending public schools compared with boys not classified as low income? Thus, when sampling is being considered, the art of planning research requires that you understand the reciprocal relationship between framing the research question and accessing a sampling frame. Research planned with rigor has little value if access to the sampling frame is not practical or feasible.

Sampling Techniques. Effective sampling from the sampling frame referred to as the selection process is predicated on a thorough understanding of techniques. The overarching goal of this selection process is to maximize the *representativeness* of the sample with respect to the sampling frame and ultimately the population that is represented by the sampling frame. This goal is ostensibly simple and has been illustrated in Figure 11.1.

The extent to which the sample, denoted by the small circle, mirrors the exact composition of the population, depicted by the larger circle shown in Figure 11.1, will increase the degree of representativeness. Because gauging the representativeness of the sample relies on determining the extent to which the sample mirrors the population, an important consideration is, How do you determine the exact composition of the population? It must be stated that it is not possible to know

**FIGURE 11.1.   THE RELATIONSHIP OF A SAMPLE
TO A POPULATION.**

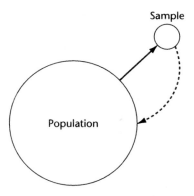

A sample is selected from a population (——►)
Inferences about a population are based on findings from the sample (- - - -►)

with certainty the infinite parameters of any given population. Thus, the best we can do in science is to use rigorous sampling techniques that enhance the likelihood that the sample represents the population.

◆ ◆ ◆

In a Nutshell

It must be stated that it is not possible to know with certainty the infinite parameters of any given population. Thus, the best we can do in science is to use rigorous sampling techniques that enhance the likelihood that the sample represents the population.

◆ ◆ ◆

The lack of correspondence between the sample and the population *not* attributed to chance represents the sampling bias in a research study. Because chance alone cannot be controlled, it is critically important to eliminate other factors that may introduce sampling bias. As with other forms of bias in research, sampling bias may yield inaccurate results that are not generalizable. Thus, choosing the most rigorous and appropriate sampling technique will ensure that sampling bias is reduced to as close to "zero" as possible. Reducing sampling bias provides the ability to *extrapolate* the findings to the population. Extrapolation implies making an inference based on the quality of the sampling technique. These inferences are an accepted and expected product of the research process. Indeed, health promotion research is very much about achieving large-scale change, and it is therefore necessary to think far beyond the relatively small numbers of people who make up the sample.

Common Probability Sampling Techniques

Several textbooks can be obtained that provide extensive discussion of probability sampling techniques (for example, Babbie, 2001; Shi, 1997). In the behavioral and social sciences, this category of sampling techniques is the most rigorous because the sampling strategies employ a *random selection* technique (a technique that ensures that each element has an equal probability of being selected), which greatly reduces the probability of sampling bias. Random selection is key to minimizing sample bias and therefore enhancing generalizability of the findings. A word of caution: random selection should not be confused with random assignment! (see Chapter Six for description of random assignment). The different types of probability sampling techniques are described in the following section.

Simple Random Sampling. The guiding principle behind this technique is that each element must have an equal and nonzero chance of being selected. This can be achieved by applying a table of random numbers to a numbered sampling frame. Another approach involves drawing numbers from a container. The product of this technique is a sample determined entirely by chance. It should be noted, however, that chance is "lumpy" (Abelson, 1995), meaning that random selection does not always produce a sample that is representative of the population. Imagine, for example, a sampling frame comprising 10,000 people. Furthermore, consider that race is a critical variable, and that the composition of the sampling frame is as follows: 1,500 are African American; 7,500 are white, and 1,000 are Asian. You are going to select a sample of 500 people from this sampling frame using a simple random sampling technique. Unfortunately, the simple random selection process may or may not yield a sample that has equivalent racial proportions as the sampling frame. Due to chance, disproportionate numbers of each racial category may be selected.

Systematic Random Sampling. As opposed to simple random sampling, systematic random sampling does not ensure that every element has an equal and nonzero probability of being selected. The systematic random sampling technique begins with selecting one element at random in the sampling frame as the starting point; however, from this point onward, the rest of the sample is selected systematically by applying a predetermined interval. For example, in this sampling technique, after the initial element is selected at random, every "*N*th" element will be selected (*N*th refers to the size of the interval—such as the twentieth element in the sampling frame) and becomes eligible for inclusion in the study. The "*N*th" element is selected through the end of the sampling frame and then from the beginning until a complete cycle is made back to the starting point (that is, the place where the initial random selection was made). Of note, all of the selections become predetermined as soon as the first selection is made. Thus, for example, if element 29 is the initial selection (and the interval equals 20), elements 30 through 48 have zero chance of being selected.

◆ ◆ ◆

In a Nutshell

As opposed to simple random sampling, systematic random sampling does not ensure that every element has an equal and nonzero probability of being selected.

◆ ◆ ◆

One important question is, When is systematic random sampling more appropriate than simple random sampling? The answer involves the term *periodicity*. Periodicity refers to bias caused by particular characteristics arising in the sampling frame (for example, if the list is ordered by date of birth). Sampling frames that are arranged in any meaningful fashion may possess periodicity, meaning that an inherent order exists. For example, a sampling frame of women receiving abnormal Pap test results may be arranged by date of the test (that is, women with abnormal Pap results in 1997 might be listed first, followed by those having abnormal Pap results in 1998, and so on). Systematic sampling from this sampling frame would ensure that each year of diagnosis is proportionately represented in the selected sample. Box 11.1 provides a comparison of simple random sampling to systematic random sampling with respect to this example. Note that the periodicity of the sampling frame is an advantage of systematic random sampling in comparison with simple random sampling in this instance.

Stratified Random Sampling. Stratified random sampling begins with the identification of some variable, which may be related indirectly to the research question and could act as a confound (such as geography, age, income, race or ethnicity, or gender). This variable is then used to divide the sampling frame into mutually exclusive *strata* or subgroups. Once the sampling frame is arranged by strata, the sample is selected from each stratum using random sampling or systematic sampling techniques. Imagine, for example, the following research goal: Identify key nutritional risk factors among adults living in New York State. Through conversations with people in the State Health Department, the researcher has learned that people in the southeastern part of the state (New York City and surrounding areas) are likely to be quite different than those in the northeastern part of the state and, furthermore, that people in the remaining part of the state (central and western New York) will be different from people in the east. Thus, a sample that does not fairly represent each of these three regions will have sampling error. This error can be controlled by dividing the sampling frame into three strata (southeastern, northeastern, and the remaining state). Each stratum becomes its own independent sampling frame, and a simple random sample or a systematic random sample is taken from each frame. It is important that the sample selected within each stratum reflects proportionately the population proportions; thus, you can employ *proportionate stratified sampling*. In this case, if 40 percent of the adults reside in the southeastern stratum, then 40 percent of the total sample should be selected from this stratum.

Box 11.1. A Comparison of Two Techniques to Sample Women with Abnormal Pap Test Results in the Past Five Years

Technique 1 (Simple Random Sampling)

Given a sampling frame of 650 women and a desired sample size of 100, the corresponding quantity of random numbers were drawn. This yielded 12 women diagnosed in 1997, 37 diagnosed in 1998, 7 diagnosed in 1999, 16 diagnosed in 2000, and 28 diagnosed in 2001. The proportions of women selected, by year, in comparison to those diagnosed were

1997:   105 (16.1 percent of 650) were diagnosed—11.4 percent ($n = 12$) were selected

1998:   155 (23.8 percent of 650) were diagnosed—23.8 percent ($n = 37$) were selected

1999:   73 (11.2 percent of 650) were diagnosed—9.6 percent ($n = 7$) were selected

2000:   110 (16.9 percent of 650) were diagnosed—14.5 percent ($n = 16$) were selected

2001:   207 (31.8 percent of 650) were diagnosed—13.5 percent ($n = 28$) were selected

Comment: By chance, the proportion selected in 1998 matched the proportion diagnosed in 1998. However, in 2001 the proportion selected (13.5) dramatically underrepresented the proportion diagnosed (31.8 percent).

Technique 2 (Systematic Random Sample)

Given a sampling frame of 650 women and a desired sample size of 100, a sampling interval of 6.5 was used. The first woman selected was selected at random (#456). The next woman selected was #462 (rounding down from 6.5 to 6.0) and the next woman was #469 (rounding up from 6.5 to 7.0). The sampling procedure continued until 100 women were selected (which brought the sequence back to the starting point of #456). The proportions of women selected, by year, in comparison to those diagnosed were

1997:   105 (16.1 percent of 650) were diagnosed—16.0 percent ($n = 16$) were selected

1998:   155 (23.8 percent of 650) were diagnosed—24.0 percent ($n = 24$) were selected

1999:   73 (11.2 percent of 650) were diagnosed—11.0 percent ($n = 11$) were selected

2000:   110 (16.9 percent of 650) were diagnosed—17.0 percent ($n = 17$) were selected

2001:   207 (31.8 percent of 650) were diagnosed—32.0 percent ($n = 32$) were selected

Comment: By design, the proportion selected in each of the five years matched the proportion diagnosed in each corresponding year. The periodicity of the sampling frame was used to ensure proportional representation for women in each of the five diagnostic years.

Cluster Sampling. Cluster sampling is *a* technique used when the research question is about organizational behavior or policy rather than the health behavior or disease status of individuals. Application of the technique is simple. First, a sampling frame of clusters is developed or obtained. Then, a random sample of clusters is selected (simple random sampling or systematic random sampling could be used to achieve this goal). Thus, the cluster itself is the intended unit of analysis for the research being conducted. Examples include research goals such as the following:

- To assess the established exercise programs in nursing homes
- To determine whether worksite health promotion programs provide financial incentives to employees for wellness indicators
- To assess the proportion of Nevada counties that treat their municipal water supplies with fluoride
- To identify the presence or absence of counseling protocols designed to promote proper infant hydration practices for women being discharged from maternity wards

In each case, data from individuals would not be appropriate. Instead, the unit of analysis (that is, the source of data) is the cluster. This type of research is especially applicable to health services research and to formulating policy related to health promotion.

Multistage Cluster Sampling. Multistage cluster sampling is used when an appropriate sampling frame does not exist or cannot be obtained. Rather than revert to a nonprobability sampling technique, multistage cluster sampling uses a collection of preexisting units or clusters (such as health districts, counties, voluntary health agencies) to "stand in" for a sampling frame. The first stage in the process is selecting a sample of clusters at random from the list of all known clusters. The second stage consists of selecting a random sample from each cluster. Because of this multistage process, the likelihood of sampling bias increases. This creates a lack of sampling precision known as a design effect. Of interest, specialized statistical programs are available to account for (and therefore control) design effects. One such example is SUDAAN (Shah, Barnwell, and Beiler, 1997).

An inflated design effect (see Henry, 1990, p. 108, for a computational formula) can be avoided by selecting a larger number of clusters. Clusters are likely to be homogenous (meaning that people within the clusters are relatively similar to one another) and homogeneity reduces sampling error. Given that sample size is always limited by financial or practical constraints, the question at hand is whether to select more clusters or to select more people within a smaller number of clusters. Thus, by sampling more clusters (as opposed to more people within clusters) the likelihood of sampling error can be reduced and the design effect can be minimized.

Two relatively common terms must be understood when reading or reporting research that used a multistage cluster sampling technique. The *primary sampling unit* (PSU) is the first set of clusters used in the process of obtaining a sample. For example, counties may be the PSU in a study designed to assess the prevalence of farm accidents in the state of Montana. Perhaps a second set of clusters could also be employed. For example, after randomly selecting a group of counties (that is, the PSU) from a list of all rural counties, perhaps the research team could then select zip code areas to be the second set of clusters. In this case, zip code areas would be the *secondary sampling unit* or the SSU. The final sampling unit might be cattle producers and would be selected at random from the zip code areas. The final sampling unit becomes the intended unit of analysis. At each stage, selection of sampling units (whether PSU or SSU) is made at random.

Stratified Multistage Cluster Sampling. An extension of multistage cluster sampling is stratified multistage cluster sampling. Contrary to a rather complicated sounding name, this technique is nearly identical to multistage cluster sampling. The only difference is that the clusters may be divided into strata before random selection occurs. As previously noted, stratification reduces sampling error to "zero" for variables that may otherwise introduce sampling bias into a study.

An important note: Probability sampling does not need to be overwhelming! To the contrary, the techniques used are simply variants of three basic tools. Box 11.2 illustrates the logic of probability sampling by showing that basic techniques (see step 1) can be applied in numerous ways to create a sample that best fits the needs of the research question.

Box 11.2. Probability Sampling Made Easy

Step 1. Consider three basic options:

    A. Simple random sampling
    B. Systematic sampling
    C. Cluster sampling

Use any of these options (*alone*) to meet the needs of your research question.

Step 2 (if needed). For some research questions, you may need to begin by dividing the sampling frame into strata. This creates three possibilities based on the options in step 1:

    Stratified random sample = stratification + a

    Stratified systematic sample = stratification + b

    Stratified multistage cluster sample = stratified c + a or b

Step 3 (if needed). In some cases you may need to *combine* the options listed in step 1:

    Multistage cluster sample = c + a or c + b

Common Nonprobability Sampling Techniques

Although the benefits of probability sampling are tremendous, it is nonetheless important to note that whenever the population being studied is narrowly defined, it may be difficult to employ these techniques. The term *narrow* signifies that certain distinguishing parameters are used to delineate the target population such as those highlighted in the following research questions:

- To examine associations of perceived parental monitoring with biologically confirmed tobacco cessation among *adolescents with severe mental illness*
- To identify factors that may preclude people in high-risk populations (*gay men, injection drug users,* and *low-income African American men*) from accepting an AIDS vaccine when one is approved for use
- To compare HIV-associated sexual health history, risk perceptions, and sexual risk behaviors of *unmarried rural and non-rural African American women*

As indicated, the population is narrowly defined in each of the three research goals. Because the existence of sampling frames for each of these three narrowly defined

DINCUS WORRIES ABOUT THEIR "SAMPLE"
OF NUTS FOR THE WINTER.

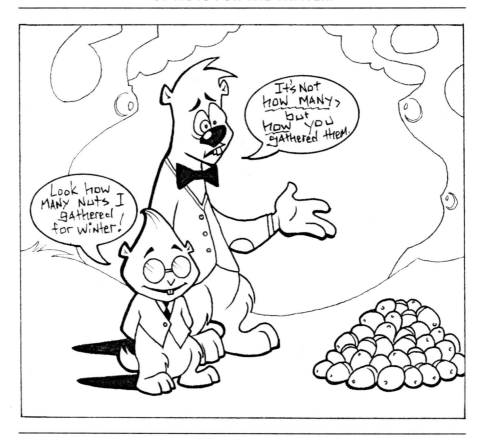

Copyright 2005 by Justin Wagner; reprinted with permission.

populations is unlikely, using a probability sampling technique is not feasible. In these instances, although a probability technique would be more rigorous, a non-probability sampling technique may be more realistic.

Convenience Sampling. Convenience sampling, perhaps the most widely used technique in health promotion research, uses preexisting groups such as a classroom of students, a support group for people with cancer, people in a waiting room of a clinic, people celebrating gay pride at a public event, and employees at work to facilitate recruitment. People in these groups can then be asked to volunteer for the study. Of course, the simplicity of this technique is attractive, but it comes with a high risk of yielding sampling bias. For example, imagine that the research question is, What are the correlates of condom use among gay men in long-term monogamous relationships? Using a convenience sample of gay men recruited from a gay bar or a gay pride event, for example, may provide a skewed view of the population in that gay male couples who attend public events may be quite different from those who stay at home.

When using a convenience sample, the key issue to consider is how well the preexisting group represents the population. Substantial and identifiable differences between the preexisting group and the population may result in study findings that misrepresent the population. Box 11.3 provides several examples of this problem. In each example it is important to note that the conclusion (despite intuitive appeal) is quite broad in scope—reaching far beyond the limitations imposed by a convenience sample.

Purposive Sampling. Purposive sampling is a technique that is targeted and specifies preestablished criteria for recruiting the sample. The need for purposive sampling is dependent on the research question. For example, "men who test positive for an STD to determine the correlates of condom use" is a research question that necessitates purposive sampling techniques. Of course, when a preexisting group is available to recruit the sample (for example, men attending an STD clinic), then

---

Box 11.3. Examples of Convenience Samples with "Large Conclusions"

Sample	*Conclusion*
952 low-income women in San Francisco	The involvement of male partners in decision making about condoms ensures greater protection against HIV infection.
789 adults recruited from a comprehensive service center in a Southeastern city	Clinicians working with adolescents should explore risk taking and prevention measures with their clients.
1,000 adolescents receiving prenatal care at one clinic	The experience of family violence is correlated with rapid repeat pregnancy among U.S. adolescents.
569 men recruited from one university	Prevention-intervention programs in high school and college reduce risk behaviors for chronic disease.

purposive sampling becomes a variant of convenience sampling. A preexisting group may not always be available, however. For example, to select a sample of delinquent youths, we may need to use a classroom as the recruitment venue and then recruit only those youths who meet the criterion for delinquency.

Quota Sampling. Quota sampling entails (1) identifying characteristics of the population to be reflected in the sample, (2) determining the distribution of these characteristics in the population ("setting the quotas"), and (3) selecting the sample based on those characteristics and their proportion in the population. These characteristics are usually sociodemographic factors such as gender, race, and age. Quota sampling can be useful if (1) the researcher determines that demographic factors such as age, gender, and race or ethnicity are critical components of representativeness, and (2) the demographic profile of the population is known. By characterizing the population and matching the sample to these characteristics sample bias is reduced.

Studies that designate college students as the target population are a good example of an opportunity to apply this technique. Suppose the research question is to identify determinants of binge drinking among undergraduates attending UCLA. Beginning with records from the registrar's office, a researcher could identify the distribution of demographics among the undergraduate population (that is, gender and race or ethnicity). Using these proportions, a matrix can be developed and would contain cells that represent the intersection between gender and race or ethnicity. One cell in the matrix is needed for each possible combination. For example, "Hispanic females" would be one cell. The quota of UCLA undergraduates, then, who are female and Hispanic would be determined based on sample size and the proportion of these characteristics in the undergraduate population (see Box 11.4). The reason for this extensive work is to have a guide for a variant of purposive sampling. The sample will be assembled to match the proportions shown in the matrix that was built from the records obtained in the registrar's office.

Box 11.4. Example of a Matrix for Quota Sampling

	Female	Male
African American/ Black	10.0 percent of enrolled students	9.0 percent of enrolled students
Asian	3.5 percent of enrolled students	1.5 percent of enrolled students
Hispanic	8.3 percent of enrolled students	6.2 percent of enrolled students
White	25.7 percent of enrolled students	35.8 percent of enrolled students

The primary problem with this technique is that the research question may or may not be one that lends itself to the assumption that demographic equivalence alone is sufficient to ensure representativeness. Perhaps, for example, binge drinking is a function of sorority and fraternity membership rather than age, gender, or race or ethnicity? Thus, representativeness is best achieved by selecting a sample that mirrors the population with respect to sorority and fraternity membership. Unfortunately, the idea that binge drinking is a function of sorority and fraternity membership may not materialize before the study is conducted; thus the researcher will not know what information should be used to build the selection matrix.

Variants of Snowball Sampling. Just as quota sampling is a specific application of purposive sampling, snowball sampling (and its variants) is also a specific application of purposive sampling. Snowball sampling is most useful in identifying and recruiting hard-to-reach populations (such as injection drug users or runaway teens). The basic technique is to begin with a "seed" (a person who qualifies to be in the study) and perform the interview (or administer any other part of a research protocol). The researcher asks the participant to identify others who meet the eligibility criteria and would possibly like to participate in the study (direct facilitation), or the researchers ask participants to contact others who meet the eligibility criteria so that they can refer them to the researcher (indirect facilitation).

Access Issues

As noted in Chapter Five, gaining access to a population is the primary starting point for health promotion research. Irrespective of the sampling technique employed, gaining access to the population may be a challenge and requires a plan to overcome obstacles and obtain the approval of certain gatekeepers that may restrict access.

The "Accounting Process"

Frequently, published reports of quantitative data will include a section that systematically accounts for the possibility of sampling bias. For nonprobability samples, such text usually begins by noting how many people were screened for eligibility and how many were found to be eligible. This first step is far less critical than the second step, which involves listing the reasons why eligible people chose not to participate and (possibly) comparing those who refused with those who agreed with respect to key demographic variables such as age, race, and sex.

FIGURE 11.2.   AN EXAMPLE OF A FIGURE USED TO REPRESENT RECRUITMENT SUCCESS.

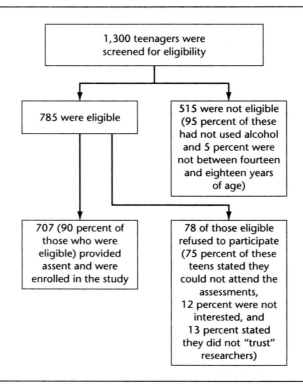

Most important, a participation rate is provided. Low participation rates suggest the possibility that *participation bias* may have occurred, while higher rates minimize participation bias. Participation bias is introduced into a sample when there may be differences between those who are eligible and participate and those who are eligible and refuse. The probability of participation bias is inversely related to the participation rate. An example of this accounting process follows and is depicted graphically in Figure 11.2.

A convenience sample of adolescent males was selected. The sample was intended to represent a broad cross-section of adolescents residing in low-income neighborhoods of Little Rock, Arkansas. Recruitment sites comprised three adolescent medicine clinics, two health department clinics, and health classes from seventeen high schools. From December 1996 through April 1999, project recruiters screened 1,300 adolescent males to assess their eligibility for participating in the study. Adolescents were eligible to participate if they were male, fourteen to eighteen years old, unmarried, and reported using alcohol at least once in the previous six months. Of those screened, 515 adolescents were not eligible to participate in the study; the majority (95 percent) did not meet the criterion of alcohol use, and 5 percent did not meet the age criterion. Of the 785 eligible adolescents, 90 percent ($n = 707$) agreed to participate and subsequently provided their assent. Of the teens who refused participation, the majority (75 percent) stated that their employment schedules would preclude them from making a time commitment (three consecutive Saturdays) to the study. Other reasons cited included lack of interest (12 percent) and a distrust of researchers (13 percent). Differences between those who refused and those who accepted the offer to participate were not found with respect to being a racial or ethnic minority ($P = .92$), age ($P = .53$), or level of education ($P = .81$).

Several points from the preceding paragraph warrant explanation. First, the participation rate of 90 percent is high and strongly suggests that participation bias is unlikely. Nonetheless, a reader who continues to suspect participation bias can be assured that refusal was mostly a function of Saturday work commitments. Three demographic comparisons between participants and "refusers" provided further assurance that participation bias was minimal. Although this process of collecting reasons for refusal and making simple demographic comparisons appears to be straightforward, an important principle of research is at odds with these practices: data cannot be collected from people who refuse study participation (see Chapter Three). Yet some researchers will argue that merely asking, "Can you please tell me why you do not want to be in the study?" is not a form of data collection. Furthermore, it can be argued that "observable" demographics (race and sex) do not qualify as collected data. Asking adolescents their age and grade level, however, is clearly a form of data collection, and engaging in this practice without their assent is a grey area with respect to ethics.

◆ ◆ ◆

In a Nutshell

Although this process of collecting reasons for refusal and making simple demographic comparisons appears to be straightforward, an important principle of research is at odds with these practices: data cannot be collected from people who refuse study participation.

◆ ◆ ◆

This accounting process is similar for probability samples except there may not be a need to determine what proportion of the people was eligible (if the sampling frame defined eligibility). Alternatively, if the sampling frame did not define eligibility, then this step in the accounting process is essential.

An Introduction to Sample Size

Before learning about the principles that guide sample size determinations, please consider the following scenario. One study ($N = 1,000$) is conducted, and the findings support the hypothesis that teens belonging to gangs will report a higher frequency of marijuana use in the past thirty days. The hypothesis was tested by performing a t-test and had a corresponding t-value of 7.5, which was significant at $P < .01$. Another study was conducted to test the same hypothesis. In this study, the sample size was much smaller ($N = 100$); however, the statistical findings were nearly identical ($t = 7.4$; $P < .01$). Knowing nothing else about the samples, determine which study had the bigger difference between means (please give this some thought before reading the next two paragraphs).

The answer to the question lies in the study's calculated effect size. Without exception, sample size and effect size are interrelated elements of any quantitative study. In the example provided, effect size can be conceptualized as "distance between group means." In the study of a thousand participants, the effect size was the difference between groups in the mean number of days that teens smoked marijuana. Teens who belonged to gangs smoked marijuana 3.7 days on average, and teens who were not in gangs smoked marijuana 1.5 days on average. In contrast, in the study of one hundred participants, the effect size was much greater. The teens who belonged to gangs smoked 9.4 days on average compared with teens not in gangs, who smoked 1.7 days on average. Figure 11.3 provides an illustration of effect size relative to this example. In this figure, effect size is portrayed as a slope. A lack of slope (a flat—horizontal—line) would represent a complete lack of effect. Conversely, an increasing slope represents an increasingly greater effect size. Note that the slope in the study of a thousand teens is quite gentle in contrast to rather dramatic slope in the study of one hundred teens.

An important (and often ignored) point is that effect size is invariant to sample size. Sample size influences the level of statistical significance only (that is, P-value). All things being equal, as sample size increases, significance is more likely to be achieved. (See Box 11.5 for an illustration of this principle.) A larger sample size (along with several other determinants) gives a study an extra "boost" to find

FIGURE 11.3. EFFECT SIZE IN TWO SIMILAR STUDIES.

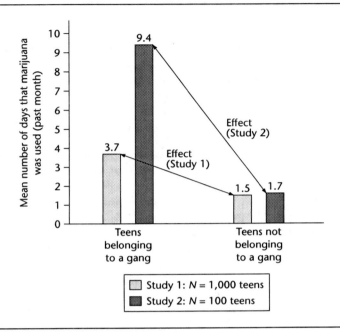

significance for modest to small effect sizes. Conversely, this boost is lacking with small samples (such as $N = 100$); thus, only large effect sizes can be detected with small samples. This point leads to a critical principle of sampling: plan for a sample size that is adequate to detect (with statistical significance) the anticipated effect size. A more thorough treatment of sample size, effect size, and statistical power is provided in Chapter Twelve.

◆ ◆ ◆

In a Nutshell

Plan for a sample size that is adequate to detect (with statistical significance) the anticipated effect size.

◆ ◆ ◆

Box 11.5. As Sample Size Goes Up, Significance Is Easier to "Find"

This principle is shown by an example. Consider an experimental program delivered to high-risk men that was designed to promote annual cholesterol testing. An index of intent to have a cholesterol test annually was constructed. The highest possible rating was 10.0 and the lowest was 0.0.

Using a pretest, posttest experimental design, with fifteen men in each of two groups, the researchers obtained posttest means as follows: Control = 6.0; Intervention = 6.9.

A significance test was conducted to determine whether the observed means were different beyond differences that could be expected by sampling error alone. The researchers used a two-tailed t-test and set their alpha at .05. The P-value achieved was .094; thus the null hypothesis was retained.

One member of the research team had a hard time accepting the finding (this person could not get over the idea that the intervention did not "change" men with respect to the measure of intent). Hence, this person suggested that the sample size "should be doubled and another study should be conducted." After the study was repeated with thirty men assigned to each of the two conditions, the same t-test was conducted (this time $N = 60$, rather than $N = 30$). This time the mean in the control group was 6.0 and the mean in the intervention group was 6.9 (exactly the same means that had been found in the study of only thirty men!). However, the obtained P-value in the test of sixty men was .001. The previously disgruntled researcher was now quite satisfied and proceeded to publish the findings.

Applied Examples

Between February and May of 1998, the Centers for Disease Control and Prevention (CDC) surveyed adolescents attending U.S. alternative schools (Grunbaum and others, 2000). Given the existence of a sampling frame, CDC used a multistage cluster sampling technique. The primary sampling unit was 121 geographical clusters of alternative high schools. Forty-eight of the PSUs were selected. For the second stage, 142 alternative schools (SSUs) were selected from the 48 PSUs. Schools with substantially greater enrollments of black and Hispanic students were purposefully oversampled. Finally, classes within the 142 selected schools were randomly chosen for study participation. Participation rates were 81.0 percent (schools) and 81.9 percent (students). A total of 8,918 students from 115 schools constituted the sample.

This preceding description illustrates the utility of a multistage cluster sample. Note that three stages were involved, thus a design effect is clearly likely. Despite this "cost" of the sampling technique, the final sample of nearly nine thousand students has a very good chance of representing the population of adolescents who attended U.S. alternative schools in 1998. The PSU is particularly important in that the CDC apparently grouped alternative schools into geographic clusters. Similar to stratification, this practice was useful in ensuring that adolescents were selected from a representative sample of geographic areas. Note that the PSUs were created by the CDC—they existed only for purposes of the sampling protocol and thus (as nonentities) they could not "refuse" or "accept" participation (hence only two participation rates were reported).

Preventive Service Utilization

A recent study investigated the effect of demographic and socioeconomic factors on elderly men's use of preventive services such as influenza vaccination, colorectal cancer screening, and testing for prostate-specific antigens (Morales and others, 2004). More than 19,000 men enrolled in Medicare health maintenance organizations and in traditional (fee for service) Medicare programs composed the sampling frame. To draw a sample that represented both high- and low-income groups, the research team used a stratified random sampling technique. In each plan (HMO and fee for service) three strata were formed: (1) men who were also Medicaid eligible and one for the remaining men, (2) remaining men who resided in a low-income zip code area, and (3) all remaining men. Men in the first and second strata were oversampled. The final sample consisted of 942 men from strata 1, 700 from strata 2, and 5,354 from strata 3.

The example clearly shows the utility of stratification. Given what appears to have been a fairly detailed sampling frame (in other words, it contained much more than names), the researchers were able to ensure that three distinct groups of men were selected into the sample. This logic is an extension of the research question (that is, the research was designed to compare men in these three groups relative to their use of preventive services). Note then, that stratification was not used for its traditional purpose of eliminating sampling error for an identified variable. Instead, stratification was used to define analytic groups! This innovative use of stratification typifies the potential of using sampling techniques in a creative manner— the ultimate principle of this creativity is to serve the research question.

◆ ◆ ◆

In a Nutshell

This innovative use of stratification typifies the potential of using sampling techniques in a creative manner—the ultimate principle of this creativity is to serve the research question.

◆ ◆ ◆

Barriers to Flu Vaccination

A study reported by Armstrong and colleagues (2001) was designed to assess perceived barriers to influenza vaccination among low-income African American urban dwellers. Health system billing records served as the initial sampling frame. Selecting only people who reside in one of twelve zip code areas that defined West Philadelphia then refined this initial sampling frame. Subsequently a random sample of 825 people was drawn from this modified sampling frame.

This example is instructive on many levels. First, it illustrates that a sampling frame can be modified to suit the research question. (In this case, West Philadelphia was selected to ensure a high likelihood of selecting low-income African American urban dwellers, thus serving the research question.) Second, the example serves as a reminder that the study conclusions should never exceed the boundaries of the sample. In this case, only people receiving medical services were represented in the initial sampling frame; thus, the findings cannot be generalized to people who do not receive medical services. Furthermore, the research question was addressed only by surveying people in West Philadelphia, thereby precluding generalization to the general population of "low-income African American urban dwellers." In short, the example serves as a reminder that not all probability samples can be used as a basis for population-level conclusions. Finally, this example raises the question of why a purposive sample was not used. Given that the intent was to identify barriers to influenza vaccination among low-income African American urban dwellers, a purposive sample might have been equally effective and perhaps far less labor intensive. If recruitment for such a purposive sample occurred in nonmedical settings, then persons not receiving medical care would not have been excluded from the study. Our intent is not to "second guess" the work of this research team. Instead, this example is used here to show that probability sampling is not always an automatically superior choice to nonprobability sampling.

Integration with the Research Process

This chapter has presented basic concepts involved with step 6 of the research process (see Figure 1.2). The appropriate selection of a "parsimonious sampling technique" is indeed a critical determinant of study rigor. Although simple rules do not apply (for example, probability techniques are always better), the general principle of parsimony is very applicable. In turn, parsimony is a function of the progress in the chain of research; studies found early in the chain probably can be quite valuable based on the use of nonprobability methods. Alternatively, studies that are in advanced positions on the research chain may or may not benefit from the use of the more elaborate forms of sampling (that is, probability techniques).

◆ ◆ ◆

In a Nutshell

Although simple rules do not apply (for example, probability techniques are always better), the general principle of parsimony is very applicable.

◆ ◆ ◆

As noted previously in this chapter, formulation of the research question (step 2) may be dependent upon ability to access the sample necessitated by the question. This iterative process of asking if a research question can be fairly addressed given realistic options for sampling must occur in conjunction with step 2. Thus, sampling is very much part of the planning process rather than simply being an implementation step.

The single most important determinant of selecting a sampling technique is the selection of a priority population (step 1 in the research process) for the research. In fact, the selection of a population immediately defines and limits the sampling options. In turn, steps 8 and 9 of the research process (data analysis and interpretation followed by dissemination of the findings) are dependent on the selection of the sampling technique. For example, inferential statistics (in theory) are meant to be applied only to data collected from a probability sample. Interpretation of any study is also very much a function of the sampling—this is because the findings cannot be generalized beyond the ability of the sample to represent the population. As sampling becomes increasingly representative of a population, the ability to generalize study findings to that population also increases. Finally, it should be noted that an unfortunate reality often exists with respect to publishing (that is, disseminating) findings from research studies—probability samples are often considered "preferred" products by virtue of their ability for generalization. However tempting, this reality does not justify selecting a probability technique simply because it may facilitate publication of a manuscript.

◆ ◆ ◆

In a Nutshell

The selection of a population immediately defines and limits the sampling options.

◆ ◆ ◆

Summary

Sampling can make or break a research study. The pinnacle of success in sampling is perfect representativeness. Unfortunately, this pinnacle is rarely achieved. However, the barriers that preclude full achievement are often inevitable. One important example is the necessary compromise that must occur to protect the rights of people to refuse study participation. Another important example is extremely practical in nature: researchers are not always granted access to a potential sample of people or organizations, and they may be denied access to useful sampling frames. Once access is achieved, sampling techniques should be chosen to parsimoniously address the research question and fairly represent the selected priority population. Sampling can select elements comprising "people" or representing organized units (clusters). Again, the selection of people versus clusters is dictated by the nature of the research question. Creative use of these techniques is not only acceptable but is also encouraged—as none of the techniques has perfect utility for all research questions.

◆ ◆ ◆

In a Nutshell

The pinnacle of success in sampling is perfect representativeness.

◆ ◆ ◆

Issues to Consider

1. An important issue can be conceptualized by the following question: What constitutes a confound in the test of the research question? A confound is a measurable factor that can produce bias. For example, imagine a study that is designed to assess the protective value of condoms against the acquisition of chlamydia. The research question is largely tied to physiological processes (for example, the porosity of the latex, the size and infectivity of the pathogen, and the biology of chlamydia transmission). Thus (with the exception of sex differences, in other words, male versus female anatomy) a sample of any kind might be justifiable as the results of this study should not vary as a function of the population. In other words, if condoms "work" for one population then they should also work for another. Although this proposition is attractive, what if a factor such as "condom skill" plays a role and the sample selected has an unusually high-level of skill? Of course, the confound (skill) will create a bias

that favors condom effectiveness. Yet, if skill is measured it can be accounted for statistically; thus, the confound no longer applies. This issue then is whether a sample inherently creates confounds that cannot be controlled. When such confounds do not exist, is the use of "any sample" justifiable in studies that address largely nonbehavioral outcomes?

2. A consistently important principle in health promotion is that ethics must always take precedence over rigor. This principle, however, is often violated by even the best-intentioned researchers. For example, the "accounting process" described in this chapter suggests that knowing the reasons nonparticipants refused to be part of the study is an important aspect of gauging rigor. Yet once a person says "no," do researchers violate this principle by proceeding to ask a question and then recording the answer and treating it as data?

3. Does providing study participants with financial compensation lead to participation bias? This is perhaps one of the most contemporary issues in health promotion research. Simply stated, the use of incentives (financial or otherwise) will be a greater enticement to some people compared with others, and the reasons for this greater enticement may be a marker for a study confound. For example, offering men $20 to complete a three-hour interview about their risks of cancer may be effective at producing a high participation rate, but many of the men who say "yes" may do so simply because they cannot in good consciousness turn down this "easy money." By comparison men who say "no" may be quite different (perhaps not perceiving $20 as a substantial amount of money). Thus, the sample may have an inherent bias of low-income men. Conversely, if financial incentives are extremely low (for instance, $5) or nonexistent, it is entirely conceivable that only men with a preexisting interest in cancer risks would volunteer, thereby creating a bias sample of men who are seemingly very concerned about cancer risks. Although striking a happy median between "too much" and "too little" incentive is an apparent answer to this issue, the question becomes how much is too much and how little is too little?

For Practice and Discussion

1. After much thought and discussion, you have developed the following research question: Are immigrant Latinas in the U.S. who have not been *acculturated* (cultural modification of an individual, group, or people by adapting to or borrowing traits from another culture) less likely to receive gynecological care than their counterparts who are more acculturated? You decide that fluency in English will be a valid proxy measure for acculturation. Thus, you need a

sample of immigrant Latinas who do and do not speak English. Alone, please list your top three choices for a sampling technique and then rank these in order of desirability—be prepared to explain your thinking! Then (if possible) find another student who has also completed this exercise and compare your list with his or her list. Try to engage in discussion about the pros and cons of the selections until your lists (and your rankings) match.

2. For the articles listed below (or any other article that you may select), please answer the following questions: (1) What type of sampling technique was employed (be careful not to simply restate what the authors have said—name the technique they used based on what you learned in this chapter; (2) Are the conclusions of the article within the boundaries of the sample? Or have the authors generalized beyond the ability of the sample?; and (3) Have the authors misused the sampling technique in any way and, if so, how?

Sources for This Exercise

1. Rosenberg, S. D., and others. (2001). Prevalence of HIV, hepatitis B, and hepatitis C in people with severe mental illness. *American Journal of Public Health, 91*, 31–37.
2. Blake, S. M., and others. (2003). Condom availability programs in Massachusetts high schools: Relationships with condom use and sexual behavior. *American Journal of Public Health, 93*, 955–962.
3. Tang, H., and others. (2003). Changes of attitudes and patronage behaviors in response to a smoke-free bar law. *American Journal of Public Health, 93*, 611–617.

References

Abelson, R. P. (1995). *Statistics as principled argument.* Hillsdale, NJ: Lawrence Erlbaum Associates.

Armstrong, K., Berlin, M., Sanford-Swartz, J., Propert, K., and Ubel, P. A. (2001). Barriers to influenza immunization in a low-income urban population. *The American Journal of Preventive Medicine, 20*, 21–25.

Babbie, E. (2001). *The practice of social research* (10th ed.). Belmont, CA: Wadsworth.

Grunbaum, J. A., and others. (2000). Youth risk behavior surveillance: National Alternative High School Youth Risk Behavior Survey, United States, 1998. *Journal of School Health, 70*, 5–17.

Henry, G. T. (1990). *Practical Sampling.* Thousand Oaks, CA: Sage.

Morales, L. S., and others. (2004). Use of preventive services by men enrolled in Medicare+ choice plans. *American Journal of Public Health, 94*, 796–802.

Shah, B. V., Barnwell, B. G., and Beiler, G. S. (1997). *SUDAAN: User's manual, release 7.5.* Research Triangle Park, NC: Research Triangle Institute.

Shi, L. (1997). *Health services research methods.* Albany, NY: Delmar Publishers.

CHAPTER TWELVE

ANALYTIC TECHNIQUES FOR OBSERVATIONAL RESEARCH

Richard A. Crosby, Ralph J. DiClemente, and Laura F. Salazar

S tudents often experience a great deal of anxiety over the topic of data analysis. Although a modest level of anxiety may be helpful, this chapter is designed to alleviate the anxiety associated with statistics. Indeed, statistical methods applied to health promotion research do not need to be highly sophisticated (or complicated) to be effective. Although the research process is often labor-intensive and time consuming, data analysis can be a fairly short process that is straightforward by comparison. The caveat, however, is that the selection of analytic tools must be exact and the analyses must be precise. Without these two conditions, selection and precision, the entire research process is jeopardized.

A s noted in Chapter One, parsimony is a critical concern with respect to data analysis. Data that tell a story worth hearing need not be "tortured" to achieve a valuable analysis. On the contrary, data analyses require the application of three basic procedures. First, the data should be described. This initial procedure is nothing more than a representation of the data in the form of frequency counts and, if applicable, means with their standard deviations. Some research questions do not require data analysis beyond this point. Second, *bivariate* associations between variables should be calculated. The term *bivariate* means that the calculated association is only between two variables. Typically, in health promotion research, the bivariate association would be between one *Y* variable (the outcome variable) and one *X* variable (the predictor variable); however, you may be interested in calculating bivariate associations between two predictor variables. Again, some research questions do not require further analysis. The problem, though, is that bivariate relationships seldom capture the complexity of health behaviors. Most health behavior is rarely, if ever, predicted by only one predictor variable. In fact, health behaviors often have complex determinants that can only be understood when a large number of *X* variables are taken into consideration. Studies of behaviors such as condom use (Sheeran, Abraham, and Orbell, 1999), teen pregnancy (Crosby and others, 2003), and being vaccinated against influenza (Armstrong, Berlin, Sanford-Swartz, Propert, and Ubel, 2001) involve multiple predictor variables as they relate to these single outcome variables. Thus, the third and final basic procedure is to conduct a *multivariate* analysis of the data. In this chapter, the term *multivariate* will be used to represent a statistical analysis involving multiple predictors or *X* variables and a single outcome or *Y* variable. Some scholars reserve the term *multivariate* for analyses that involve multiple *Y* variables, however.

◆ ◆ ◆

In a Nutshell

Data that tell a story worth hearing need not be "tortured" to achieve a valuable analysis.

◆ ◆ ◆

After presenting these three basic procedures, the chapter will also provide an overview of other related statistical issues such as power, sample size, and effect size, as these affect testing the research question. This presentation will be modest in scope. Readers who are interested in a more comprehensive treatment of these topics are encouraged to consult a text authored by Cohen (1988). The overall approach of this chapter is to provide a conceptual basis for applying analytic procedures that are commonly used in health promotion research. This chapter will serve as a springboard into statistics for observational research. Fortunately, a large number of very well-written statistics textbooks are readily available (for example, Pagano and Gauvreau, 2000; Siegel and Castellan, 1988; Tabachnick and Fidell, 1996).

Illustration of Key Concepts

Analyses generally begin with basic descriptive techniques and then proceed to employ tests for bivariate associations and, finally, for multivariate associations. When testing for bivariate and multivariate associations, it is important to understand the use of *P*-values. Last, but certainly not least, issues pertaining to statistical power and effect size must constantly be considered in the analytic process.

Descriptive Analysis

Observational data analysis seeks to describe and explain characteristics of defined groups. Ideally, these are representative samples of priority populations. (See step 1 in Chapter One.) Thus, an initial goal of descriptive analysis is to characterize the group through the use of appropriate statistics. In this section, we will use an example of an observational study of adolescents residing in detention facilities, which was conducted by the editors of this textbook, to highlight the different descriptive statistics. In this particular example, one of the research questions involved assessing the prevalence of thirty-four different health risk behaviors. After collecting the data, we produced the graphic shown in Figure 12.1. The

FIGURE 12.1.   DISTRIBUTION OF HEALTH-RISK BEHAVIORS FOR 569 DETAINED ADOLESCENTS.

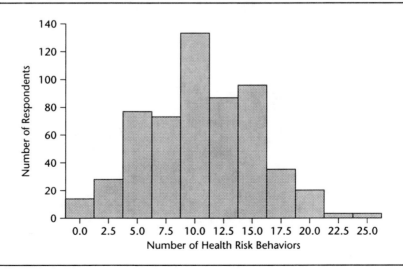

figure shows the distribution of scores and thus provides a useful overview of the data.

The Normal Curve. Scores that are distributed normally produce a distribution that, when graphed, create a specific, symmetrical curve shaped like a bell that follows a particular mathematical function. Often the normal curve is referred to as a bell-shaped curve, although, strictly speaking, not all bell-shaped curves are normal, but any distribution that is not symmetrical cannot be a normal curve. It is important to determine whether or not your data are approximately normally distributed, as this characteristic is an assumption that must be met for many statistical analyses to be performed correctly and accurately. Statistical analyses that require data to be normally distributed (for instance, linear regression) fall under the category of parametric tests. Other tests that do not require the data to be normally distributed (for example, a chi-square test) are deemed nonparametric.

A curve's deviation from normality can be judged based on two properties: *skewness* and *kurtosis*. Skewness is the degree to which scores in the distribution fall disproportionately on one side creating a curve with a long "tail." Although by graphing and visually inspecting a distribution we have a gross indicator of a distribution's skewness, it should be evaluated statistically. Most statistical software programs will determine whether or not skewness exceeds that of a normal distribution. The distribution shown in Figure 12.2 illustrates a positively skewed

FIGURE 12.2.   NUMBER OF SEX PARTNERS (LIFETIME) REPORTED BY DETAINED ADOLESCENTS.

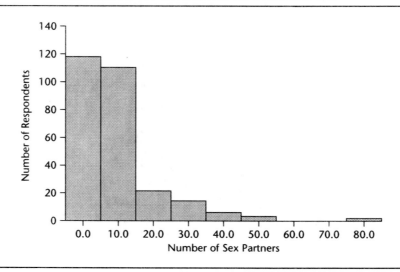

**FIGURE 12.3.   NUMBER OF PAP TESTS (LIFETIME)
REPORTED BY 273 WOMEN.**

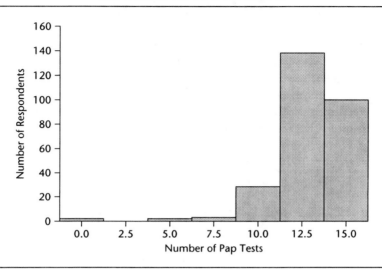

distribution in that most of the scores fall to the left side (in other words, most of the study participants reported having sex with ten or fewer partners), creating a long tail extending to the right. Whether or not a distribution is positively or negatively skewed depends on the direction of this tail. Therefore the distribution in Figure 12.2 is positively skewed. Many variables assessed in health promotion research will have a positive skew. Some examples include number of pregnancies, number of times diagnosed with a sexually transmitted disease, use of illicit substances, and frequency of driving while intoxicated.

An example of a distribution that is negatively skewed is shown in Figure 12.3. As indicated, the majority of scores are clumped together on the far right, leaving a long tail that extends to the left (the negative direction of the number line). Thus, most women in the sample reported having approximately twelve or more Pap tests in their lifetime.

Kurtosis refers to the shape of the distribution from top to bottom rather than side-to-side. A distribution with a preponderance of cases clustered in the middle—making a very tall spike-like shape—is called *leptokurtic*. Conversely, a distribution with a relatively flat shape (an absence of scores grouped around the mean) is called *platykurtic*. Again, by graphing and visually inspecting a distribution we can have a gross indicator of a distribution's kurtosis; however, it should be evaluated statistically. Most statistical software programs will also determine whether or not kurtosis exceeds that of a normal distribution.

The Mean. A mean can be calculated for any distribution assessed using ratio-level or interval-level data. *Ratio-level* data are assessed such that the distance between possible values is always equal and an absolute (rather than arbitrary) zero point exists. Age is a good example of a ratio-level measure. *Interval-level data* assume an equal distance between values but an absolute zero point is not present (see Box 12.1 for more information about levels of measurement). The obtained distribution portrays the health risk behavior profile of the entire sample of 569 adolescents (Figure 12.1). Of thirty-four possible risk behaviors, some adolescents engaged in no risk behavior, whereas others engaged in as many as twenty-five. The arithmetic average, or the *mean*, was 10.6. It is important to note

---

Box 12.1. Four Levels of Data

1. Nominal data represent discrete categories that are not ordered in any particular way.
Examples: sex, religion, reasons for not having a mammogram, types of illicit substances used in the past thirty days, and outcome of health promotion program (for example, improved or did not improve).

2. Ordinal data represent a value, category, or level that can be ranked or ordered in some particular way. Distances between categories are not assumed to be equal.
Examples: questionnaire responses coded as "strongly agree," "agree," "unsure," "disagree," or "strongly disagree"; decisional focus for contraceptive use (response option might be "my partner decides without my input," "I provide some input into these decisions," "I provide an equal amount of input," "I decide without my partner's input").

3. Interval data represent numerical values that are ordered, and distances between values are assumed to be equal. The value for zero is arbitrary.
Examples: psychological measures such as intelligence, special abilities, personality, and so on; temperature measured on Fahrenheit or Celsius scales.

4. Ratio data represent numerical values that are ordered, have equal distances between values, and have an absolute zero-point.
Examples: age, inches, weight, dollars, number of times a person used alcohol in the past month, number of times a person has had their blood serum cholesterol checked, number of vaccinations given by voluntary health organizations, percentage of body fat.

Note: Sometimes data can be converted from one type to another. For example, age (a ratio measure) can be converted to an ordinal measure by assigning scores that fall below 45 to a category named "young" and scores that equal or fall above 45 to a category named "old."

that the mean does not pertain to any one person; instead, it represents the average score of the group. Because it is an average score of the group, the mean is vulnerable to any extreme scores or outliers. For example, in a study of 141 high-risk men, frequency of crack (cocaine) use was assessed for the past six months. The mean number of uses was 29.1. Of interest though, one man indicated using crack a thousand times. Upon converting this score to "system missing" (as it is quite difficult to place full confidence in this extremely high value) the mean is reduced to 22.1 (a much truer representation of the group).

Spread. One important aspect of the group scores is characterized by their distribution or spread. It is important to understand two elemental indicators of spread: the *range* of the scores (in other words, the lowest score subtracted from the highest score) and the *dispersion* (that is, how much each score differs from the mean). Both the range and the dispersion are sensitive to extreme scores. For example, the initial range in the study of men who use crack was 1,000 (1,000 − 0). After excluding the extreme score of 1,000, the range decreased to 250 (250 − 0), indicating a much more narrow degree of spread.

The Standard Deviation. Because the goal is to characterize the group, it is useful to calculate an average measure of dispersion. This is called the standard deviation and can be derived by first summing each of the squared deviations (all 569) from the mean. Because negative deviations will cancel out positive deviations, the sum of all deviations will always produce a value of zero. Thus, the deviations are squared. Then, to obtain an average of the deviations, the sum of the squared deviations must be divided by the number of study participants, minus 1 (that is, 568). To return to the original metric, the square root is then calculated. The obtained value is known as the standard deviation and is always a positive value.

Like the mean, the standard deviation provides a great deal of clarity to the description of a group. It too is sensitive to influence of extreme scores. In the example of men who use crack, before excluding the score of 1,000 the standard deviation was 88.4 (this is a very large standard deviation). After excluding the extreme score, the standard deviation became much more reasonable (32.2). It is important to note that size does matter. When the standard deviation is small, this statistic indicates that the group is very similar relative to the variable being studied. This similarity is also called *homogeneity.* Conversely, when the standard deviation is large, this statistic indicates that the group is very diverse relative to the variable being studied. This level of diversity is also called *heterogeneity.*

The standard deviation can be used as a tool to characterize distributions that are relatively symmetrical. Returning to the previous example, recall that the mean is 10.6 and the standard deviation is 4.8. Moving in both positive and negative directions from the mean by one standard deviation (in other words, ± 1 SD) will account for approximately two-thirds of the scores (about 68 percent). Stated differently, slightly more than two-thirds of the sample will have scores between a low value of 5.8 (10.6 − 4.8) and a high value of 15.4 (10.6 + 4.8). Furthermore, moving in both directions from the mean by two standard deviations accounts for 95 percent of scores. Thus, 95 percent of the scores would fall between scores of 1.0 (10.6 − [4.8 × 2]) and 20.2 (10.6 + [4.8 × 2]).

The Median. The median is the score occurring at the midpoint of a ranked distribution of scores and should be used when data are skewed or when the data are measured using an *ordinal scale* (ordinal measurement means that the scores can be ranked from low to high, but that the distance between scores is not known to be equal; see Box 12.1 for more information about levels of measurement). For example, in the United States a distribution of income would have a strong positive skew, meaning that most people have low income levels whereas a small minority has extremely high income levels. Thus, the mean is not an accurate indicator of the "middle" income level for all people residing in the United States. In this instance, the median would be a better statistic to use to describe income distribution levels, as it separates the ranked order distribution at the middle. In health promotion research, many health-related variables are not always amenable to interval- or ratio-level measurement. Instead, ordinal-level measures are quite common. For example, to characterize a group with regard to satisfaction levels of physician-patient relationships when the difference between satisfaction levels are unknown and should not be assumed to be equal is conducive to the use of the median to describe the distribution of scores.

Frequency Distributions. When nominal-level data are collected, statistics are not available to characterize a distribution. *Nominal-level* measurement means that discrete categories are being assessed (such as male and female; black and white; former smoker, current smoker, never smoked); therefore, ranking from low to high or ordering in a particular way is not possible nor is it logical (again, see Box 12.1 for more information about levels of measurement). Because nominal data are not ranked, a median would be an inappropriate statistic for describing these distributions (a mean, standard deviation, or other statistic is also not applicable). Instead, simply enumerating the number of occurrences for each attribute of the nominal measure is appropriate. An example of a computer-generated frequency distribution is shown in Table 12.1. Notice that four columns appear in this table. The first provides the actual number of study participants categorized into each of the listed attributes. For example, 219 adolescents self-identified as black and

TABLE 12.1.   FREQUENCY DISTRIBUTION OF RACE OR ETHNICITY FOR A SAMPLE OF 569 DETAINED ADOLESCENTS.

Race or Ethnicity	Frequency	Percentage	Valid Percentage	Cumulative Percentage
White-not Hispanic	223	39.2	40.1	40.1
Black-not Hispanic	219	38.5	39.4	79.5
White-Hispanic	32	5.6	5.8	85.3
Black-Hispanic	42	7.4	7.6	92.8
Asian American	4	.7	.7	93.5
Native American	6	1.1	1.1	94.6
Other	30	5.3	5.4	100.0
Total	556	97.7	100.0	
Missing	13	2.3		
Total	569	100.0		

non-Hispanic. Notice in this column that data are missing for 13 adolescents. This observation is important because it suggests that converting the frequency counts into percentages could be achieved by using one of two possible denominators. The second column shows percentages based on the entire sample as the denominator (in this case 569). The third column also shows the percentages, but these are based only on the number of valid cases (meaning that the thirteen missing cases are not included in the denominator). Thus, when data are missing (which is generally unavoidable) the values in the third column will always be greater than the values in the second column. The fourth column is merely a running subtotal of the third column. This can be useful for descriptive purposes. For example, inspection of this column reveals that 92.8 percent of the sample self-identified as either white or black.

Bivariate Analysis

Before we describe a few selected types of bivariate analyses, it is important to clarify in general why statistical tests are performed. The tests yield two critical pieces of information that must be considered to answer the research question. First, the test informs us whether or not a finding may have occurred by chance. In this context, chance is determined by a probability value that when conducting statistical tests is judged against *alpha*. Alpha can be conceptualized as a cut-off point to determine the statistical significance of a test and by convention is set at .05 or less. Alpha is the probability that given the null hypothesis is true (for example, no effect) the results observed were by chance. Uppercase *P* and lowercase *p* are both used to denote the probability level associated with a particular statistical test. The second piece of critical information that statistical tests provide is a quantitative indicator of strength in relationships.

When embarking on a bivariate analysis, a key step is to select an appropriate statistical test. Three of the most basic options in health promotion research are (1) a *t*-test, (2) a chi-square test, and (3) the Pearson Product Moment Correlation. The *t*-test is used when the research question has a grouping variable that identifies only two groups (the predictor) and an outcome variable measured at an interval- or ratio-level. The chi-square test could be used with the same grouping variable (with two or more levels), but only when the outcome variable is nominal (both variables might also be ordinal, especially if only a few values are used). Finally, the Pearson Product Moment Correlation is used when both variables are represented with interval- or ratio-level measures.

T-*Test Example.* A common goal of observational research in health promotion is to compare subgroups of a sample (defined by a "grouping" variable) with respect to a second variable. Imagine, for example, that your research question involves comparing males and females on an index of health risk behavior. The grouping variable would be sex and the second variable would be the score on an index. Consider the distribution shown in Figure 12.1. Because this was assessed with a ratio-level measure, a *t*-test would be an appropriate method of addressing a research question involving sex differences. The test answers a basic question that is essential to all statistical tests: Are observed differences between the two groups "real" or due to chance? By convention real differences can be attributable to chance no more than five times out of one hundred tests. This corresponds to an alpha of .05. In some research studies, a more restrictive *P*-value may be used, such as .01. Of interest, the *P*-value of .05 corresponds to values of the test statistic that are greater than two standard deviations above or less than two standard deviations below the mean. This relationship is explained in Box 12.2.

The *t*-test will compare a mean risk score for females to the mean risk score for males. Dispersion of each distribution (one pertaining to females, the other to males) plays an important role in the calculation of *t* (small standard deviations will produce a larger *t* value). The number of study participants in each group also plays an important role in the calculation of *t*; larger numbers of participants will produce a larger *t* value. In this example, 283 females had a mean risk score of 9.9 (SD = 5.0) and 276 males had a mean of 11.3 (SD = 4.5). The obtained value for *t* was 3.4. This value was significant (that is, the probability associated with this test was less than .05). In fact, the obtained *P*-value of .001 suggests that given no sex differences, the findings would be attributable to chance only 1 out of 1,000 times! So, what can be concluded from this bivariate analysis? Given that the test was significant, it can be said that the mean for males is significantly greater

Box 12.2. Confidence Intervals

Intervals—defined by lower and upper boundaries, can be used to define a given level of confidence that a mean (or a similar estimate) is accurate. For example, a statement might read, "The mean was 19.2 (95 percent CI = 9.2 − 29.2)." The statement provides a range of confidence for the mean—implying 95 percent confidence that it is, in reality, a value that falls between 9.2 and 29.2. Values beyond this range (in either direction) would be attributable to chance—note then, that chance is set at 5 percent (corresponding to a *P*-value of .05). If a 99 percent confidence had been reported, then chance would be set at 1 percent (corresponding to a *P*-value of .01).

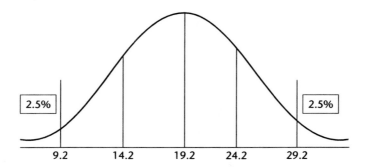

The confidence interval is defined by standard deviations. Adding and subtracting two standard deviations from the mean defines the 95 percent confidence interval (three standard deviations defines the 99 percent CI). Given a standard deviation of 5.0, the 95 percent CI would be defined according to the picture shown here. The 2.5 percent of the cases that fall at either extreme would be "outside" of the defined interval. Wide intervals imply less precision (or confidence) in the estimate. Thus, narrow confidence intervals are a desirable standard. For example, what if the standard deviation had been 2.0 rather than 5.0 percent?

Confidence intervals can also be applied to test statistics. An odds ratio, for example, is always shown with a corresponding 95 percent CI. Again, narrow intervals are desirable. The interval can be used to compare the relative strength of two odds ratios. If the lower limit of the interval with the higher odds ratio "laps" into the higher limit of the lower odds ratio, then the two odds ratios are not significantly different from each other. However, if they do not have overlapping values between their confidence intervals, they are indeed "different," and the value of the larger odds ratio is significantly greater than that of the lower odds ratio.

DINCUS IS UNSURE OF HIS STATISTICAL PLAN.

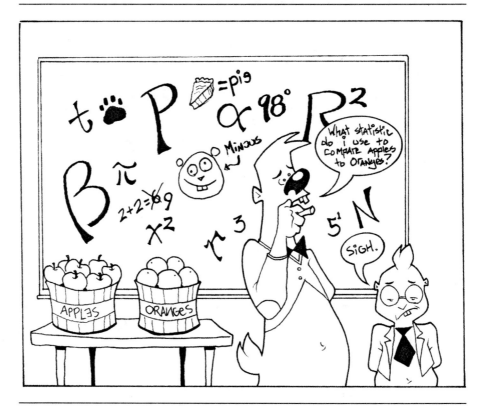

Copyright 2005 by Justin Wagner; reprinted with permission.

than the mean for females (in other words, the observed difference between 11.3 and 9.9 has a low probability of being a chance occurrence). Thus, the conclusion might read, "The average level of risk was significantly greater for males as compared to females."

Chi-Square Example. Suppose that a research study is examining whether family history of breast cancer (that is, the predictor) is related to practicing breast self-exams on a regular basis. The nature of the research question demands that women with a history be contrasted to all other women (these are two discrete categories). Those women practicing breast self-exam on a regular basis—perhaps defined as once a month—would then be compared to those engaging in the practice less frequently (again, these are two discrete categories). The public health

TABLE 12.2. CONTINGENCY TABLE OF DATA PERTAINING TO A STUDY OF BREAST SELF-EXAMINATION PRACTICES.

	Frequency of Breast Self-Examination		
	Monthly	Less Than Monthly	Total
Family history of breast cancer	79	14	93
No family history of breast cancer	66	19	85
Total	145	33	178

outcome of interest here is clearly breast self-exam; thus the predictor variable is family history of breast cancer (none vs. some). Table 12.2 displays a contingency table that contains data addressing this research question.

As shown in Table 12.2, the contingency table has four cells. These tables have an endless array of uses in health promotion research and therefore deserve extensive study by the new investigator. The outcome is shown in columns and the predictor is shown in rows. Each column and row has a total. The row totals and the column totals must, by definition, sum to the same value (in this case the value 178; this is a "grand total"). The most basic function of the table is purely descriptive. Notice, for example, that among the ninety-three women with a family history, fourteen (15.1 percent) did not practice breast self-exam on a monthly basis. Among the eighty-five women without a family history, nineteen (22.9 percent) did not practice breast self-exam on a regular basis.

Although the descriptive value of a contingency table is important, the question that arises is identical to that posed earlier in the t-test example: How likely is the difference between 15.1 percent and 22.9 percent due to chance alone? This question can be addressed by the chi-square statistic (shown as χ^2). Using the row and column totals, a value expected by chance can be calculated for each of the four cells. For example, the upper left cell has a corresponding row total of 93 and a corresponding column total of 145. To obtain the value expected by chance for this cell, multiply 93 by 145 and divide the product by the grand total of 178. Thus, the chance value for the upper left cell is 75.75. The obtained value for the upper left cell was 79. Herein lies the key to the chi-square test: the difference between the obtained value of 79 and the value expected by chance is 3.25. Across the four cells, these differences form the *conceptual* basis for the calculations needed to arrive at the χ^2 value.

After obtaining the χ^2 value, the final step is to evaluate the value for statistical significance. Again, a corresponding *P*-value of .05 or less would typically be counted as evidence that the difference between 15.1 percent and 22.9 percent is not readily attributable to chance. In the example shown in Table 12.2, the χ^2

value is 1.77 and the corresponding P-value is .18. Thus, 15.1 percent and 22.9 percent are not significantly different values. The conclusion for this study might then read: "The chi-square test revealed that the percentage of women who practiced breast self-exam and had a family history of breast cancer was not significantly different from the percentage of women who do not have a family history of breast cancer."

Before leaving this discussion of the chi-square test, it is useful to discuss the concept of a median split (as "splitting" a distribution at its median can be a useful procedure and results in the ability to apply a chi-square test). The median can be used to split a non-normal distribution of interval- or ratio-level data into two distinct parts (for example, high versus low, healthy versus unhealthy, more frequent versus less frequent). This median split can be a very useful tool for describing a group in relationship to a second variable. Consider the following research questions:

- Does a measure of attitude toward preventive practices predict ever having a colonoscopy?
- Does a measure of attitude toward preventive practices predict ever being tested for HIV?
- How do people diagnosed with depression differ from those not having this diagnosis with respect to whether they use tobacco?

In each question, the predictor variable (that is, attitude toward prevention or, in the latter question, depression level) necessitates the use of a scale measure (see Chapter Nine). However, as noted previously in this chapter, the obtained distribution for such measures may be markedly skewed (as shown in the examples displayed in Figures 12.2 and 12.3). In such cases, the lack of a normal (or nearly normal) distribution violates typical assumptions of statistical tests that might be used for these ratio-level measures. Moreover, the people represented by the skew (the long tail) are a potentially important focal point. Thus, if a median split was performed on each of these predictor variables, then the analyses could all be addressed by chi-square tests. (Note: in each test a contingency table with four cells—like that displayed in Table 12.2—could be created.)

Correlation Examples. When interval- or ratio-level data are available, the Pearson Product Moment Correlation is an efficient method of representing the strength of a linear relationship (correlation) between variables. The correlation coefficient is represented by a lower case r. The values of r range from -1.0 to $+1.0$, with a perfect correlation being found at either extreme (in other words, both -1.0 and $+1.0$ are perfect correlations). A positive and significant value of r means that the two variables being compared each increase together; this is known as a *direct relationship*. Consider, for example, self-efficacy for engaging in aerobic exercise (X) and the average number of aerobic workouts per week (Y). As scores on the measure of X (presumably a paper-and-pencil assessment) increase, an increase (to some corresponding degree) in Y would be expected. Because the value of r provides an indicator of how strong the correspondence is between X and Y, an r of $+1.0$ would mean they rise in perfect synchrony. However, this is only a theoretical possibility; in reality the two variables may rise together at a level of .20 or .30 or higher. Note also that r does *not* address causality; that is, X may be influencing the corresponding rise in Y, or Y may be influencing the corresponding rise in X. Sometimes, a researcher can rule out the possibility that Y could be "causing" X by knowing that X cannot be changed (age, gender, and race are good examples). However, if X and Y are related, this still does not establish that X must cause Y (as there could be unknown variables that actually cause Y—see Chapter Four).

◆ ◆ ◆

In a Nutshell

A positive and significant value of r *means that the two variables being compared each increase together; this is known as a* direct relationship.

◆ ◆ ◆

A negative and significant value of r means that an increase in one variable corresponds to a decrease in the other variable; this is known as an *inverse relationship*. Consider, for example, a relationship between age (X), ranging from fourteen to forty-five, and the average number of health risk behaviors (Y) assessed by an index. A study may have obtained an r-value of $-.35$ for this correlation. Given that this value was significant (it had an acceptably low probability of occurring by chance), the value provides an indicator of how strongly (strength) the two variables are connected inversely. The direction of this relationship (that is, negative or inverse) is not surprising, and the magnitude (that is, .35) is modest. This latter point regarding magnitude, however, warrants further consideration.

◆ ◆ ◆

In a Nutshell

A negative and significant value of r *means that an increase in one variable corresponds to a decrease in the other variable; this is known as an* inverse relationship.

◆ ◆ ◆

FIGURE 12.4.   SCATTERPLOTS ILLUSTRATING DIRECT
AND INVERSE CORRELATIONS.

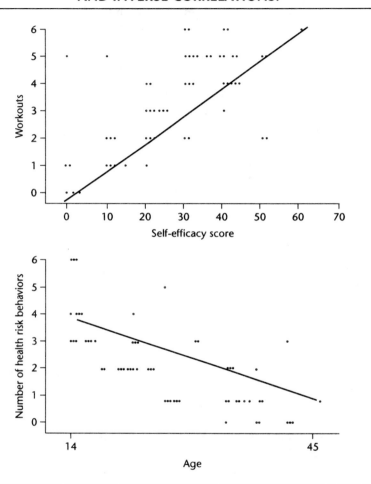

Figure 12.4 displays two scatterplots. A scatterplot is a collection of bivariate data points. A bivariate data point represents the intersection of locations on an *X*-axis (an abscissa) and a *Y*-axis (an ordinate). Through visual inspection of these data points, two observations can be made related to determining the magnitude of the linear relationship. First, a conceptual line should be "drawn" that indicates whether the two variables may be linearly related. Second, the conceptual

line may be steep or flat, indicating a perfect linear relationship or no linear relationship, respectively.

In the first scatterplot in Figure 12.4, it can be seen that a conceptual line superimposed on the data rises from left to right at a relatively sharp increase. Because the purpose of the line is to depict a linear relationship and compare how close the corresponding data points are to the line, it appears that the correlation is quite high: the closer the data points are to the line, the greater the correlation; data points that are quite distant from the conceptual line indicate a low correlation. In the second example in Figure 12.4, although the data points are close to the conceptual line, the line is not as steep as in the first example. Consequently, the correlation must be lower. Notice also that the line descends as it moves from left to right. This means that the correlation is inverse.

A caveat to each of the bivariate procedures is in order. After the two variables have been identified, it is critically important to determine which one is the outcome measure and which one is the predictor variable. (Note: the term *predictor variable* technically only applies to prospective studies; in cross-sectional studies a preferred term is *correlate*.) This determination is made based on the research question and the nature of the variables. In this example, the determination is simplified because sex cannot possibly be a logical outcome variable (that is, we could not possibly expect scores on the health risk index to be a determinant of sex, but we could fairly expect that sex would be a determinant of health risk behavior). Thus, we urge that great caution and careful logic be applied when interpreting bivariate findings; causality is often elusive and difficult to determine!

◆ ◆ ◆

In a Nutshell

After the two variables have been identified, it is critically important to determine which one is the outcome measure and which one is the predictor variable.

◆ ◆ ◆

A second caveat is in order. Imagine a graphic display of bivariate data points that takes the shape of an inverted "U." In this case, the correlation may be nonsignificant and very weak—approaching zero. This does not mean that X and Y are unrelated! This is true because not all relationships are linear. In this example, the relationship could be *quadratic*. A quadratic relationship between variables means that the two variables do not rise or decline in synchrony; rather, at some point along the X axis the relationship changes. A classic example of a quadratic relationship is anxiety (X) and performance (Y): at low levels of X, performance is low; at medium levels of X, performance is high; at high levels of X, performance is low.

Multivariate Analysis

Although several forms of multivariate analyses are available, two of the most widely selected are linear and logistic regression. Linear regression is appropriate for outcomes comprising interval-level data or ratio-level data. Conversely, logistic regression is used when the outcome is a dichotomy.

Linear Regression. The Pearson Product Moment Correlation forms the basis for simple linear regression. In simple linear regression, you are calculating an equation that determines the Y-intercept and slope of *the best fitting line.* The best fitting line refers to an actual line generated from the data and that minimizes the distance from the data points to the line. The Y-intercept and slope are termed *parameter estimates* of this equation. In turn, multiple linear regression is an extension of this test. As opposed to only one predictor variable, multiple linear regression involves several predictors.

Basically, regression serves several purposes: the first is to test the nature of the linear relationship between X variable(s) and a given outcome Y; a second purpose is to test the strength of the relationship; and a third purpose is to formulate prediction equations based on sample data that can be applied to the population. All three purposes can be achieved by generating the equation for the regression line.

One key concept in regression is the parameter estimation of the slope that reveals what the association is between X variable(s) and Y. The slope estimate, which is referred to as b, gauges how much Y would increase given a one-unit increase in X. This involves a brief understanding of *rise-to-run.* The estimate for slope is an unstandardized estimate, meaning that it is read in the original metric of the variable. Interpretation of slope estimates is as follows: "a one-unit change in X corresponds to a change in Y of b units." For example, a regression equation that was generated to examine the relationship between self-efficacy and number of days per week people exercise had a slope of 1.5. In practical terms this means that for every 1 unit increase in self-efficacy (the X variable shown on the abscissa, the run), people exercised 1.5 more days (the rise). Alternatively, if the relationship is inverse, the question becomes, How much does Y *decrease* for a one-unit increase in X?

Another function of regression is to provide standardized values of the slope estimate. Standardizing a variable places the measure on a common metric. The standardized regression coefficient is a measure of the strength of the association between X variable(s) and the outcome Y. The standardized parameter estimates are known as Beta (β) weights. Imagine three X variables: self-efficacy, age, and depression. An important question might be which of these three variables has the strongest relationship with an outcome of "attitudes toward getting a colonoscopy." Imagine further that the obtained Beta weights are .30, .21, and .15 respectively. Because they are standardized, these Beta weights can be directly compared with each other. Thus, the strongest variable in this case would be self-efficacy, followed by age, and then depression.

Another purpose of linear regression is to generate equations used for prediction. It should be noted that multiple linear regression models will generate a value for a "constant" and unstandardized parameter estimates (symbolized as b) that can be used to construct an equation that will predict Y. The assumption here is that the sample data can be applied to make inferences about the population. The equation may look familiar to anyone who can recall taking a high school math class: $Y = \text{constant} + b_1 (X1) + b_2 (X2) + b_3 (X3)$, and so on. Using the constant and the unstandardized parameter estimates, the information from this model could then be applied to persons who were not included in the sample to make predictions of Y.

Multiple linear regression is also used to determine how well a set of variables collectively is related to Y. Specifically, multiple linear regression can be used to judge the collective strength of the X-variables in explaining *variance* in Y. Accounting for variance is an important goal of multiple regression. The statistic used to represent this value is R^2.

◆ ◆ ◆

In a Nutshell

Multiple linear regression can be used to judge the collective strength of the X*-variables in explaining* variance *in* Y.

◆ ◆ ◆

R^2 ranges from 0 to 1.0. The value of R^2 typically does not exceed the sum of the r^2-values representing the bivariate relationships between the assessed X-variables and the given Y-variable, at least when the X-variables are intercorrelated. Figure 12.5 provides an illustration of this principle, using three X-variables: level of gang involvement, level of parental monitoring, and age (the outcome of interest [Y] is number of health risk behaviors). Although the Pearson

FIGURE 12.5.   THE SUM OF PEARSON *r* VALUES DOES NOT NECESSARILY EQUATE WITH R^2.

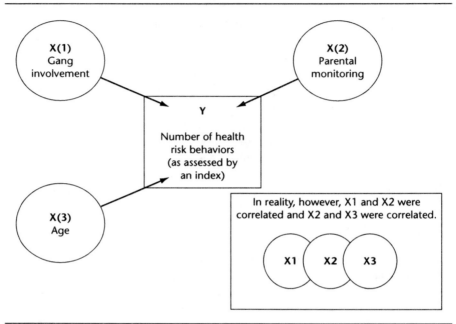

Note: Bivariate correlations: $X(1)r = .33$, $r^2 = .11$; $X(2)r = .30$, $r^2 = .09$; and $X(3)r = .10$, $r^2 = .01$ (all are significant at $P < .05$).

correlations were all significant, two were modest while the magnitude for age was very weak.

◆ ◆ ◆

In a Nutshell

The value of R^2 *typically does not exceed the sum of the* r^2*-values representing the bivariate relationships between the assessed* X*-variables and the given* Y*-variable, at least when the* X*-variables are intercorrelated.*

◆ ◆ ◆

While a quick glance at the *r*-values might suggest that R^2 would be about .21, the box in the lower right-hand corner of Figure 12.5 shows the common, multivariate reality. In fact, the R^2 for this model was .09. The diminished value occurs because of intercorrelation between the X-variables. Parental monitoring was significantly correlated (inverse) with the level of gang involvement. Parental monitoring was also significantly correlated with age (direct). Thus, the three X-variables exert a collective effect on Y but overlap between variables represents joint influence on Y. Of course, the overlap cannot be counted twice. Thus, the question becomes one of determining which variable (X_1 versus X_2, for example) is "credited" for explaining variance in Y relative to the region of overlap. The answer is determined by the research team and takes the form of an analytic decision relative to the order of entering X variables into the regression model. Although entry methods are beyond the scope of this introductory chapter, the curious reader should consult an excellent textbook authored by Tabachnick and Fidell (1996).

Logistic Regression. In linear regression, the Y-variable must be an interval- or ratio-level measure. Analyses that rely on outcomes that are assessed with interval- or ratio-level measures are termed *parametric*. Conversely, nonparametric analyses use outcome measures that are assessed with a categorical variable. A common form of nonparametric analysis in health promotion research is logistic regression. Logistic regression is used when the outcome variable is dichotomous. Of course, the number of research questions in health promotion that necessitate a dichotomous outcome measure is nearly infinite. Assessing the presence or absence of a disease, condition, or risk behavior, then, is clearly part of a research question that will lend itself to the use of logistic regression.

For the purposes of this introductory chapter, it can be said that the basic principles of multiple linear regression apply to multiple logistic regression. The principle behind the procedure is that an exponent (a constant value) is raised to a power of Beta (β), yielding an adjusted odds ratio. The model will then classify a given percentage of the cases correctly, based on the collective X-variables that achieve multivariate significance. Keep in mind, however, that the odds of classifying the outcome correctly are 50 percent by chance alone. Thus, for example, classifying 60 percent of the cases correctly would result in classifying only 10 percent beyond that expected by chance alone.

◆ ◆ ◆

In a Nutshell

The principle behind the procedure is that an exponent (a constant value) is raised to a power of Beta (β), yielding an adjusted odds ratio.

◆ ◆ ◆

Interpreting odds ratios is an important prerequisite to understanding research findings from logistic regression. Odds ratios are an estimate of added risk for Y based on the knowledge of an X-variable. For example, text in a manuscript might read as follows: "Adolescents identifying as members of a minority group were more than three times as likely to test positive for an STD (AOR = 3.12; 95 percent CI = 1.31 − 7.43)." This adjusted odds ratio can be judged for significance based on its 95 percent confidence interval. Simply put, confidence intervals that exclude the value of 1.0 are significant. An odds ratio of one has to be nonsignificant because it means "one time as likely," which, of course, means the same as or equally likely. (Recall that 1 times anything is itself.) In prospective studies, the odds ratio can be called a relative risk ratio. In either instance, a higher value represents a greater degree of risk for Y. An exception to this occurs when an X-variable is inversely associated with Y. Consider, for example, parental monitoring (from the previous example used in Figure 12.5). A high-level of parental monitoring might be associated with a decreased risk of teen pregnancy. Therefore, the obtained odds ratio would be protective (meaning that high monitoring would equate with *lower* risk of a negative outcome). Protective odds ratios range from 0 to .99. A protective odds ratio of .50, for example, would mean that teens with high monitoring were one-half as likely as those with low monitoring to become pregnant or (if male) cause a pregnancy. As before, the significance of a protective odds ratio is judged by whether its 95 percent confidence interval excludes 1.0.

A Warning About *P*-Values

Even seasoned researchers sometimes become confused about the meaning of a significant *P*-value. Simply stated, a *P*-value less than the established alpha level means that the related finding was statistically significant, indicating that the association had a low probability of occurring by chance alone, assuming that there is in fact no association. The *P*-value is *not* a measure of substantive effect (that is, strength of association between X and Y).

The confusion comes from a tendency to equate diminishing *P*-values (those such as .01, .001, and .0001) with progressively larger associations. This is not the case. Indeed, a large (and important) association may have a high probability of occurring by chance (yielding a nonsignificant *P*-value). Conversely, a rather weak (and unimportant) association may have a very low probability of occurring by chance alone (thus, the *P*-value would be significant). How is this possible? The difference is a function of sample size. The lesson here is quite simple: *P*-values only speak to the question of the probability or likelihood that an association can be attributed to chance alone. To understand this concept in greater detail, it is important to have a basic understanding of statistical power and effect size.

Statistical Power and Effect Size

When considering observational research, power is the ability of a statistical test to detect true associations (effects) between variables. Power is influenced by

- Sample size (this is a "direct relationship")
- Effect size
- Dispersion or variance (this is an "inverse relationship")
- The alpha level selected for the study (a lower, more stringent *P*-level gives less power)
- The use of a one-tailed versus two-tailed test of significance (more power with one tail)

Effect size can be conceptualized as the magnitude of association between two variables. For example, suppose that 22 percent of teens who reported low parental monitoring had ever been pregnant. In comparison, only 11 percent of those reporting high parental monitoring had ever been pregnant. Teens who had low parental monitoring were two times as likely to get pregnant than teens with high parental monitoring. The "two-times" is the odds ratio and is a measure of effect size in this example.

As empirical values, effect sizes allow readers to judge whether statistically significant results are also meaningful at a practical level. Stated differently, effect size captures the "true impact" of an association, whereas significance testing merely provides a determination of whether or not the association is a chance occurrence. Unlike other determinants of power, effect size is not influenced by anything other than the observations that are collected from the research participants. Power, on the other hand, can be affected by the researcher and can be increased (for example, by using a very large sample size or a high alpha level). By the same token, power may be low due to a small sample size.

◆ ◆ ◆

In a Nutshell

Effect size captures the "true impact" of an association, whereas significance testing merely provides a determination of whether or not the association is a chance occurrence.

◆ ◆ ◆

Large effect sizes require less power than medium or small effect sizes. Conversely, small effects require a great deal of power to detect them. Thus, an important and perhaps never-ending question in health promotion research is,

When are small effects that are deemed statistically significant, substantive? The flipside to this question is, When are large effects mistakenly declared nonsignificant due to low levels of power? These questions correspond to two classic forms of error in analysis. When an effect is deemed significant but is not real (false positive), the result is termed a *Type 1 error* and is in fact represented by alpha. Recall that alpha is the probability of results occurring by chance given that there are no real effects. When large effects are mistakenly declared nonsignificant (based on problems with low power), the result is termed a *Type 2 error* (false negative). Both types of error unfortunately are common. Studies with very large sample sizes (for example, greater than a thousand participants) may be prone to Type 1 errors and, of course, studies with very small sample sizes (for example, less than two hundred participants) may be prone to Type 2 errors.

This somewhat abridged discussion of power and effect size is important for several reasons. First, a fair test of a research question implies that the power is not too high and not too low (by convention, 80 percent power is considered a "fair test" criterion). Of note, power can be adjusted before the study begins (by planning sample size) or after the study has concluded (by adjusting alpha upward). Second, power problems in small studies that have already been completed may not be resolved; thus, effect size may be an especially important value to report. Third, as previously mentioned, in studies that have high power due to a large sample size, the effect size is an important indicator of whether the findings have substantive significance. Finally, studies should be planned to detect a reasonable effect size that is not unrealistically large but substantive, and this planning should culminate in an empirical estimate of the sample size requirement. Several software packages are available (many are freely obtained over the Internet) that can calculate sample size requirements based on estimated effect sizes and the determinants of power shown in the previous bulleted list. Furthermore, after a study is done these programs can be used to calculate the available power (based on effect sizes obtained) and the determinants of power shown in the bulleted list on page 339.

Applied Examples

This chapter provides two applied examples. The first illustrates the use of linear regression and the second illustrates the use of logistic regression.

Correlates of Unprotected Vaginal Sex

A study published in the *Archives of Pediatrics and Adolescent Medicine* provides a good application of linear regression to observational research in health promotion.

Crosby and colleagues (2000) selected a priority population for the prevention of HIV, sexually transmitted infections, and pregnancy of low-income African American adolescents residing in a risky urban environment. Using social cognitive theory as a framework, the researchers investigated correlates of engaging in unprotected vaginal sex (UVS) among 522 adolescent females.

The correlates were largely composed of scale measures (each assessed using interval- or ratio-level data). The outcome variable was frequency of UVS as reported by adolescents during a six-month recall period (a ratio-level measure). Pearson correlation was used to assess the direction and magnitude of the bivariate associations between each correlate and UVS. Several correlates achieved bivariate significance. These were then entered into a multiple linear regression model. UVS was regressed on fourteen correlates in a model restricted to UVS with steady partners. Subsequently, UVS was regressed on five correlates in a model restricted to sex with casual partners. The R^2 for the first model was .235 and the R^2 for the second model was .22. The strongest predictor of UVS in the first model was the average amount of time spent with the steady boyfriend during any given week ($\beta = .26$). Several other correlates retained multivariate significance in this model (their Beta coefficients ranged from $-.10$ to $.15$). In the second model, three correlates achieved multivariate significance: (1) pleasure barriers to condom use ($\beta = .23$); (2) history of STD infection ($\beta = .28$), and (3) partner control over sexual decisions ($\beta = .23$).

Correlates of Colorectal Cancer Screening

A study published in the *American Journal of Preventive Medicine* illustrates an application of logistic regression in health promotion. Mandelson and colleagues (2000) surveyed 931 women who were fifty to eighty years of age. The study was designed to identify correlates of fecal occult blood testing (FOBT) in the past two years. Demographic, attitudinal, perceptual, and physician-based variables were examined for their relationship to recent FOBT.

First, the study reported the strength of the bivariate relationships between the assessed correlates and FOBT. The bivariate relations were based on a contingency table (like the one shown in Table 12.2) and expressed as unadjusted odds ratios. (These are odds ratios that have not been "adjusted" for the influence of variables outside of the bivariate relationship.) For example, 38.5 percent of the women in their fifties had been screened in the past two years compared with 52.5 percent of those in their sixties and 56.5 percent of those in their seventies. Women in their sixties were about 2.75 times more likely to be screened in the past two years compared with women in their fifties (OR = 2.76; 95 percent CI = 1.85 − 4.11). Women in their seventies were about 4.5 times more likely to be screened in comparison with women in their fifties (OR = 4.47; 95 percent CI = 2.91 − 6.86). Note that the odds ratios are significant (in other words, their 95 percent confidence intervals exclude 1.0), and that the range encompassed by the intervals is relatively narrow. In contrast, women who reported having a mammogram two years or less before the survey were more than nine times as likely to be screened compared with women who had never had a mammogram (OR = 9.21; 95 percent CI = 3.72 − 22.8). Notice here that the confidence interval is quite wide.

Next, a multivariate analysis was used to test variables achieving bivariate significance. Three variables achieved significance using multiple logistic regression to calculate adjusted odds ratios: (1) the extent that physicians encourage screening, (2) the degree of comfort women had in discussing FOB testing with a physician, and (3) perceptions that the unpleasant aspect of the screening is justified based on the risk of colorectal cancer.

Integration with the Research Process

Good research is brought to life by a fair analysis; the same cannot be said for poor research. Stated differently, the decision points and planning steps that lead to data analysis (step 8 in the nine-step model) are, in essence, the most important elements of an analysis. Measurement (step 5) and sampling (step 6) are particularly critical, as these steps determine, in part, the quality of the variables and the power of the analysis, respectively. Of course, the nature of the research question (step 2) is perhaps the most critical determinant of a successful analysis. A carefully crafted study will be designed to identify effect sizes that can be detected without having to sample an unduly high number of participants. More important, this careful planning will result in findings that go beyond statistical significance into the realm of practical significance.

Although a fair analysis can bring good research to life, judging what constitutes a fair analysis is problematic. Certainly, assurances that Type 1 and Type 2 errors have been avoided are important. Moreover, parsimony is important, but some research questions will demand quite complex analytic approaches. For example, data from a panel study with multiple waves of data collection cannot be fairly analyzed without controlling for the inherent correlation of responses over time within each of the study participants. These repeated-measures data sets must be analyzed using advanced tools such as Generalized Estimating Equations. Similarly, data from an observational study that is based on sampling from clusters (that is, preexisting and well-defined groups or communities of people) cannot be fairly analyzed without accounting for the unavoidable correlations found within the various clusters of participants. In such an instance, a software program called SUDAAN can be used to control for this intercorrelation effect. Although numerous other examples could be provided, the main point is that fair analyses can be complicated to a point far beyond the capacity of the few analytic tools presented in this chapter. Vigilance in analysis, then, sometimes requires the assistance of qualified statisticians. This assistance may also be needed as the findings are interpreted in the early phase of step 9 (dissemination).

Finally, it should be noted that observational research is quite distinct from experimental research. In the latter, analyses are prescribed by the study design. In observational research, however, analyses can be conceived before and after the data has been collected. Furthermore, observational research can be used to answer two distinct varieties of research questions. First (and probably most common), the research can be designed to predict Y (meaning that correlates or predictors of one given outcome are identified). Most examples provided previously in this chapter have been patterned using this approach. The hallmark here is that only one outcome variable is investigated. Second, the research can begin with only a single X-variable and then determine the relationship of this variable to multiple outcomes that are pertinent to public health. Although less common, this approach can be an effective means of addressing a broad range of health promotion outcomes as opposed to a monolithic goal. For example, a recent study found that infrequent parental monitoring of adolescent females was associated with increased risk for marijuana use, greater levels of alcohol consumption, recent arrest, having multiple sex partners, not using condoms, the acquisition of sexually transmitted diseases, and not using contraceptive methods (DiClemente and others, 2001).

Summary

Data analysis is a turning point in the research process. This chapter has presented a few of the most basic techniques that are applied to the descriptive, bivariate, and multivariate analyses of data collected in the field of health promotion. One key thread that deserves attention is that not all data are created equal. In fact, data typically follow a divide between parametric and nonparametric camps. The former involves interval- or ratio-level outcome measures and is generally based on means, standard deviations, and variance. A t-test is a common example of bivariate parametric analysis, and multiple linear regression is a common example of a multivariate parametric analysis. Alternatively, nonparametric analyses are used for data with nominal- or ordinal-level outcome measures. Frequency distributions and medians are quite useful for describing nominal and ordinal data, respectively. A common example of a bivariate nonparametric analysis is the chi square test. Logistic regression is often used to handle nonparametric multivariate analyses pertaining to health promotion research. These tools should be used with great caution to precision and with careful attention to issues relevant to power and effect size.

Issues to Consider

1. A somewhat inflammatory and certainly important issue involves Type 1 error. The essence of this issue is that effect size can be lost in the context of other factors that may ultimately have an undue influence on whether a given finding achieves statistical significance. A good example of this can be found in the analysis of a CDC study known as Project Respect (Kamb and others 1998). This study found, for example, that incidence of sexually transmitted infections (assessed six months after study enrollment) among those assigned to an enhanced counseling condition was significantly lower ($P = .0001$) than incidence among those in the control condition. Incidence was approximately 7 percent versus 10 percent. Statistically, the finding seems quite promising. However, the obtained effect size was very small, suggesting that significance may have been an artifact of an extremely large sample size (that is, greater than three thousand participants). The issue is not easily resolved. On one hand, the difference between 7 percent and 10 percent could represent a substantial number of cases averted if the enhanced counseling protocol was widely applied; yet the potential case for the operation of Type 1 error is clear. Indeed, the larger question is, "What are the ethical obligations that researchers have to disclose the liability of a study to Type 1 error?"

2. After pondering the first issue, another related issue involves the difference between statistical significance and practical significance. A case in point is the common practice of discussing significant r-values as though they represent findings in their own right. It is imperative to know that P-values do not reflect strength in a relationship; instead they merely reflect the likelihood of a chance occurrence. Significant Pearson r-values of less than .20 are commonly discussed in manuscripts as though they have great value in understanding a given outcome variable. The problem is that an r-value of .20, for example, only explains 4 percent of the variance! (This can be easily calculated by squaring r.) The ultimate value of observation research to health promotion is that it can inform practice. Investigation of X-variables, then, implies that the findings can have implications for improving practices. Yet

research that explains such a small amount of the variance can hardly be said to have value with respect to changing (or sustaining) practice. Thus, the issue becomes, How can research findings be judged for practical as opposed to statistical significance?

3. An all-too-common analytic issue is whether a skewed distribution should be transformed into a simple dichotomy. Recall that skewness implies that an interval- or ratio-level variable has a distribution that "clumps" to the right or left rather than being centered. Recall also that the "tail portion" of a skewed distribution typically represents those people who may be at greatest risk for negative health outcomes. Critics of the median split suggest that a great deal of precision is lost when an interval- or ratio-level distribution is converted to a simple dichotomy (for example, low versus high). Proponents suggest that the conversion can create a dichotomy with a great deal of utility. The utility may derive from the nature of health promotion practice. For example, the regular practice of breast self-examination (BSE) may confer a protective measure against mortality from breast cancer, whereas women who practice BSE infrequently have no more protection against breast cancer–induced mortality than do women who never practice BSE. Thus, a natural dichotomy (formed from a ratio-level measure) could be warranted. The final question may be phrased, When (if ever) is the artificial creation of a dichotomy justified?

For Practice and Discussion

1. You have been presented with a data set that addresses one research question. The question seeks to identify predictors of HIV testing in a high-risk sample of gay men. You first examine the outcome measure (frequency of having HIV tests in the past ten years) and discover that the distribution has a strong positive skew. Also, you observe that the mean is 6 and the standard deviation is 4.5. What "tools" will you use to describe the outcome measure? What tools will you use to identify the predictors of HIV testing? Most important, please justify your selection of these tools.

2. You are reading a manuscript that reports findings based on observational research of an elderly population. The research question involved determination of differences in health behaviors (nutrition, rest, exercise, and abstinence from tobacco use) between those residing and those not residing in nursing homes. Without knowing anything else about this study, what type of bivariate analysis do you suppose would be used? Again, please justify your answer.

References

Armstrong, K., Berlin, M., Sanford-Swartz, J., Propert, K., and Ubel, P. A. (2001). Barriers to influenza immunization in a low-income urban population. *The American Journal of Preventive Medicine, 20,* 21–25.

Cohen, J. (1988). *Statistical power analysis for the behavioral sciences* (2nd ed.). Hillsdale, NJ: Lawrence Erlbaum Associates.

Crosby, R. A., and others. (2000). Correlates of unprotected vaginal sex among African American female teens: The importance of relationship dynamics. *Archives of Pediatrics and Adolescent Medicine, 154,* 893–899.

Crosby, R. A., and others. (2003). Psychosocial predictors of pregnancy among low-income African American adolescent females: A prospective analysis. *Journal of Pediatric and Adolescent Gynecology, 15,* 293–299.

DiClemente, R. J., and others. (2001). Parental monitoring and its association with a spectrum of adolescent health risk behaviors. *Pediatrics, 107,* 1363–1368.

Kamb, M. L., and others (1998). Efficacy of risk-reduction counseling to prevent human immunodeficiency virus in sexually transmitted diseases: A randomized controlled trial. *Journal of the American Medical Association, 280,* 1161–1167.

Mandelson, M. T., and others. (2000). Colorectal cancer screening participation by older women. *American Journal of Preventive Medicine, 19,* 149–154.

Pagano, M., and Gauvreau, K. (2000). *Principles of biostatistics* (2nd ed.). Pacific Grove, CA: Duxbury Thompson Learning.

Sheeran, P., Abraham, C., and Orbell, S. (1999). Psychosocial correlates of heterosexual condom use: A meta-analysis. *Psychological Bulletin, 125,* 90–132.

Siegel, S., and Castellan, N. J. (1988). *Nonparametric statistics for the behavioral sciences* (2nd ed.). Boston: McGraw-Hill.

Tabachnick, B. G., and Fidell, L. S. (1996). *Using multivariate statistics* (3rd ed.). New York: HarperCollins.

CHAPTER THIRTEEN

BASIC PRINCIPLES OF STATISTICAL ANALYSIS FOR RANDOMIZED CONTROLLED TRIALS

Ralph J. DiClemente, Laura F. Salazar, and Richard A. Crosby

The aim of this chapter is to provide an overview of the main statistical principles and data analytic techniques useful in the analysis of randomized controlled trials (RCT). Many of these principles and techniques, while specifically applied to RCTs, are also applicable to the broader category of studies incorporating an experimental research design.

To begin we would like to remind you of two terms that pertain only to experimental research. These are the *independent variable* and the *dependent variable*. The independent variable is the variable manipulated by the investigator. In the context of a health promotion RCT, the independent variable is the health promotion program (HPP) and the goal is to determine its effect on the *dependent variable*. The dependent variable is the outcome of interest and is measured by the investigator, but not controlled or manipulated by the investigator.

The primary focus of the chapter is to describe the underlying purposes of statistical techniques, develop an understanding of selecting an appropriate statistical technique, and enhance understanding of the interpretation of data derived from an RCT. This chapter is deliberately written to be statistical-lite; that is to say, nonmathematical.

Illustration of Key Concepts

We will provide an overview of the data analytic process, which will entail planning for the data analysis, describing the data, assessing the comparability between groups, and understanding different types of dependent variables. Finally, and perhaps most important, we will describe a process for selecting the appropriate statistical analysis and describe those analyses as applied to an RCT.

Planning for the Data Analysis

Statistical analysis of data, while usually conducted after all data have been collected, is in reality a process that should begin much earlier in the research enterprise. The data analysis is directly related to the design of the study and how well the study has been implemented. Indeed, no matter how well designed, clever, or sophisticated a data analytic plan, it cannot compensate for a poorly designed study. A poorly conceived data analytic plan may obscure the detection of meaningful findings, obscure interpretation of the resultant findings, or both. A data analytic plan entails conducting a power analysis to determine the appropriate sample size needed to detect a statistical difference, ensuring that measurements are administered in a timely and appropriate fashion, specifying a procedure for handling participant attrition, and selecting the statistical techniques most appropriate for the design and research question. Thus, proper planning and execution of the study as well as the statistical analysis is critical to yielding reliable and valid results. Throughout this book, we have described various research designs (see Chapters Four, Five, and Six); however, without the appropriate attention on the front end of the study (the design and implementation), the data analysis on the back end will not be as useful.

In a Nutshell

No matter how well designed, clever, or sophisticated a data analytic plan, it cannot compensate for a poorly designed study.

Describing the Data

Once the data are obtained by following the data analytic plan, it is useful to examine the underlying characteristics of the scores for the variables collected before proceeding to more complex analyses. The first analytic activity is usually the generation of simple descriptive statistics (for example, mean, median, standard deviation, range, frequencies). These descriptive statistics are used to evaluate how scores on various variables are distributed. These variables include the dependent variables, the participants' sociodemographic characteristics, and other key predictors (in other words, hypothesized mediators of the dependent variables). Summary statistics for all of the measures should be computed separately for each arm of the trial. A visual inspection of the data, especially histograms, may reveal underlying deviations from normality of which the investigator should be aware prior to progressing to the selection of statistical techniques for the data analysis. Generation of these statistics also serves as the last quality control and quality assurance activities in data management.

Assessing the Comparability Between the Study Groups

The concept of assessing comparability between the HPP group and the control group is, at times, difficult for novice investigators to understand. An often-asked question, for example, is, Why assess comparability between groups that were created through randomization of participants in the first place? Doesn't the fact that participants were randomized, using appropriate allocation techniques, obviate the need to assess comparability? This is a common refrain. Randomization does not ensure that the study groups are equivalent, only that there is no systematic bias in the assignment of participants to the two study conditions. Indeed, for relatively small samples, it is likely that the groups will not be comparable on all variables (dependent variables, sociodemographics, and other predictors). Thus, a critical step in the data analytic plan is to assess the comparability between the study groups with respect to sociodemographics, dependent variables, and other predictors of interest. An example from our research may be illustrative.

◆ ◆ ◆

In a Nutshell

Randomization does not ensure that the study groups are equivalent, only that there is no systematic bias in the assignment of participants to the two study conditions.

◆ ◆ ◆

We conducted an RCT to test the efficacy of a behavioral intervention to increase condom use among African American female adolescents, fourteen to eighteen years of age. As participants completed their baseline assessment they were randomized to one of two study conditions using a computer-generated randomization algorithm, complying with established concealment of allocation techniques (see Chapter Six). Comparisons between the study conditions were made for a host of variables, including sociodemographic characteristics, other potential predictors of sexual behavior, psychosocial mediators of sexual behavior, and sexual behaviors. We compared the conditions using t-tests for continuous dependent variables (such as age) and chi-square tests for categorical variables (for instance, whether participants received public assistance). Results of these analyses are presented in Table 13.1.

Examination of Table 13.1 reveals that randomization was effective. The HIV risk-reduction condition and the general health education control condition were similar with respect to sociodemographic characteristics, psychosocial mediators that serve as secondary dependent variables, and sexual behaviors that serve as the primary dependent variable. In general, it is valuable to include a range of variables when assessing comparability between study conditions. If there are imbalances between the groups (for example, in this case, if there were a statistically significant mean difference for the variable "age" between conditions), then it is important to control for this age difference in the analysis. Differences between the study groups for other variables that may be potential confounders (that is, variables theoretically or empirically associated with the dependent variables) could also be controlled for in subsequent data analyses.

Understanding Different Types of Dependent Variables

In all studies there are different types of dependent variables. Two types often collected as part of an RCT are categorical and continuous variables.

Categorical Dependent Variables. Categorical dependent variables refer to the classification of participants into one of several categories according to some predefined evaluation criteria. In its most elemental form, categorical data can assume a binary format. These categories might be labeled as "has a disease or is disease-free," "changed behavior or did not change behavior," or "consistent or inconsistent condom use," and are based on a participant's responses, test scores, or medical examinations. For example, in a study of vegetable consumption, a primary dependent variable could be "heart attack" over the follow-up period. The research question is whether or not there were more heart attacks observed among participants in the control group relative to the HPP group. Thus, for any participant in the study, the range of potential values for the dependent variable "heart attack" is 1 = Yes (experienced a heart attack over the course of the follow-up) or 0 = No (did not experience a heart attack over the course of the follow-up). In

TABLE 13.1. COMPARABILITY OF THE HIV RISK REDUCTION AND GENERAL HEALTH PROMOTION CONDITIONS.

Characteristic	HIV Prevention Condition			General Health Promotion Condition			P
	Mean (sd)	Percentage	(N)	Mean (sd)	Percentage	(N)	
Sociodemographics							
Age	15.99 (1.25)			15.97 (1.21)			.87
Education (did not complete tenth grade)		45.80%	(251)		48.70%	(132)	.51
Recipients of public assistance		17.90%	(45)		18.50%	(50)	.86
Living in single-family home		74.10%	(146)		72.30%	(162)	.68
Living with someone other than a parent		21.50%	(54)		17.30%	(47)	.23
Employed		16.10%	(40)		19.70%	(53)	.28
Psychosocial Mediators							
HIV Knowledge	8.88 (3.25)		(248)	9.13 (3.03)		(267)	.38
Condom attitudes	36.02 (4.22)		(250)	35.62 (4.42)		(271)	.29
Condom barriers	42.23 (14.16)		(243)	43.13 (14.30)		(267)	.48
Communication frequency	8.61 (4.10)		(251)	8.37 (4.50)		(271)	.54
Condom use self-efficacy	30.74 (9.30)		(249)	30.52 (9.73)		(264)	.79
Condom use skills	2.91 (1.30)		(248)	3.03 (1.18)		(268)	.25
Put condom on partner	1.49 (1.01)		(232)	1.46 (0.98)		(246)	.77
Sexual Behaviors							
% Condom use, past thirty days	0.79 (0.38)		(232)	0.77 (0.38)		(246)	.68
% Condom use, past six months	0.72 (0.37)		(232)	0.70 (0.38)		(245)	.53
Unprotected vaginal sex, past thirty days	1.12 (2.84)		(226)	0.84 (2.01)		(241)	.22
Unprotected vaginal sex, past six months	4.81 (16.01)		(232)	4.23 (10.25)		(245)	.64
Consistent condom use, past thirty days		40.27%	(60)		43.35%	(75)	.58
Consistent condom use, past six months		43.53%	(101)		48.57%	(119)	.27
Condom use, last time had sex		31.90%	(74)		32.11%	(79)	.96

**MINCUS USES "NO HEAD LUMP = 0" AND
"HEAD LUMP = 1" FOR THE DEPENDENT VARIABLE.**

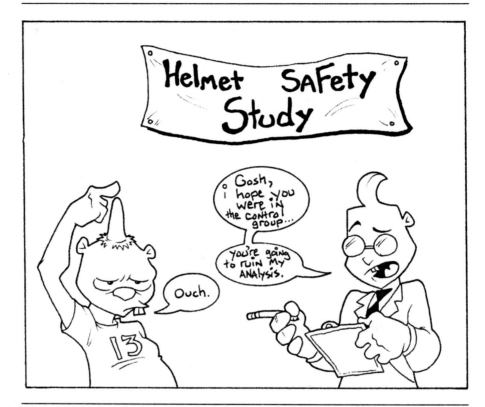

Copyright 2005 by Justin Wagner; reprinted with permission.

a study designed to test the effects of an HPP on reducing alcohol use among adolescent drivers and, as a consequence, reducing the risk of an automobile accident,
we could have a categorical dependent variable of alcohol-related vehicular accidents. In this case, for any participant in the study, the range of potential values
that could be obtained for the dependent variable "alcohol-related auto accident"
is 1 = Yes (experienced an alcohol-related automobile accident over the course
of the follow-up) or 0 = No (did not experience an alcohol-related automobile accident over the course of the follow-up).

There are circumstances when it may be desirable to have multiple levels of
the categorical dependent variables. This is a logical extension of the binary
categorical dependent variable described above. For example, it is possible to have

an ordered categorical dependent variable—usually called an ordinal variable. This ordered categorical dependent variable would assume the form of a hierarchy or gradient. For example, in a study designed to test the effects of a stress reduction class (the HPP) on reducing headaches among college students during final exams, we could have an ordered categorical dependent variable of "headaches." In this case, for any participant in the study, the potential values for the dependent variable "headache" could range from 0 to 2 with 0 = Did not experience a headache during final exam week; 1 = Experienced a mild headache during final exam week; and 2 = Experienced a severe headache during final exam week. Oftentimes we would be tempted to treat these data as continuous when in fact the data are ordinal and should be treated as categorical.

Continuous Dependent Variables. A second type of dependent variable is a continuous variable. Continuous variables are distinct from categorical variables in that the data represent a continuous scale of measurement assessed using interval or ratio scale metrics (such as temperature, height, blood pressure, weight). Often in health promotion research, our interest is in enhancing mental health. Let's return to our study of how stress reduction may reduce headaches among college students during final exam week. RCTs, in general, have primary dependent variables; in this case, "preventing headaches." They may also have secondary dependent variables. Secondary dependent variables could include a host of other variables that the HPP is hypothesized to effect. In this study, for example, we may hypothesize that participation in a stress-reduction class (the HPP) not only would reduce headaches (the primary dependent variable) over the course of final exam week (the follow-up period) but also may have the collateral benefit of reducing depressive symptoms (a secondary dependent variable). In this example, we could collect participants' self-reports of depressive symptoms with a depression inventory at baseline, randomize them to the stress-reduction-class or no stress-reduction-class condition, then administer the same depression inventory at the scheduled follow-up assessment at the end of the final exam week. The depression inventory thus provides a continuous dependent variable, with the hypothesis that participants in the HPP will have fewer depressive symptoms during the final exam week than participants in the control condition.

Continuous dependent variables can also be transformed into categorical variables. One reason for transforming a continuous dependent variable is that the underlying distribution of the continuous variable violates assumptions of normality necessary for performing certain statistical analyses. For example, if we were also interested in hypothesizing that participation in a stress-reduction class (the HPP) would not only reduce the risk of having a headache and depressive symptoms but also result in less weight gain over the course of final examinations week, we could measure a participant's weight at baseline and at follow-up and examine changes in his or her weight as a function of his or her group assignment. While we have a continuous dependent variable, weight in pounds, this variable can be transformed into a categorical dependent variable with the following dependent variable categories: "gained weight," "lost weight," or "no change in weight." Thus, what was a continuous dependent variable is now a categorical dependent variable. However, there are some issues to consider in categorizing a continuous dependent variable. In general, use of a categorical dependent variable derived from continuous data may entail some loss of detail in describing each participant as a range of scores is reduced to only two or three categories. The issue is potential loss of statistical power. A continuous variable implies certain statistical tests that rely on variability within the data for performing those tests. When a continuous variable is transformed into a categorical dependent variable, the variability in the dependent variable is markedly reduced. Thus, when a reliable continuous dependent variable exists and it meets statistical assumptions necessary for certain statistical analyses, it is usually best *not* to transform the data.

Selection of Statistical Techniques

In health promotion research, while there are numerous statistical techniques for testing whether an HPP is effective relative to a control group, we will focus on those that are most readily applicable. More complex research designs, by their very nature, require the use of more complex statistical techniques. Thus, we propose a decision strategy based on the type of dependent variable (categorical or continuous) as an overarching framework to facilitate understanding, identifying, and selecting the most appropriate statistical technique.

Data analysis is a process. At each juncture in the data analytic process the investigator (that is, you) will be faced with making decisions regarding what statistical technique is most appropriate for analyzing the type of dependent variable collected. The decision-mapping approach is based on an understanding of the types of data to be analyzed and the qualities and characteristics of those data. The type of statistical approach used is directly dependent on the type of data represented by the dependent variable.

The Case of Categorical Dependent Variables. Categorical dependent variables in RCTs are often dichotomous, meaning that there is a possibility of the data assuming only two levels or categories (although dependent variables can be classified into multiple levels, in which case they are polychotomous). For example, in a long-term study (let's say it's a ten-year follow-up) of the health-promoting effects of stress-reduction classes for men, ages fifty to fifty-nine, at high-risk for a heart attack (low density lipoprotein (LDL) over 250; overweight by twenty pounds, and reporting no regular physical exercise), the primary dependent variable is a dichotomous variable representing "heart attack." Thus, for any participant in the study, the range of potential values on the variable "heart attack" is 1 = Yes (experienced a heart attack over the course of the follow-up) or 0 = No (did not experience a heart attack over the course of the follow-up).

The hypothesis is that participation in the HPP would reduce the risk of heart attacks relative to the control group. The basic approach to testing this hypothesis is to compare the proportion of participants in each condition experiencing a heart attack over the follow-up period. This can be done using a nonparametric technique (nonparametric techniques do not make distributional assumptions about the underlying normality of the distribution of dependent variables) such as a simple chi-square test of proportions. If we compare the proportion of participants in each condition experiencing a heart attack and find statistically significant differences, with the HPP group having a lower proportion of participants experiencing a heart attack, we can conclude that the HPP was effective in reducing the risk of a heart attack. Let's see Figure 13.1.

As Figure 13.1 indicates, five men in the HPP group reported having a heart attack compared with twenty men in the control group. This corresponds to 2.5 percent of the HPP participants compared with 10 percent of the control participants. The question is whether this proportional difference is statistically significant. In analyzing the study, the investigator is required to make a determination as to what statistical technique is most applicable to these data. To assist you, we have developed a simple decision map to guide the selection of a statistical test. This map is depicted in Figure 13.2.

FIGURE 13.1. NUMBER OF PARTICIPANTS EXPERIENCING A HEART ATTACK IN A STRESS-REDUCTION PROGRAM AND A CONTROL CONDITION.

		Heart Attack		
		Yes	No	
	Yes	5	195	200
Stress reduction class (HPP)				
	No	20	180	200

FIGURE 13.2. STATISTICAL DECISION MAP.

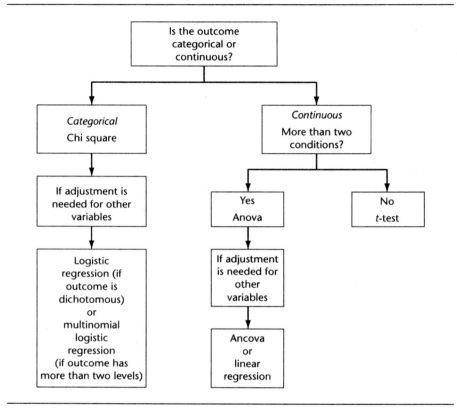

Let's use our decision map and see where it takes us. We have a categorical dependent variable (heart attack, "yes" or "no"), and there is no need for adjustment for other sociodemographic or predictor variables based on our examination of the baseline data (essentially, the groups are comparable). Thus, following our guide, a simple chi-square test would be the test statistic. The chi-square can determine whether the difference observed in the proportion of participants having a heart attack between conditions is statistically significant. Statistical significance is expressed as a probability (P), relative to chance. The customary criterion for determining statistical significance is $P < .05$.

In our example, the results are statistically significant ($P < .05$). The findings support the hypothesis that stress-reduction classes can reduce the risk of a heart attack among high-risk men fifty to fifty-nine years of age. Please note the specificity of reporting the result. We may not be able to generalize the findings to populations with different sociodemographic characteristics, such as women, younger men, men of a particular ethnic or racial group, or men without risk indicators. External validity or generalizability is an issue related to how we select our sample and not to the type of test statistic used or the validity of the findings.

While the P-value is useful, it does not provide a full assessment of the effects of the HPP. Indeed, it describes the findings relative to chance. To capture more fully the effect of the HPP on the risk of a heart attack, it is useful to consider calculating a measure of effect size (ES). Effect size measures the strength of association between the HPP and the dependent variable (heart attack). In this case there are two measures that could be calculated. One is an absolute measure, the percent (or, if preferred, the proportion) difference that entails subtracting the percentage of participants with a heart attack in the HPP (2.5 percent) from the percentage with a heart attack in the control condition (10 percent), resulting in difference of 7.5 percent. A second measure of effect size is a relative measure called the relative risk (RR). The RR is defined as the risk of a heart attack in one group relative to the other group. In this example, RR = 20/200 divided by 5/200 = 4, indicating that participants in the control group had four times the risk of having a heart attack relative to the HPP. Alternatively, the RR could be expressed as .25 (5/200 divided by 20/200), indicating that participants in the HPP condition had only one-quarter the risk number of having a heart attack compared with participants in the control condition. Either calculation of RR is correct depending on how you prefer to present your findings.

The RR as a measure of intervention (or treatment) effect has a number of advantages. First and foremost, it is readily interpretable. We commonly refer to "risk" for a dependent variable. For example, dependent variables might include the risk for a heart attack, the risk of having an automobile accident while driving under the influence of alcohol, and the risk of developing cancer. Second, the RR is a "true" measure of the strength of the effect of the HPP, not a measure of chance. Third, the RR is invariant with respect to sample size. This latter advantage may require some further discussion. Thus, if the sample size was increased in each group, but the same proportions of participants in each study condition were identified with a heart attack, the RR would be exactly the same!

In addition to measuring the magnitude of the HPP effect (the RR), it is also recommended that the confidence interval around the RR be calculated. The confidence interval provides a measure of the precision of the effect. What does this mean? Well, let's illustrate. Suppose we did the exact same study one hundred times; the 95 percent confidence interval (the customary statistic) would inform us that ninety-five of those one hundred times, the RR would be between the lower and upper limits. When the confidence intervals are relatively narrow, we have more confidence that our RR calculation is precise. Conversely, relatively wider

TABLE 13.2. EFFECTS OF AN HIV RISK-REDUCTION INTERVENTION ON ADOLESCENTS' SEXUAL BEHAVIORS.

	6-Month Follow-Up Assessment		
	RR	**(95% CI)**	**P**
Consistent condom use, (past thirty days)	1.76	(1.07–3.19)	.04
Consistent condom use, (past six months)	2.46	(1.44–4.21)	.001
Condom use, last time had sex	3.94	(2.06–6.42)	.0001
Sex with new partner, (past thirty days)	0.30	(0.11–0.78)	.01

intervals detract from our confidence that our RR calculation is precise. For example, an RR of 2.1 with a confidence interval of 1.7, 2.5 suggests that the estimate is very close to its limits. An RR of 2.1 with a confidence interval of 1.2, 3.0 would not equate with the same degree of confidence.

In summary, in analyzing and interpreting data from an RCT to test the efficacy of an HPP, three statistics should be calculated: (1) the appropriate statistical test to determine if differences between conditions were statistically significant, (2) the RR as a measure of intervention effect size, and (3) the confidence interval around the RR as a measure of precision of effect. In keeping with our advice, in Table 13.2, note that we have calculated all the statistics necessary to describe the HPP effects for an HIV risk-reduction program designed to enhance consistent condom use and reduce number of sex partners. All three of these statistics should be presented when describing the results.

Interpreting the Results of an HPP with Categorical Dependent Variables. Now that we have calculated the appropriate statistics to describe the effects of the HPP, let's interpret them. The findings would be interpreted as follows: relative to participants in the control condition, participants in the HIV risk-reduction intervention were 1.76 times (95 percent CI = 1.07 − 3.19, P =.04) more likely to report using condoms consistently in the thirty days prior to assessment, 2.46 times (CI = 1.44 − 4.21, P = .001) more likely to report using condoms in the prior six months, 3.94 times (CI = 2.06 − 6.42, P = .0001) more likely to report condom use at last sexual intercourse, and .3 times (CI = .11 − .78; P = 0.1) as likely to have a new sex partner in the prior thirty days. Thus, the use of all three statistics provides a richer description of effects of the HIV intervention (the HPP); one that includes a measure of the strength of the HPP effect that is invariant with respect to sample size (the relative risk), one that provides a measure of precision of the effect size (the confidence limits around the relative risk), and, of course, one that includes the traditional measure of statistical significance, the *P*-value.

Multivariable Models with a Categorical Dependent Variable

As we noted earlier, a key step in preparing for the analysis of any RCT is to examine the distribution of sociodemographic and other predictor variables between the HPP and the control group to assess whether the groups are comparable at baseline. In the event that differences between groups are found on sociodemographic variables or other study variables, we would want to control for them statistically. Otherwise our findings may not be valid. Including multiple variables in a model that predicts a singular dependent variable is considered to be a *multivariable* analysis. In intervention analyses, this implies the independent variable plus any identified *covariates*. Covariates are factors that vary in conjunction with the dependent variable. An analytic strategy that controls for the effects of these covariates while testing for intervention effects could be logistic regression. Logistic regression is used for categorical dependent variables that are dichotomous (Hosmer and Lemeshow, 1989); other analyses (for example, multinomial regression) would have to be employed for categorical dependent variables with more than two categories or levels (see Figure 13.2).

Logistic Regression. Logistic regression is a statistical technique that allows for the testing of an independent variable (in other words, the HPP intervention) in the presence of identified covariates. This process "controls" statistically for the effect of the covariates on the categorical dependent variable. "Controls for" in this context essentially means that the influence of intervention on the dependent variable is determined in addition to any effect the covariates may have on the dependent variable. Thus, differences between groups on the covariates are addressed.

Like linear regression, a logistic regression yields several parameter estimates. However, the primary estimate of interest is the odds ratio. The odds ratio is similar to the RR and is comparably interpreted (a 95 percent confidence interval is also derived from the analysis). For example, if a logistic regression equation that had condom use as the dependent variable, and a variable representing the HPP condition, along with several covariates, yielded an odds ratio of 3.9, it would be interpreted as "the likelihood that participants in the HPP group would report condom use at last sexual intercourse were 3.9 times the likelihood that participants in the control group would report such condom use." In addition to the odds ratio for the HPP, we would also like to calculate the 95 percent confidence interval and the corresponding *P*-value for the HPP.

Multiple Follow-Up Assessments

While the pretest-posttest RCT is the basic research design to assess change as a function of an HPP, there are, as might be expected, a number of more complex designs, and, of course, comparably more complex statistical approaches to analyze data derived from these complex designs. While it is beyond the scope of this chapter to address the range and complexity inherent in these advanced RCTs, we think it's important that students of health promotion be aware of them.

One way to extend the basic pretest-posttest design is to incorporate multiple follow-up assessments. Often investigators are curious about the sustainability of the HPP. Although we may expect that people would change their behavior, attitudes, and beliefs related to some health topic as a function of an HPP, these changes may begin to show decay over time. We might want to assess people on several occasions over a protracted time period. This design could be diagrammed as shown in Figure 13.3.

Analysis of this design with a categorical dependent variable can be accomplished through a variety of statistical techniques. One statistical approach that is gaining popularity is the use of generalized estimating equations (GEE). The GEE logistic regression model is an extension of the simple logistic regression model discussed in the previous section and can be used when the categorical dependent variable is dichotomized. With the GEE logistic model, all variables are measured on multiple occasions. Because repeated observations (measurements) collected for the same participant (for instance, measuring a participant's weight at two or more time points) are not independent of each other, a correction must be made for these within-participant correlations. This approach permits an adjustment for repeated within-participant measurement and the correlation between any one participant's measurements over time (Hardin and Hilbe, 2003).

The overall model design includes a time-independent variable, which in an RCT is the variable representing the program such as the HPP, as well as time-dependent variables (these are other predictors as well as the dependent variable that are expected to change). Additionally, a variable representing the number of time periods involved is also included in the model to differentiate the temporal order of the repeated measures. The resultant statistics are adjusted odds ratios and 95 percent confidence limits.

FIGURE 13.3.   STANDARD PRETEST-POSTTEST DESIGN.

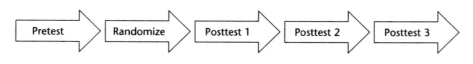

Pretest Randomize Posttest 1 Posttest 2 Posttest 3

Thus, while we have simplified, for heuristic purposes, the rationale and format of a GEE logistic model, it is important to note that not all popular computer statistical packages offer this statistical routine as part of their package.

Analysis with a Continuous Dependent Variable. Analysis with a continuous dependent variable is often more familiar to investigators in health promotion and health education research. In this case, the dependent variable assumes a range of scores rather than a binary response. For instance, commonly used dependent variables in health promotion research could be blood pressure (either diastolic or systolic), a person's weight, a score on an aptitude test, a score on a scale measuring depressive symptoms, number of servings of fruits and vegetables consumed, and so on. As you can see, the range of dependent variables is almost limitless.

The test statistic is one that is familiar, often learned in Introductory Statistics, the student's *t*-test. In the case of an RCT, the student's *t*-test provides a statistic that compares the means of two samples. Let's use an example to illustrate a simple analysis. In the HIV risk-reduction intervention described previously, a secondary dependent variable was to increase positive attitudes toward condom use (a continuous secondary dependent variable) among the participants in the intervention group. Attitude was assessed using a well-established scale with higher scale scores reflecting more positive attitudes toward using condoms during sexual intercourse. Participants were then randomized to either the risk-reduction group or a control group. Subsequent to completing the intervention or control group, six months later we asked all participants to return and complete a follow-up (posttest) assessment. The goal, of course, was to determine if condom attitude scores were different in the HIV risk-reduction group relative to the control group. The question is, How do we test for this important difference?

Let's assume that at follow-up (posttest), the participants in the HIV risk-reduction group had a mean condom attitude score of 32.65 (the scale range from a low of 10 to a high of 40). The control group had a mean condom attitude score of 22.40. The *t*-test assesses whether these observed means for the two study groups are statistically different from each other. It is important to note that, in the case of the RCT above, we are using an independent groups *t*-test. In our example, the results were statistically significant ($P < .05$). The findings support the motivator hypothesis that HIV risk-reduction intervention increases participants' positive attitudes toward condom use. A hypothesis may be proposed as either a *null hypothesis* (that is, there are no differences between groups) or as a *motivator* or *alternative hypothesis* (that is, differences exist between groups). However, as we noted in previous sections describing analysis of RCTs with a categorical dependent variable, while the *P*-value is useful, it does not provide a full assessment of the effects of the HPP. Indeed, it describes the findings relative to chance. To capture more fully the effect of the HIV risk-reduction intervention on condom attitude scores (continuous secondary dependent variable), it is useful to calculate a measure of effect size.

As noted earlier, but bears reiterating, an effect size provides an index of the strength of the association between the HPP and the dependent variable. In this case, a measure that could be calculated is the mean difference (D) between the group's condom attitude scores. Let's refer back to our example by examining Table 13.3.

Thus, we have calculated an absolute measure of effect on mean condom attitude scores attributable to the HIV risk-reduction intervention. On average, condom attitude scores in the HIV risk-reduction group are 10.25 units greater compared with the control group. As noted earlier, in measuring the magnitude of the HPP effect (the mean difference), and the corresponding P-value to assess its statistical significance, it is also recommended that the confidence interval around the mean difference be calculated. The confidence interval provides a measure of the *true* effect of the HPP in the population. In other words, if the study was repeated one hundred times, the 95 percent confidence interval would indicate that ninety-five of those one hundred times the mean difference would be between the lower and upper limit. In Table 13.4 we have calculated all the statistics necessary to describe the HPP effects for an HIV risk-reduction designed to enhance condom attitude scores.

Although Table 13.4 conveys a great deal of information about the effects of the HIV risk-reduction intervention on participants' condom attitude scores, it is important to understand that the statistic D is not a standardized measure of

TABLE 13.3.   DIFFERENCES ON CONDOM ATTITUDE SCORES BY STUDY GROUP.

Group Assignment	Mean (at follow-up)	Mean Difference
HIV risk-reduction	32.65	+10.25
Control	22.40	

TABLE 13.4.   EFFECTS OF AN HIV RISK-REDUCTION INTERVENTION ON CONDOM ATTITUDE SCORES.

Group Assignment	Mean (at follow-up)	D	95% CI	P
HIV risk-reduction	32.65	10.25	(7.38–13.86)	.03
Control	22.40			

Notes: D = mean difference (HPP – Co).
95% CI = 95 percent confidence limits around D.

TABLE 13.5. EFFECTS OF AN HIV RISK-REDUCTION INTERVENTION ON HIV KNOWLEDGE AND SELF-ESTEEM.

Dependent Variable	Mean Posttest Scores Intervention	Control	D	95% CI	P
HIV knowledge	8.0	6.0	2.0	1.5–2.5	.04
Self-esteem	4.0	2.0	2.0	1.5–2.5	.04
Condom attitude	32.65	22.40	10.25	7.38–13.86	.03

Notes: D = mean difference (HPP – Co).
95% CI = 95 percent confidence limits around D.

effect size. If we wanted to compare a number of continuous dependent variables with different scale ranges, it would be problematic (similar to comparing apples to oranges). For example, the condom attitude scale used had a range from 10 to 40. Perhaps we want to examine another two scales as continuous secondary dependent variables (not an unreasonable thing to do). One scale measures HIV prevention knowledge and has a range from 1 to 10 (higher scores indicate greater knowledge) and another scale measures self-esteem and has a range from 1 to 5 (higher scores indicate greater self-esteem). Table 13.5 has information regarding these new scales.

Examining the differences between the HIV knowledge score and the self-esteem score, we note that the mean difference (D) = 2 in both instances. Hence, should we conclude that the effect of the HPP is identical for both of these dependent variables? Well, yes; if we focus only on the absolute differences. However, it is important to note that the HIV knowledge scale has a much larger range of potential scores (1 to 10) compared with the self-esteem scale (1 to 5). Thus, the same difference (D = 2) observed for each of the scales may have a markedly different magnitude of effect if we consider the relative difference. One measure that permits a relative assessment of change is called percent relative difference (RD). The RD statistic provides a common metric for measuring the magnitude of change across different scale measures. The RD is calculated by dividing the value for D by the mean posttest score for the control group. Below we demonstrate the calculation and utility of this statistic. In this example, the RD for HIV knowledge would be equal to 2/6 = .33. Likewise, for the dependent variable, mean self-esteem scores, the RD would be 2/2 = 1.00. It may be easier if the RD is then converted to the percent RD by multiplying the value by 100. Thus, as the example demonstrates, the percent RD for knowledge was 33 percent and for self-esteem, 100 percent. Thus, the HPP had a relatively greater effect on improving mean self-esteem scores compared with HIV knowledge scores. However, examining only the absolute differences in mean scores would obscure this potentially important finding. As with the other measures of HPP effects, the 95 percent confidence interval can also be calculated around the percent RD.

Interpreting the Results of an HPP with Continuous Dependent Variables. Now that we have calculated the appropriate statistics to describe the effects of the HPP, let's interpret them. The findings would be interpreted as follows: relative to participants in the control group, those in the HIV risk-reduction intervention had significantly higher scores on condom attitudes, HIV knowledge, and self-esteem. We concluded this based on the significant *t*-test. Moreover, the effect sizes indicated that the greater proportional difference was found for self-esteem, as assessed by the percent RD. Thus, the use of these statistics provides a richer description of significant effects of the HIV intervention (the HPP).

Multivariable Models with Continuous Dependent Variables

As we noted earlier, a key step in preparing for the analysis of any RCT is to examine the distribution of sociodemographic and other predictor variables between the HPP and the control group to assess whether the groups are comparable at baseline. In the event the groups are not comparable with respect to several key variables of the primary dependent variable or secondary dependent variables, we would want to control for these differences. Otherwise, our findings may not be valid. In addition to controlling for group differences revealed on baseline measures, it is important to control for the baseline measure of the dependent variable when performing analyses on the posttest data. To control for baseline measures, enter them into the analysis as covariates. This analysis strategy provides a more rigorous test of the intervention effects, such that differences between groups on posttest means are adjusted for baseline measurement. The statistical analysis used to control for both the effects of covariates and the baseline value of the dependent variable is either linear regression or its algebraic equivalent, analysis of covariance (ANCOVA).

◆ ◆ ◆

In a Nutshell

In addition to controlling for group differences revealed on baseline measures, it is important to control for the baseline measure of the dependent variable when performing analyses on the posttest data.

◆ ◆ ◆

Linear Regression and ANCOVA. Linear regression and ANCOVA are statistical techniques that allow for two or more variables to be included in a model with a continuous dependent variable. The HPP variable is included as the independent variable as well as covariates and the baseline measure of the continuous dependent variable. While the computation of the linear model is beyond the scope of this chapter, the interested reader is referred to Kleinbaum, Kupper, Muller, and Nizam (1998) for an eminently readable discussion of this approach. Linear regression and ANCOVA can adjust for the effects of group differences that would otherwise obscure intervention effects as well as adjusting for the baseline value of the continuous dependent variable. Linear regression and ANCOVA permit computation of adjusted means and mean differences (D) for continuous dependent variables similar to that discussed earlier in this section as well as constructing the 95 percent confidence interval around these effect sizes (D).

Multiple Follow-Up Assessments

As noted in earlier sections of this chapter, for categorical data with multiple assessments, the use of GEE was recommended. GEE are recommended also for continuous dependent variables, and can be used to construct a model adjusting for the correlations between the repeated measures. GEE control for autocorrelations that could distort the true effect of the HPP.

Applied Example

A study published in the *Journal of the American Medical Association* reported findings from an RCT designed to test the effects of an Internet-based behavioral intervention program. The goal of the behavioral intervention program was to promote weight loss among people with type 2 diabetes (Tate, Jackvony, and Wing, 2003). Volunteers were randomly assigned to receive an Internet-based weight loss program or the same program with the addition of an e-mail-based counseling component. Weight was assessed at baseline, three, six, and twelve months postintervention. Forty-six people were assigned to each of the two conditions ($N = 92$).

A repeated measures analysis was conducted. The continuous outcome variable suggested that a *t*-test or analysis of variance (ANOVA) could be used to test the study hypothesis (see Figure 13.2). The example is quite instructive because it illustrates a point that is not included in Figure 13.2. The *t*-test is the most parsimonious data analytic technique when the independent variable has only two levels. However, ANOVA can also be used when the independent variable has only two levels. So, why would ANOVA be a better choice? The answer involves ease of testing for the influence of covariates. Although a "controlled *t*-test" can be conducted, the more commonly accepted approach is to control with ANCOVA. Thus, the initial selection of ANOVA allows for an easy "switch" to ANCOVA. The authors used a repeated measures ANOVA to assess the Group (intervention or control) X Time (baseline through the multiple follow-ups) interaction. Ideally, there should be greater positive change, over time, for those randomized to the condition designated as being the treatment (in this case the Internet plus the e-mail counseling service) as opposed to the control (in this case, the receipt only of material and messages provided by Websites).

Using data collected at baseline, the authors first determined that the two groups did not differ as the study began (in other words, randomization worked). Because likely covariates were not identified, the use of ANCOVA was not necessary. The ANOVA produced the desired Group X Time interaction, showing greater weight loss among persons receiving the addition of e-mail-based counseling.

Integration with the Research Process

The analysis of an RCT is indeed an important undertaking. The amount of time and resources devoted to the RCT certainly warrant careful attention to every aspect of this analysis. However, it is critical that the analysis be constructed on a solid foundation. In particular, the RCT should have a sound design (step 4 of the nine-step model described in Chapter One), and it should include reliable and valid measurement of all variables (step 5 of the research process), including potential covariates. Of course, a great deal of attention should be devoted to measurement of the dependent variable(s); this is the primary outcome variable of interest. A well-planned analysis cannot make up for lack of planning in either of these two steps.

The quality of analysis for the RCT is highly dependent on how well the study protocol was implemented (step 7 of the research process). For example, if contamination occurred between study conditions (that is, intervention and control group participants had frequent contact) even the best statistician will not be able to rescue the analysis from this threat to internal validity. Day-to-day study procedures are also important. Consider, for example, the decline of study quality that would occur if research staff failed to collect information relative to the number of people who refused to participate in the study. Or consider the decline in quality that could occur if study participants frequently skipped large sections of the assessment questionnaires (research staff can easily help remind participants that it is important to answer all of the questions). In essence, the procedures described in Chapter Six are critical building blocks for the RCT. The subsequent analysis, then, is merely a "crowning achievement."

Fortunately, the analysis is unique in the research process because it can be reconceptualized. Consider an article published in the journal *Preventive Medicine* (Maxwell, Bastani, Vida, and Warda, 2003). The article reported findings from an RCT of a breast and cervical cancer screening program designed for Filipino American women. In a sample of 444 women, the intervention program was not significantly different from the control program in producing change in the dependent variable. However, the analysis was changed to assess intervention effects among only a sub-sample of women Filipino American women who had immigrated to the United States within the past ten years. In this subgroup analysis, intervention effects were observed.

Summary

This chapter has provided an overview of the logic and process involved in data analyses pertaining to testing whether an HPP is effective. A decision map can be used to determine the type of analytic technique appropriate for the type of dependent variable and for when other adjustments are necessary. It is critical that the decision map be followed, given the necessity to provide an accurate and valid test of the HPP, thereby avoiding biased results. In addition to choosing the appropriate statistical technique for testing of intervention effects, we also emphasized the importance of moving beyond the reporting of basic significance associated with the statistical test to include measures of effect size and confidence intervals. Including these additional statistics provides a breadth to the analysis that enhances the precision of the results while allowing for their comparability across other studies.

Issues to Consider

1. The first issue is an extension of the previous paragraph. The study was designed to test an intervention program among Filipino American women. A distinction between those residing in the United States for more versus less than ten years was not part of the a priori study hypotheses. Thus, a question that can be asked would be, Is it "fair" to conduct post-hoc analyses of an RCT when the original null hypotheses are not rejected? A skeptical position on this issue would include mention that a post-hoc analysis may be a "search" for something meaningful that can be used to vindicate the study. Alternatively, the tremendous value of the RCT to the science of health promotion could be justifiable grounds for a post-hoc analysis.

2. The issue of missing data is tremendously important to consider when analyzing an RCT. One common strategy has been to estimate the value of missing data by calculating a mean from the rest of the data. This process seems fair when the amount of missing data is small in comparison with the amount of data that is not missing. As noted in Chapter Six, the adage "once randomized always analyzed" implies that people cannot be dropped

from the analysis of an RCT on the grounds of missing follow-up data. Thus, this remedy of *imputing* data seems logical. The issue, however, becomes one of how much imputation should be consider too much?

For Practice and Discussion

1. Locate three examples of RCTs by doing an electronic search. Be sure that your examples relate to health promotion rather than medical advances. You will notice that most RCTs are indeed designed around questions in medical care such as drug effects or the effects of a new treatment procedure. Using the Decision Map shown in this chapter, determine if the authors of each study used an analytic strategy that is consistent with the map.

2. Again, using the Decision Map select an analytic approach for each scenario listed below.

   - The dependent variable is blood serum cholesterol level.
   - The dependent variable is having a Pap test in the past two years (women answered "yes" versus "no").
   - The dependent variable is an ordinal measure of cigarette use (participants answered using one of three options: "none," "less than one pack per day," "at least one pack per day."
   - The dependent variable is a scale measure of depression.
   - The dependent variable is a scale measure of depression, and several covariates are critical to the analysis.
   - The dependent variable is contraceptive use (dichotomized as "yes" versus "no"), and several covariates are critical to the analysis.

References

Hardin, J. W., and Hilbe, J. M. (2003). *Generalized estimating equations.* New York: Chapman and Hall/CRC.

Hosmer, D. W., and Lemeshow, S. L. (1989). *Applied logistic regression.* New York: John Wiley and Sons.

Kleinbaum, D. G., Kupper, L. L., Muller, K. E., and Nizam, A. (1998). *Applied regression analysis and other multivariable methods.* New York: Duxbury Press.

Maxwell, A. E., Bastani, R., Vida, P., and Warda, U. S. (2003). Results of a randomized trial to increase breast and cervical cancer screening among Filipino American women. *Preventive Medicine, 37,* 102–109.

Tate, D. F., Jackvony, E. H., and Wing, R. R. (2003). Effects of Internet behavioral counseling on weight loss in adults at risk for type 2 diabetes. *Journal of the American Medical Association, 289,* 1833–1836.

PART FOUR

CORE SKILLS RELATED TO HEALTH PROMOTION RESEARCH

CHAPTER FOURTEEN

INTRODUCTION TO SCIENTIFIC WRITING

Richard A. Crosby, Ralph J. DiClemente, and Laura F. Salazar

Students, practitioners, and researchers in the discipline of health promotion often experience a great deal of anxiety when they hear the phrase "publish or perish." The term *publish* should actually be thought of as an extension of the research enterprise, in which publishing is viewed as a necessary and logical endpoint. In reality, then, publishing is an artifact of the larger and more important process of health promotion research. Nonetheless, the published report is indeed a critical piece of dissemination (see step 9 of the nine-step model in Figure 1.2). Thus, researchers should be well versed in the "art of scientific writing." The phrase includes the word *art* because few universal standards exist with respect to the construction of manuscripts that report findings from health promotion research.

This chapter will introduce the basic structure of a manuscript and describe in detail how each section of the manuscript should be written and formatted to meet journal expectations of content and style. Moreover, we also provide guidance in how researchers can tailor their work to "fit" the intended journal to which the manuscript will be submitted. The chapter will expand on the basic themes that publishing is essentially an extension of the research enterprise and

MINCUS AND DINCUS FACE REJECTION.

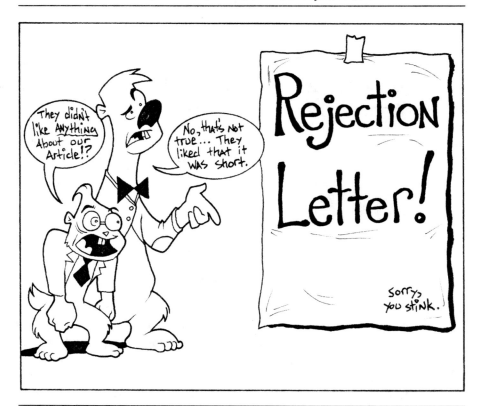

Copyright 2005 by Justin Wagner; reprinted with permission.

that producing acceptable manuscripts from rigorous research does not need to be a challenging process. Of course, no matter how well the research manuscript is prepared, publishing findings based on research severely lacking in rigor is a challenge. Thus, the chapter assumes that the "would be" authors are summarizing a rigorous research process.

◆ ◆ ◆

In a Nutshell

Of course, no matter how well the research manuscript is prepared, publishing findings based on research severely lacking in rigor is a challenge.

◆ ◆ ◆

Illustration of Key Concepts

Before the writing begins it is imperative that members of the research team carefully deliberate the question, To which journal will we submit? Once this step is complete, the remaining process is to simply begin composing the manuscript—one section at a time!

Finding the Right Fit

Three considerations are paramount when authors begin to assemble a research manuscript. First, the authors should select a journal that will provide the *maximum impact* for the topic and practical significance of the study findings. Impact ratings are frequently determined by (1) the number of journal subscribers, (2) how often journals are cited, and (3) indices related to the breadth of electronic distribution.

Second, the journal should be selected for a readership that is interested and invested in the outcomes of your study. In a discipline as diverse as health promotion, this consideration is particularly important in that the spectrum of health promotion research is vast, and, therefore, the research findings seldom appeal to a general audience. Instead, the conclusions of the manuscript may have greater impact if the manuscript is targeted to a well-defined audience. Ideally, the audience should share a common interest in the research and its findings. For example, professionals in preventive medicine may benefit tremendously from a study conclusion that has implications for clinical practice (such as "Physicians and other health professionals who counsel pregnant adolescent females should be aware that marijuana use may be common among those in their first trimester."). Professionals who have dedicated their careers to improving health practices such as fostering exercise behavior may benefit from research that supports the efficacy of a novel approach (for example, "Findings suggest that changes to the physical environment of the workplace can have a favorable impact on the exercise behavior of employees.").

Third, the nature of the study and the analyses should be understandable to the intended readership. Health promotion is multidisciplinary. Indeed, one measure of the growing strength of health promotion is the degree to which people from social sciences, behavioral sciences, law, education, nursing, and medical disciplines are mutually engaged in health promotion research. This diversity brings a welcome and critical mass of expertise to bear on a large number of disparate research questions. The drawback to this high-level of diversity is that not all researchers "speak the same language." For example, psychologists often are well versed in analysis of variance, whereas epidemiologists ply their trade with contingency table analyses. Sociologists may have a tremendous appreciation for community-level interventions, whereas physicians may be far more interested in clinic-based approaches to health promotion. One quick and efficient strategy for ensuring this fit is to know as much as possible of the professional organization sponsoring the journal (although not all journals are sponsored by a professional organization).

Once the authors have agreed upon a journal, the next task is to locate the "Instructions for Authors" (also called "Author Guidelines" or "Submission Requirements") located on the journal's Website or in a designated issue of the journal. These requirements usually change when the journal hires a new editor-in-chief; thus, authors should consult the instructions immediately prior to writing. Figure 14.1 displays a sample of journals that typically publish health promotion research.

Instructions are explicit and provide authors with a number of manuscript categories for reporting empirical findings, such as a letter, a report, a brief report, or a full-length original article. Again, the authors must strive to find an ideal fit; selecting the wrong manuscript category may severely hamper the odds of acceptance. Once the manuscript category has been identified, the authors

FIGURE 14.1. EXAMPLES OF JOURNALS THAT PUBLISH ARTICLES RELEVANT TO HEALTH PROMOTION.

Journal Name

Addiction
The American Journal of Health Behavior
The American Journal of Health Education
The American Journal of Health Promotion
American Journal of Preventive Medicine
American Journal of Public Health
Canadian Journal of Public Health
Ethnicity and Disease
Health Education and Behavior
Health Education Research
Health Promotion International
Journal of Adolescent Health
Journal of Consulting and Clinical Psychology
Journal of Health Care for the Poor and Underserved
Journal of School Health
Journal of the American Medical Association
Patient Education and Counseling
Prevention Science
Public Health Reports
Social Science and Medicine

should painstakingly adhere to the instructions that are specific to that category. Such instructions are typically broken down by section of the manuscript.

Sections of the Manuscript

The manuscript is typically divided into several discrete sections.

Abstract. The abstract is your one and only chance to make a good first impression. Often the only portion of an article that is widely available, accessible, and read in its entirety is the abstract. In fact, most journals that publish health promotion research will make article abstracts freely available through on-line search engines such as Medline®. Accessing the abstract only is often the initial goal of readers, as doing so can subsequently provide enough information to readers that they can determine whether they will benefit from reading the full article. Abstracts are also the medium for judging the quality of research that has been submitted for oral or poster presentations at professional conferences. Often the conference organizers will print the abstracts in the conference program and make them available on their Website. As is true for any first impression, a good-quality abstract can greatly enhance the odds that readers will ultimately seek (and benefit from) the full article or attend the conference presentation.

◆ ◆ ◆

In a Nutshell

Abstracts are also the medium for judging the quality of research that has been submitted for oral or poster presentations at professional conferences.

◆ ◆ ◆

Typically an abstract comprises 250 words or less. Within this limited number of words, the abstract must concisely describe the objective(s), methods, results, and conclusion(s) of the research. The abstract should convey essential information such as

- The research question(s)
- Sample size and sampling technique
- Participation rate
- Study design (retention rates if applicable)
- Key measures

- Data-collection methods
- Descriptive, bivariate, and multivariate findings (with test statistics)
- A one-sentence conclusion that addresses the research question(s)

Quick inspection of the items in this list suggests that the abstract is a "stand alone" unit within the manuscript. Indeed, the abstract should always be prepared as a digest of the complete story; it should *not* dilute the story through the use of vacuous phrases such as "implications will be discussed" or "a few examples of the findings are." Remember, space is limited so make every word count!

The important and very demanding requirements of an abstract may at first seem impossible to meet given a word limit of 250 or less. However, the judicious selection of words and the elimination of any superfluous information can greatly aid the writer in bringing the word count down within limits. Traditionally, abstracts do not have to adhere to essential rules of grammar. (See Box 14.1 for several examples.) Of course, even with a stringent selection of words and thoughts, abstracts may seem impossible to create given their strict word limits. One way to create abstracts that meet word limits is to reduce the number of findings presented. For example, it may be better to focus on the findings related to the primary research question. If space permits, then you could include the ancillary findings.

Unfortunately, universal standards for the structure of abstracts are nonexistent in the discipline of health promotion research. Some journals require that the abstract should not have specific headings, but most journals specify the headings that are mandatory and those that are optional. Knowing these requirements (based on the published "Instructions to Authors") is therefore a prerequisite to creating an acceptable abstract.

Introduction. The scope and depth of a well-written introduction is a function of journal requirements. For example, typically, journals that cater to a largely medical audience (such as the *Journal of the American Medical Association*) prefer very short introductions (two to three paragraphs), whereas journals that fall under the umbrella of behavioral and social science disciplines (for example, *Health Education & Behavior*) prefer and encourage introductions that provide a great deal of detail and allow more space. The difference between these two "camps" is not only a matter of degree but also of substance.

As described in Chapter One (steps 2 and 9), the research enterprise is focused on identifying and addressing key gaps in the existing literature. Thus, one purpose of the introduction is to describe the chain of research that led to the current

Box 14.1. Examples of Abridged Grammar in Abstracts

For the purposes of writing and submitting an abstract, the grammar used is considered correct and acceptable.

A. **Study Objectives**

This study was designed to identify factors that may preclude people from accepting an AIDS vaccine when one is developed and approved for use.

or

To identify factors that that may preclude people from accepting an AIDS vaccine when one is developed and approved for use.

B. **Study Design**

The study used a prospective design with assessments at baseline, three months, six months, and twelve months.

or

A prospective study with assessments at baseline, three months, six months, and twelve months.

C. **Study Sample**

The sample comprised 679 adult volunteers recruited from cardiac outpatient units.

or

679 adult volunteers recruited from cardiac outpatient units.

D. **Conclusion**

The study findings provide support for the hypothesis that men are less likely than women to initiate cigarette use after the age of twenty-one years.

or

Findings suggest that men are less likely than women to initiate cigarette use after the age of twenty-one years.

---

study—this description sets the stage for the remainder of the manuscript and clearly prepares readers for a conclusion (or conclusions) that will represent the next link in this chain. Short introductions provide this information in summary form. Consider, for example, the one paragraph hypothetical introduction that follows:

Although intensified HIV testing efforts and behavioral interventions may greatly contribute to reducing the incidence of HIV,[ref] the anticipated advent of a vaginal microbicide may represent a substantial turning point in the epidemic. Unfortunately, only two studies have investigated social and behavioral correlates pertaining to microbicide acceptance among female partners of injection-drug-using men, a population greatly at risk for HIV infection. The first study focused solely on the identification of demographic factors (such as race, ethnicity, and income),[ref] and the second investigated a large number of partner-related barriers to potential microbicide use.[ref] Related studies of other high-risk populations have found that self-efficacy for microbicide application and perceived threat of HIV infection were robustly associated with intent to use microbicides.[ref] As opposed to studies investigating intent (or actual participation) to enroll in randomized controlled trials of a microbicide,[ref] this study identified factors that may preclude women from using an HIV-preventive microbicide that was approved for use in western Kenya.

◆ ◆ ◆

In a Nutshell

One purpose of the introduction is to describe the chain of research that led to the current study.

◆ ◆ ◆

The introduction succinctly conveys the chain of research and notes the gap in the literature (in other words, no studies of women whose partners are injection-drug users and no studies of actual microbicide use). Each article is cited and described just enough to allow an interested reader to find out more by retrieving a specific article. The final sentence is the logical conclusion of the paragraph (and the entire introduction).

Alternatively, longer introductions serve the same purpose, but they provide more depth to the literature reviewed. A longer version could describe each of the cited articles in greater detail. A long introduction, however, will nonetheless take on a general form that mimics the sample shown (that is, the chain of research is reviewed, a gap is identified, and the research question is stated).

Methods: Study Sample. This subsection of the manuscript should provide details related to the generation of the study sample, such as the population from which the sample was drawn and the inclusion and exclusion criteria (as well as the number of otherwise eligible participants who were excluded based on these criteria). This section also should describe the sampling technique employed and provide the rationale for its selection. This rationale is critically important because it justifies the sampling technique (see Chapter Eleven). Consider the following hypothetical example:

> To identify differences between low-income women who have and have not ever had a mammogram, we began with a sampling frame of women receiving WIC benefits in the state of Vermont. The sampling frame was a list of all women currently receiving benefits, with women receiving benefits for the longest period of time listed first through women receiving benefits for the shortest period of time listed last. Next, every twenty-fifth name on the list was selected; this created a systematic random sample. The sample therefore comprised women who had previously been categorized as low-income and it equally represented women regardless of how long they had been receiving WIC benefits.

The text states the sampling technique used (systematic random sample) as well as the reasons the research team used this approach.

Another obligation of this section is to report the participation rate. This rate is used as a gauge to judge the potential for *participation bias* (that is, whether volunteers were systematically different from those who refused to be in the study). Although a low participation rate does not necessarily mean that the sample was biased, it nonetheless suggests that this form of bias cannot be ruled out. Consider the following example:

> From December 2000 through April 2002, project recruiters screened 1,590 men attending health department clinics to assess eligibility for participating in a cancer prevention study. Of those screened, 685 were eligible to participate. Men were eligible if they were African American, eighteen to twenty-nine years old, unmarried, and had been previously diagnosed with cancer. Of those men not eligible to participate, the majority (83 percent) were either too young or too old. The current study consisted of 605 (88.3 percent) eligible men who volunteered and provided written informed consent. The majority (91.2 percent) of eligible men who did not participate in the study were unavailable due to conflicts with their employment schedules.

Note that the paragraph provides information pertaining to eligibility requirements and shows that "age" was the primary reason why screened men were not eligible. Lack of eligibility is *not* indicative of participation bias, because this is a reason for nonparticipation that is imposed by the research question rather than a self-selection phenomenon. The important numbers are 605 (the N for the study) and 685 (the number of eligible men who were asked to volunteer). By use of these numbers as the numerator and denominator, respectively, a participation rate was obtained and reported. Although universally accepted standards do not exist, participation rates in excess of 80 percent are widely considered acceptable (that is, the potential for a strong participation bias is considered sufficiently low).

In studies that have one or more planned follow-up assessments, you should also report the *retention rate* or the *attrition rate*. The retention rate is the percentage of participants who remained in the study and completed each of the follow-up assessments. Unfortunately, in prospective studies, retaining a high percentage of participants is a challenge. Consider, for example, an article that reports only a 51 percent retention rate. This information is important to report because it suggests a possibility for *attrition bias*. (Attrition bias can be assessed analytically, and these analyses should be reported in the results section—see Chapters Five and Thirteen for analyses to assess attrition bias).

This section of the manuscript also meets several other obligations. The time period of data collection should be disclosed. This information lets readers judge whether the data represent thinking or practice that may have changed in the study population. For example, a study concerning awareness of smallpox and anthrax (among U.S. residents) conducted in 2002 would provide substantially different results than the same study conducted before the events of September 11, 2001, and the subsequent media attention to bioterrorism. Also, because this is traditionally the first section of the manuscript that reports methodology, a sentence should be included informing readers that the entire study protocol was approved by an Institutional Review Board. (Indeed, journal editors will demand that this sentence be included.)

Methods: Data Collection. This section is designed to inform readers *how* the data were collected, not *what* data were collected. A subsequent section will provide readers with specific information about the measures or instruments used in the study. As described in Chapters Nine and Ten, data-collection methods span a broad range from paper-and-pencil assessments to electronic diaries. A rationale for the selected method should be provided. Consider the following example:

> Based on studies suggesting decreased reporting bias,[ref] all self-reported measures were assessed using audio-computer-assisted self-interviewing

(A-CASI). By providing a voice track that delivered each question to adolescents through headphones, A-CASI technology may have reduced problems that otherwise would have been posed by low literacy. The A-CASI technology also created a user-friendly interview method that automatically handled skip patterns in the questionnaire and provided adolescents with an interactive experience, possibly increasing their attention to the task. The private environment created by the A-CASI may also be useful with respect to the elicitation of honest responses for questions that assessed sexual and drug-use behaviors.[ref] Adolescents' responses to the computer-delivered questions were automatically encrypted to ensure confidentiality. To help facilitate accuracy, a relatively short period of time was used when asking adolescents to recall past behaviors. Adolescents were assured that their names could not be linked to the codes used to identify documents containing their responses.

This example illustrates a good match between the research questions and the selected method of data collection. The study apparently asked adolescents to disclose information about their recent sexual behaviors and their recent drug use behaviors. Complete with references to support their position, the authors justify their selection of A-CASI with respect to these research goals.

In addition to *how* the data were collected, this section should also provide information pertaining to the physical location *where* the data were collected. This information is important because the reader must have the necessary details to potentially replicate the study and because readers may want to make judgments regarding the potential effect of the setting on participants' responses. For example, collecting data from incarcerated men in prison may inadvertently affect how they respond to certain questions (for example, Have you had sex in the past seven days) as opposed to interviewing men in a community center after their release. Finally, this section should also include a sentence that describes what compensation was provided to participants to encourage their participation.

Methods: Measures. The primary obligation of this section is to justify the constructs (for example, self-esteem) (see Chapter Nine for more details on constructs) included and describe the measures employed for assessing those constructs (such as the Rosenberg Self-Esteem Scale). If the study was guided by theory, then a sentence should be included in this section that articulates the particular theory used and that the measures chosen correspond to the theoretical constructs. This approach is mainly used in medical journals; for psychological or other social science journals, you may want to include a whole section on the theory in greater detail in the introduction. In the absence of a theoretical framework, authors should justify their selection of constructs based on previously conducted research.

Informing readers how the study constructs were measured is equally important. These constructs could be organized according to their role in the study. You could first describe the measures used to assess the X-variables (correlates in a cross-sectional study, predictors in a prospective study, or independent variables in an experimental study) followed by the measures used to assess the Y-variables (outcomes in observational research and dependent variables in experimental research). Within each category, authors may want to first describe single-item measures (such as measures of race or ethnicity, income, or geographic area) and then describe the use of scales or indexes. For each scale or index, a rationale should be provided for the choice of that particular measure. Moreover, if previous psychometric data are available, this should be provided and referenced, as well as current psychometric findings. It is also important to provide a sample question from the scale or index. The number of items constituting each scale or index should also be reported. If this information is extensive, then a table can be used. Table 14.1 provides a sample of summary information that should be reported. These measures were used to assess eight constructs among a sample of high-risk adolescents. To conserve precious journal space, the table may also provide descriptive statistics for each measure. Readers can also be referred back to this table a second time when they are reading the results section of the manuscript.

When research questions necessitate the use of directly observed or biological measures, the nature and use of these measures should be described in great detail. Two samples follow:

(1) After the interview, men were asked to demonstrate the act of applying a condom to a penile model. Trained observers scored men's performance based on six criteria: correctly opens package, squeezes air from tip, places condom right side up on model, keeps tip pinched while unrolling, unrolls to base of model, and condom remains intact. Men received one point for each of the six steps they performed correctly. Those scoring three points or less and those scoring four points or more were classified as having lower and higher demonstrated ability, respectively.

(2) Two vaginal swab specimens were evaluated for *Neisseria gonorrhoeae, Chlamydia trachomatis,* and *Trichomonas vaginalis.* The first swab was placed in a specimen transport tube (Abbott LCx Probe System for *N. gonorrhoeae* and *C. trachomatis* assays) and tested for chlamydia and gonorrhea DNA by (LCR). The second swab was used to inoculate a culture medium for *T. vaginalis* (InPouch TV test; BioMed Diagnostics, Inc., Santa Clara, California). A

TABLE 14.1. DESCRIPTION OF SCALE MEASURES AND BIVARIATE CORRELATIONS OF THESE MEASURES WITH SELF-ESTEEM AMONG AFRICAN AMERICAN ADOLESCENT FEMALES.

Scale and Sample Item	# of items	α	M	SD	Range
Body image[a] *I usually feel physically attractive.*	7	.73	27.2	4.8	12–35
Perceived family support[b] *My family really tries to help me.*	4	.86	15.2	4.3	4–20
Ethnic pride[c] *I feel good about black culture.*	13	.74	42.3	4.6	20–52
Normative beliefs favoring males[d] *Your boyfriend gets angry when you don't do what he wants.*	8	.72	15.6	5.6	8–36
Perceived support from a special person[e] *I have a special person who is a source of comfort to me.*	4	.82	17.2	3.5	4–20
Traditional sex role beliefs[f] *Boys are better leaders than girls.*	7	.64	13.2	3.9	7–28
Religiosity[g] *How often do you attend religious or spiritual services?*	4	.68	10.4	2.7	4–16
Perceived support from friends[h] *My friends really try to help me.*	4	.87	15.3	4.4	4–20

[a]Higher scores represent a more favorable body image.
[b]Higher scores represent a greater perceived family support.
[c]Higher scores represent greater ethnic pride.
[d]Higher scores represent stronger beliefs favoring male decision making in a relationship.
[e]Higher scores represent greater perceived support from special persons.
[f]Higher scores represent more traditional sex-role beliefs.
[g]Higher scores represent greater religiosity.
[h]Higher scores represent greater perceived support from friends.

number of studies have established the high sensitivity (at least 97 percent) and specificity (at least 99 percent) of these assays.[ref]

For biological measures, the authors should disclose sensitivity and specificity estimates of the test used as well as providing references. Finally, it should be noted that the name and location (city and state) of the company that produced the test should be disclosed. This practice is typically required by journals, and it also allows for replication by other researchers and possible comparison of findings across studies that use identical tests.

Methods: Data Analysis. This section should be brief yet informative. The authors have an obligation to compose a paragraph or two that informs readers about the specific statistical techniques that constituted the analytic procedures. Once described, these procedures should be followed without exception; introducing a new technique halfway through the results section creates confusion.

◆ ◆ ◆

In a Nutshell

The authors have an obligation to compose a paragraph or two that informs readers about the specific statistical techniques that constituted the analytic procedures.

◆ ◆ ◆

This section must describe the rationale and procedures used to transform any of the variables if applicable. The use of descriptive statistics does not need to be included; however, the use of each kind of statistical test employed in the analyses should be disclosed at this point. A rationale for the selection of every statistical test is *not* necessary; however, a rationale should be provided if one is not readily apparent or if the statistical test was complex. If appropriate references that support the selection of statistical tests, the rationale, or both are available, then they should be included. A manuscript may also benefit from succinct explanations of relatively novel tests or tests that are otherwise likely to be unfamiliar to readers of the journal. Finally, the authors should describe how they defined statistical significance. If statistical significance does not follow convention ($P < .05$), then a justification for choosing a different value should be provided.

When writing the methods section, it is important to note that sufficient detail should be provided to allow another research team to replicate the study. Indeed, achieving this level of descriptive detail is often considered a hallmark of well-written manuscripts.

Results: Characteristics of the Sample. This section is purely descriptive. The goal is to inform readers about the composition of the study sample. Common indices include race or ethnicity, sex, age, income-level, and marital status. However, most indices reported should be selected based on the nature of the research question. For instance, if the research question concerns associations between family structure and teen pregnancy, then basic descriptive information regarding these variables should be provided. An example of this section follows:

About one-third (34.2 percent) of the sample reported ever being pregnant, with 12.5 percent reporting a current pregnancy. The majority of participants reported residence with only their mother (59.3 percent) or with both their mother and father (32.1 percent). The remainder of the sample lived with friends (5.0 percent) or in their own apartment (3.6 percent).

When multiple sites are involved or participants are recruited from different venues, sample characteristics including number of participants can be provided for each of these different sites. Also, at this juncture, descriptive statistics for measures of key constructs should be reported. Table 14.1, for example, displays the range of scores, means, and standard deviations for each of eight assessed constructs. Referring readers to this table is therefore an important aspect of this opening part of the results section.

Results: Findings. This section is the heart of the manuscript. Describing the findings is not interpretive writing. Prose is not part of this section. The findings should be reported using technical writing, that is, using terse and precise language. Your task is to report the final output from the statistical analyses. In reporting the final output using text appropriate for this section, you should present the statistical findings in terms of the research question or study hypotheses. This context is necessary for understanding the results. As an elementary example, consider output from a logistic regression analysis that yielded an odds ratio of 3.9 and an associated P level of .001. In the text, you would say, "Women who had a regular physician were almost four times more likely to get a pap test in the past year relative to those without a regular physician."

◆ ◆ ◆

In a Nutshell

Describing the findings is not interpretive writing. Prose is not part of this section. The findings should be reported using technical writing, that is, using terse and precise language.

◆ ◆ ◆

Nearly all journals require that authors use tables and figures to extend the level of detail provided by the narrative used in the results section. The act of balancing text with these visuals, however, can be quite challenging. On one hand, the text must tell a complete story (as many readers will not inspect the visuals).

On the other hand, the visuals must also tell a complete, stand-alone story that only extends and does not replicate the story told in words. This seemingly tall order can be simplified by using a few simple guidelines:

- Tables are a good place to report test statistics, confidence intervals, and P-values.
- Figures are an efficient way of displaying associations between two or three variables (for example, linear, quadratic, and cubic trends loan themselves to the use of figures).
- Tables and figures should have footnotes when these are needed to tell a complete story.
- Text should provide a "bird's eye view" of the findings—nothing should be left out, but readers can be referred to visuals for details.

Discussion: General. Up to this point the manuscript has been guided by a blueprint that delineates the content and format of the sections. By convention, this entails a description of the research and thought processes underlying the research questions. Authors should not offer opinions or state implications of the research findings as of yet. The discussion section signals the beginning of a new set of rules and far fewer constraints with less structure. The discussion allows the authors (for the first time) to have their own voice! This voice, however, should not extend beyond the reach of the study findings. Stated differently, the study findings support the authors as they offer suggestions (albeit tempered by limitations of the study) to improve health promotion practice or policy.

Because the discussion is not driven by a rigid convention, it is much more difficult to know how to proceed with the writing process. However, several guidelines may prove quite useful.

- The opening paragraph is traditionally a place to summarize the findings. In this paragraph, avoid the use of statistics and jargon; instead strive for language that is comprehensible to the lay public.
- After the opening paragraph, it is useful to examine the findings in light of previous studies that have been reported. At this juncture authors should feel free to speculate as to why their findings may have differed from findings in other studies.
- Although the discussion should highlight findings that supported the study hypotheses, it should also offer explanations as to why any one hypothesis was not supported.
- Place the findings into a practice context. First and foremost, health promotion research should serve practitioners. Write each paragraph in a way that will put the findings to work in the field. Given that your research questions were important, this task should be relatively easy.

- Offer the findings and describe their implications in humble language. There is no such thing as a definitive study. A study that is extremely high in rigor is still just one study—it has much more meaning if it corroborates and extends evidence from previous studies.
- To help find a balance between sufficient elaboration and too much elaboration, it is helpful to read several articles that appear in recent issues of the journal you have selected. Read the discussion sections in articles that have used a study design and analytic procedures similar to the study you have conducted.

Discussion: Limitations. This section is perhaps one of the most important and most difficult sections of the entire manuscript. Virtually every research study has limitations. Study limitations are recognized weaknesses in the research that detract from rigor. Figure 14.2 provides a display of common limitations that if present, need to be addressed.

◆ ◆ ◆

In a Nutshell

Virtually every research study has limitations. Study limitations are recognized weaknesses in the research that detract from rigor.

◆ ◆ ◆

FIGURE 14.2.   COMMON STUDY LIMITATIONS.

Participation bias

Attrition bias

Social desirability bias, recall bias, and other problems inherent with self-reported measures

Limitations of the sampling technique

Limitations of the study design

Misclassification

Bias introduced by the transformation of variables

In experimental studies, bias introduced from lack of blinding and from contamination

Contrary to the instinct of some authors, limitations should be exhaustively identified. Authors should keep in mind that journal reviewers will readily spot limitations as they begin reading the manuscript. A good thing to know is that reviewers seldom expect perfection and typically anticipate that authors will disclose the study limitations and their potential impact on the findings. In keeping with this expectation then, authors need to show that they are indeed aware of each and every limitation. Thus, an exhaustive list is simply smart writing.

Discussion: Conclusions. Conclusions are the pinnacle of the manuscript. To avoid diluting the message, the conclusions should be stated in a single—preferably short—paragraph. In fact, two or three sentences can be sufficient for a well-written conclusion. Because being succinct is highly valued, authors must know exactly what to say and what not to say. The conclusions should be directly relevant to the research questions and provide a straightforward answer to each of the questions. Moreover, conclusions should not be definitive, as the research process entails ruling out alternative possibilities and providing support for hypotheses; it does not entail *proving* hypotheses. Authors should also avoid restating the findings or summarizing the research process.

One way that may be helpful when constructing your conclusion is to imagine a news story based on your study. What would the headline say? What would the thirty-second report on a local television channel be like? Indeed, few people may read the published article in its entirety, but massive numbers of people may read your three-sentence conclusion. Thus, your conclusion should be strong and striking without being overly intellectual. For all practical purposes, it should be written for a lay audience and easy to understand. Finally, high-quality manuscripts are defined by the practical value of the conclusions. Indeed, health promotion research only has value when it informs health promotion practice and policy. Thus, be absolutely sure to place the findings squarely into the context of health promotion practice. Box 14.2 displays several sample conclusions.

References. A reference list is a mandatory section of any manuscript. The list may, however, be constructed using any number of different styles. The selection of any given style is made by the journal editor and the editorial board. Although this lack of a universal system can appear overwhelming to new authors, most styles of referencing can be divided into two categories. Even within these two categories, some journals deviate from these styles; authors' instructions should always be consulted before compiling the reference list.

Numbered endnotes, of which biomedical referencing is one example, are probably the most common system used in journals that publish health promotion research. This system uses numbers in the text to denote corresponding

Box 14.2. Examples of Effective Conclusions

Research Question: The purpose of this study was test the efficacy of a structural intervention designed to increase protein intake among children residing in rural areas of Tanzania.

Conclusion: Evidence from this randomized, controlled trial suggests that a structural intervention can increase protein intake among children residing in rural villages. Widespread implementation of the intervention may contribute to substantial declines in nutrition-associated morbidity among rural Tanzanian children.

Research Question: This study identified psychosocial correlates of binge drinking among college females.

Conclusions: Binge drinking was predicted by three distinct constructs: impulsivity, loneliness, and low levels of academic motivation. Campus-based intervention programs designed to reduce binge drinking may benefit female students by addressing potential issues related to impulsive drinking decisions and drinking as a way of coping with loneliness. Such intervention programs may be especially important for female college students who are not highly motivated to achieve academic success.

Research Question: The purpose of the study was to identify barriers that may preclude low-income adults from receiving a flu vaccine.

Conclusions: Low-income adults may not receive an annual flu vaccine because they perceive the time commitment and expense as being excessive. Furthermore, African American men and women may not receive the vaccine because they lack trust in the medical system. Health departments and other organizations that provide the flu vaccine to low-income adults may need to demonstrate that receiving the vaccine involves a minimum time commitment and, simultaneously, they should seek to inspire the trust of African American adults. Findings also suggest that policies directed toward reduced price flu vaccines may promote acceptance.

references in a numbered reference or endnotes list. In contrast, the other style used quite often is the author-date style, of which the American Psychological Association (APA) style (American Psychological Association, 2001) is one example. This style uses the authors' last names and the publication year to denote the citation, and the reference list is alphabetized. Samples of the two styles as they would appear in the body of a manuscript follow:

Sample 1: Adolescents' lack of self-esteem has been associated with diverse health-compromising behaviors such as alcohol and cigarette use, the early onset of sexual activity, eating disorders and general emotional distress.[1-4] Conversely, high levels of self-esteem have been identified as a protective factor against adolescents' engagement in these behaviors.[5–7]

Sample 2. Adolescents' lack of self-esteem has been associated with diverse health-compromising behaviors such as alcohol and cigarette use, the early onset of sexual activity, eating disorders, and general emotional distress (Fisher, Schneider, Pegler, & Napolitana, 1991; Gordon-Rouse, Ingersoll, & Orr, 1998; Harrison & Luxenberg, 1995; Resnick, Bearman, Blum, et al., 1997). Conversely, high levels of self-esteem have been identified as a protective factor against adolescents' engagement in these behaviors (Harter, 1990; Kawabata, Cross, Nishioka, & Shimai, 1999; Vingilis, Wade, & Adlaf, 1998).

The citation style shown in Sample 2 is described in the *Publication Manual of the American Psychological Association* (2001). APA style is used by a large number of journals that publish health promotion research. Each citation gives the reader enough information to locate the reference in the alphabetized reference list—numbers (other than dates) are not used. By convention, the text citation usually comes at the end of the sentence (before the period), and multiple citations within any single set of parentheses are arranged alphabetically. For detailed instructions and other rules regarding APA style, consult the publication manual.

Before writing a manuscript, it is wise to learn the referencing style that will be required for the selected journal. Again, the endnote and author-date styles are basic categories; each has a number of variants that may be used. As a rule, a reference should have enough information that any reader could easily retrieve it from an electronic database. Rules for truncating the number of authors shown, placement of the publication year, abbreviation of journal names, and constructing other parts of the entry vary. Examples of how the reference should be written for the reference list in both endnote and author-date style follow:

1. Kawabata T, Cross D, Nishioka N, Shimai S. Relationship between self-esteem and smoking behavior among Japanese early adolescents: Initial results from a three-year study. J Sch Health 1999;69,:280–4.

Kawabata, T., Cross, D., Nishioka, N., & Shimai, S. (1999). Relationship between self esteem and smoking behavior among Japanese early adolescents: Initial results from a three-year study. *Journal of School Health, 69,* 280–284.

Applied Example

To apply the key concepts, a brief manuscript will be shown here in its entirety. Each main section will be presented separately and each will be annotated for teaching purposes.

Abstract

Background: The purpose of this study was to identify correlates of self-esteem among a sample of African American female adolescents. ← (Note that the research question is stated immediately.)

Methods: A prospective study was conducted. As part of a larger HIV prevention study, a purposive sample ($N = 522$) of sexually active, African American female adolescents, ages fourteen to eighteen years, was recruited from low-income neighborhoods characterized by high rates of unemployment, substance abuse, violence, teen pregnancy, and STDs. Adolescents completed a self-administered questionnaire that contained the Rosenberg self-esteem scale ($\alpha = .79$) and other scale measures that assessed constructs hypothesized to be associated with self-esteem. ← (Key information includes sampling technique, the sample size (N), the inclusion criteria, assessment of the primary variable, and the study design.)

Results: The regression model explained 38 percent of the variance in adolescents' self-esteem scores. Significant correlates of higher self-esteem were having a more favorable body image ($\beta = .35$), greater perceived family support ($\beta = .19$), nontraditional sex role beliefs ($\beta = .16$), greater ethnic pride ($\beta = .15$), normative beliefs not favoring male decision making in a relationship ($\beta = .12$), and greater religiosity ($\beta = .09$). ← (In a short amount of space the research question is answered using common statistical procedures.)

Conclusion: Diverse psychosocial measures were associated with self-esteem among high-risk African American female adolescents. Programs designed to enhance the self-esteem of this population may benefit by promoting more favorable body images, greater perceptions of family support, greater ethnic pride, and beliefs supporting egalitarian decision making. ← (The conclusion is suggestive and practical, not definitive and strongly related to health promotion.)

Introduction

Self-esteem, an indicator of self-worth, has been defined as a critical index of mental health[1] and is an important construct often integrated in resiliency theories, where it has been conceptualized as a protective or buffering factor.[1,2] ←(For purposes of brevity we have not included the reference list corresponding to these endnotes.) Specifically, resiliency theories posit that adolescents in high-risk social environments may be protected from adopting health-compromising behaviors because of their high self-esteem, which is reflected in their desire and commitment to overcome negative circumstances. An important aspect of enhancing adolescents' self-esteem is tailoring program content to target those psychosocial influences associated with adolescents' high self-esteem. These influences are likely to vary depending on characteristics of the adolescents.[3–12] ← (These opening sentences are based on twelve references—thus, a chain of research is now available to the reader.)

According to the U.S. Department of Health and Human Services report titled *Healthy People 2010*, minority adolescents are a priority population for health promotion interventions.[13] An especially important population is sexually active African American adolescent girls residing in communities that predispose them to risk of infection with human immunodeficiency virus (HIV), other sexually transmitted diseases (STDs), pregnancy, delinquent behaviors, substance abuse, and a range of other risk behaviors and problems that negatively affect their quality of life.[13,14] ← (This portion justifies the selected priority population.) Research identifying the correlates of high self-esteem among this population could be a valuable source of information for developing and tailoring risk-reduction programs that include the enhancement of self-esteem as one objective. ← (Here, the practical value of the research is noted.)

The purpose of this study was to identify the psychosocial correlates of high self-esteem among a sample of sexually active African American female adolescents residing in a high-risk environment. ← (The research question is concisely stated.) Previous studies have suggested that social support,[15] particularly family support,[16] may be important to the self-esteem of adolescents. Based on a literature review, we also hypothesized that several other constructs would be positively correlated with self-esteem: favorable body image, religiosity, ethnic pride, and parental monitoring.[16–19] Additionally, we hypothesized that traditional sex role beliefs and having normative beliefs that favor male decision making in a relationship would be inversely correlated with self-esteem.[20] ← (Study hypotheses and their basis are provided.)

Methods

Study Sample. From December 1999 through April 2003 project recruiters screened 1,780 female teens in adolescent medicine clinics. Of those screened, 1,609 adolescents were eligible. Adolescents were eligible if they were female, African American, fourteen to eighteen years old, unmarried, and reported sexually activity in the previous six months. Of those adolescents not eligible to participate, the majority (98 percent) were not sexually active. Of those eligible, 1,457 (82 percent) were enrolled. ← (Enough information is provided to let the reader make judgments about the potential for participation bias.) The study protocol was approved by the University Institutional Review Board prior to implementation. ← (This sentence (expressed in some form) is mandatory.)

Data Collection. Data collection consisted of a self-administered questionnaire administered in a group setting with monitors providing assistance to adolescents with limited literacy and helping to ensure confidentiality of responses. ← (The readers are now aware how the data was acquired.) Adolescents were reimbursed $20.00 for their participation.

Measures.

Criterion Variable. The Rosenberg self-esteem scale[21] was included as part of the assessment instrument. This scale has well-established psychometric properties and has been used widely with diverse populations to assess adolescents' self-esteem. The scale contained ten items, scored using a four-point Likert format, with responses ranging from "strongly agree" to "strongly disagree." Higher scores represented greater levels of self-esteem. Inter-item reliability of the scale was satisfactory ($\alpha = .79$). ← (A great deal of attention is given to this variable because it is the outcome measure (Y).)

Correlates. Two single-item measures of parental monitoring were assessed. One measure asked adolescents how often their parents or parental figure(s) knew where they were when not at home or in school. The other measure asked how often their parents or parental figure(s) knew whom they were with when not at home or in school. Eight scales were used to assess various constructs hypothesized to correlate with adolescents' self-esteem. Table 1 displays psychometric information for the eight scales as well as a sample item for each. ← (Note, the use of a table to keep the text brief.)

Data Analysis.

Pearson product-moment correlations were calculated to assess strength and direction of the bivariate relationship between self-esteem and each of the hypothesized correlates. To assess the partial contribution of each of the hypothesized correlates working as a set in explaining the observed levels of self-esteem, multiple linear regression was used. Variables representing the correlates were entered into the regression model using a stepwise procedure with the alpha criteria set at .05 for entry and .10 for exit. The F-statistic was computed to test the overall significance of the final model. Acceptance of statistical significance was based on an alpha of .05. ← (Enough information is provided that someone else could replicate the analysis.)

Results

Characteristics of the Sample.

The average age of the adolescents was 16.0 years ($SD = 1.2$). The majority (81.2 percent) were full-time students; 9.4 percent were part-time students, and the remainder were not enrolled in school. Nearly one-fifth of the adolescents reported that their family received welfare.

The Rosenberg self-esteem scale was completed by 98.6 percent of the adolescents ($n = 515$). Scores ranged from 16 to 40 ($Md = 34.0$, $M = 33.4$, $SD = 4.8$).

Although the distribution of scores had a slight negative skew (skewness $= -.50$), the degree of skewness was not sufficient to necessitate transforming the scores so that they more closely approximate a normal distribution. ← (Note that a great deal of descriptive attention is given to outcome measure, including a consideration to transform the measure.)

Bivariate Findings. Table 1 displays the Pearson Product Moment Correlations between each of the correlates and self-esteem. ← (For brevity, the table is not shown in this example, but it should be noted that it serves dual purposes: (1) it describes the measures psychometrically and (2) it provides bivariate correlation coefficients.)

Each of the constructs was significantly correlated, in the hypothesized direction, with adolescents' self-esteem. In addition, positive correlations between the two single-item measures assessing parental monitoring and adolescents' self-esteem were observed. ← (Text describes the table.)

Adolescents' age was not significantly correlated with self-esteem ($r = .07$, $P = .11$). ← (This text provides results that are not shown in the table.)

Multivariate Findings. Table 2 displays the standardized partial regression coefficients and the proportion of unique variance accounted for by each correlate in the final model. Overall, the model explained 38 percent of the variance in adolescents' self-esteem ($F = 49.3$, $df = 6,479$, $P = .0001$). ← (These values are rarely provided in tables.) Body image was the most important correlate of self-esteem, followed by perceived family support. Ethnic pride was an important contributor to the overall model, and religiosity played a lesser but significant role in explaining the variance observed in adolescents' self-esteem. ← (Text summarizes the values shown in Table 2.)

Discussion

Findings suggest that African American female adolescents' self-esteem may be associated with at least six relevant psychosocial constructs. The strong association between self-esteem and body image is not surprising, since some researchers have suggested that physical appearance is the most important factor in determining global self-worth for adolescents.[22] These findings also suggest that even among older adolescents, family support may be an important factor in contributing to their emotional well-being. ← (Note that the text is speculative and no longer written in the past tense.)

Influencing these six constructs may in turn promote higher levels of self-esteem, thereby providing high-risk adolescents with a valuable protective factor against health-compromising behaviors. Behavioral intervention programs may benefit African American adolescent girls with low self-esteem by helping them improve their perceptions of body image and family support while affecting their ethnic pride. Additionally, programs may benefit this population by promoting more egalitarian beliefs about sex roles and decision making in the context of adolescents' relationships with male partners. ← (The practical implications for health promotion are explored.)

Limitations. These findings are limited by the validity of the measures ← (Limitation 1) and the inherent limitations of the cross-sectional design. ← (Limitation 2) In addition, the findings can only be generalized to sexually active African American female adolescents. ← (Limitation 3) Finally, the sample was limited to economically disadvantaged African American adolescents. Therefore, the findings may not be generalized to other racial or ethnic groups, or adolescents from different socioeconomic strata. ← (Limitation 4).

Conclusions. Diverse psychosocial constructs were found to be associated with self-esteem among a sample of high-risk African American female adolescents. Several of the assessed constructs may be particularly amenable to behavioral intervention. ← (Notice that the speculative language is couched as "may.") Programs designed to increase high-risk African American adolescent females' self-esteem may benefit from promoting more favorable body images, greater perceptions of family support, greater ethnic pride, and more egalitarian sex role beliefs. ← (Again, a practical value of the research is noted.)

Integration with the Research Process

A good manuscript reflects nothing more (and nothing less) than the completion of steps 1 through 8 in the research process. Leaving out any one step of this "historical description" greatly diminishes the value of the manuscript. Indeed, a manuscript should be viewed as a historical accounting of the events that led to the conclusion. The conclusion, of course, is the penultimate product of the research. Unfortunately, this product only has value when step 9 of the research process (dissemination) occurs. The preparation of a manuscript (as outlined in this chapter), then, can be viewed as the starting point for dissemination. Indeed, once the manuscript has been completed, the researcher can also disseminate the findings by making oral presentations at conferences. Such presentations may be extremely helpful in deciding what final changes to make to a manuscript before it is submitted for review and eventual publication. Figure 14.3 displays

FIGURE 14.3.   HOW A MANUSCRIPT BECOMES
A PUBLISHED JOURNAL ARTICLE.

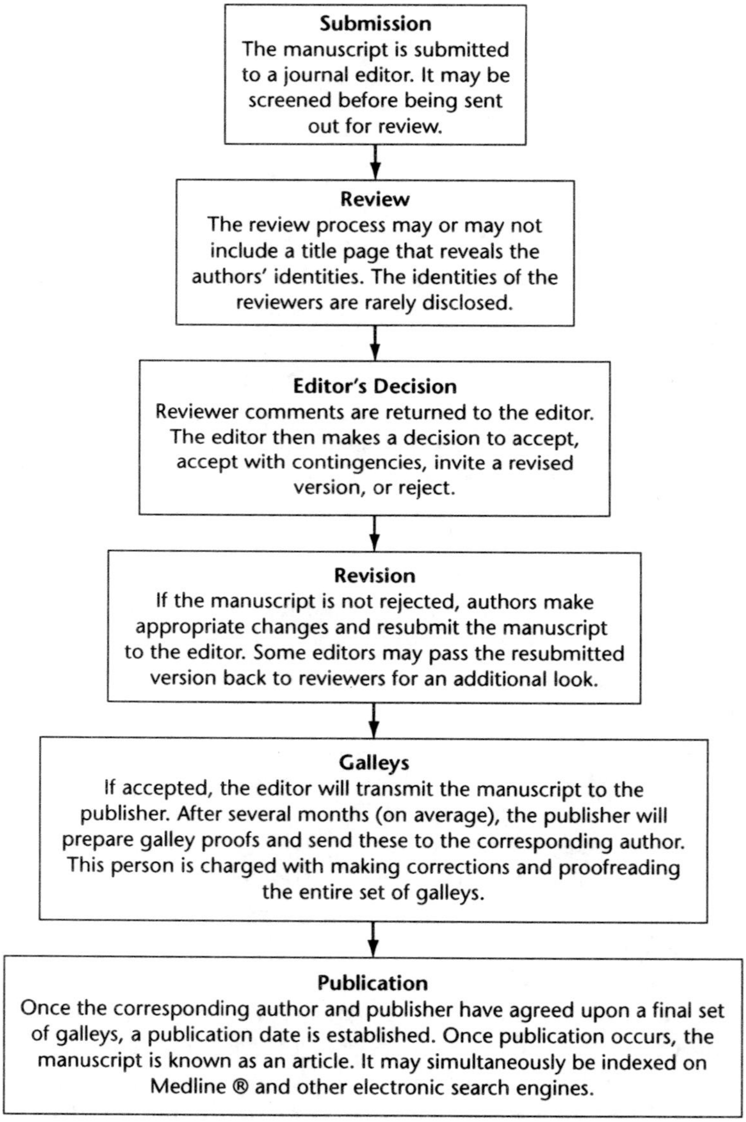

Submission
The manuscript is submitted
to a journal editor. It may be
screened before being sent
out for review.

Review
The review process may or may not
include a title page that reveals the
authors' identities. The identities of the
reviewers are rarely disclosed.

Editor's Decision
Reviewer comments are returned to the editor.
The editor then makes a decision to accept,
accept with contingencies, invite a revised
version, or reject.

Revision
If the manuscript is not rejected, authors make
appropriate changes and resubmit the manuscript
to the editor. Some editors may pass the resubmitted
version back to reviewers for an additional look.

Galleys
If accepted, the editor will transmit the manuscript to the
publisher. After several months (on average), the publisher will
prepare galley proofs and send these to the corresponding author.
This person is charged with making corrections and proofreading
the entire set of galleys.

Publication
Once the corresponding author and publisher have agreed upon a final set
of galleys, a publication date is established. Once publication occurs, the
manuscript is known as an article. It may simultaneously be indexed on
Medline ® and other electronic search engines.

the process of taking the manuscript through the review process as it becomes a published article.

◆ ◆ ◆

In a Nutshell

Leaving out any one step of this "historical description" greatly diminishes the value of the manuscript.

◆ ◆ ◆

Summary

A manuscript is a historical accounting of the entire research process. Success in publishing is therefore a direct function of success in conducting rigorous research. The preparation of this document is not an art; indeed, the majority of journals that publish health promotion research findings will provide authors a very specific set of instructions for what should and what should not be included in the manuscript, how the manuscript should be constructed, the length of the manuscript, its citation and reference style, and a host of other considerations. Although authors should be skilled in the application of simple rules for writing (grammar, paragraphing, and so on), these skills will not "carry the day." Instead, the construction of a parsimonious and poignant manuscript—one that has an important conclusion—will ensure success. Most important is to remember that the process can be fun and exciting, especially when your manuscript is accepted for publication. Give yourself a pat on the back—you deserve it! (Go ahead.)

Issues to Consider

1. Integrity is to manuscript preparation as a roof is to a house. Without integrity, the entire process (from floor to ceiling) loses all meaning. Integrity means that the authors have purposefully avoided omitting from the manuscript any information that would otherwise help readers evaluate the strength and importance of the conclusion. It means that the authors have faithfully disclosed any conflicts of interest or any potential improprieties

in their work. It clearly implies that all statistical values are transposed verbatim from the computer output files and that "close" values are not rounded up to achieve significance. Given that science as a whole suffers when a breach of integrity is discovered, a worthwhile issue to consider is how members of a research team should ensure mutual integrity among themselves.

◆ ◆ ◆

In a Nutshell

Integrity means that the authors have purposefully avoided omitting from the manuscript any information that would otherwise help readers evaluate the strength and importance of the conclusion.

◆ ◆ ◆

2. *Publication bias* is a common problem in health promotion research. This implies that editors (and reviewers) have a preference for accepting manuscripts that confirm popular thought and may therefore shy away from (1) papers that have significant findings which support an unpopular position or (2) papers that have nonsignificant findings. Thus, an important question that peer reviewers must entertain is how to avoid, even at the subconscious level, this form of bias in science.

For Practice and Discussion

A single exercise is recommended. Working with a fellow student or colleague, select a published article that is of mutual interest and make a copy of the article for each of you. In separate locations, read and evaluate the article as though it had not been published and, instead, you have been asked to serve as a peer reviewer of the manuscript. Carefully evaluate each section of the manuscript, making detailed notations on every page. When you finish, fill out the following form and then exchange forms with your colleague. How much agreement existed between the two of you?

Please rank the quality of each section from 1 (poor) to 5 (outstanding)

Abstract   1   2   3   4   5

Main weakness: _____

Introduction   1   2   3   4   5

Main weakness: _____

Methods   1   2   3   4   5

Main weakness: _____

Results   1   2   3   4   5

Main weakness: _____

Discussion   1   2   3   4   5

Main weakness: _____

Is the title *appropriate?* Please explain. _____

_____

Is the conclusion *appropriate?* Please explain. _____

_____

Is the conclusion *important?* Please explain. _____

_____

Please write a short summary of the strong points.

Please write a short summary of the weak points.

Would you recommend this manuscript for publication?

If yes, what level of enthusiasm do you have?   1 = low, 10 = high

        1   2   3   4   5   6   7   8   9   10

Reference

American Psychological Association. (2001). *Publication manual of the American Psychological Association* (5th ed.). Washington, DC: American Psychological Association.

CHAPTER FIFTEEN

CRAFTING A SUCCESSFUL RESEARCH PROPOSAL

Ralph J. DiClemente, Laura F. Salazar, and Richard A. Crosby

Unlike the preceding chapters in this textbook that have each addressed an aspect of the research process, the overarching aim of this chapter is to provide guidance in how best to craft a research proposal. Rather than being an explicit part of the research process, obtaining funding to conduct research is an implicit demand that gives rise to the entire process. Because this chapter is therefore fundamentally different from the previous fourteen chapters, we have chosen to provide only an overview, the illustration of key concepts, and a summary.

First, we need to recognize that writing a research proposal is not magic. Anyone can learn the skills needed to be proficient at proposal writing. Second, proposal writing is not a one-trial learning opportunity. It is an incremental, iterative, and calibrated learning process. We need to acknowledge that proposal writing, like any other skill, whether it's surfing, gymnastics, or playing the piano, requires practice to become proficient. This is an important point that many young (and some established) investigators fail to acknowledge. Thus, to be a skilled proposal writer requires an investment of time and energy and a willingness to be receptive to constructive feedback.

While we talk of a "research proposal" as a generic product, it is useful to acknowledge that research proposals vary markedly depending on the source of funding. For example, a National Institutes of Health (NIH) proposal will have different requirements than, perhaps, a Centers for Disease Control and Prevention (CDC) or private foundation proposal. Even within an agency, NIH for example, there is an array of application types (R01, R03, R21, and so on) as well as varying research stages, purposes, and designs. For example, a research proposal that is testing the efficacy of a health promotion program (HPP) will differ in format, scope, and design from one that is proposing to conduct an observational study or a qualitative research study (that is, using focus groups, elicitation interviews, or other qualitative methods). Notwithstanding the variability inherent in these different formats, proposals do have a common core of elements. Rather than attempt to address each variation, we will provide a template of the critical elements necessary for a successful research proposal.

Illustration of Key Concepts

There is a core set of key concepts that are germane to most research proposals. These core concepts form the proverbial "backbone" of the proposal. In this section we discuss each of these concepts.

Statement of the Problem: The Specific Aims

The desire to write a research proposal is not driven by whim. Indeed, the interest in designing any study, whether it is qualitative, observational, or interventional, does not exist in a vacuum, but rather is mobilized when we identify a problem that needs to be addressed. The "problem" can range from how best to enhance vegetable consumption among adolescents, to enhance mammography-seeking behavior among women, or to promote safer sex behavior among gay men. In the discipline of health promotion, the range of problems is as limitless as our imagination. The only stipulation is that the problem should be timely and health related.

To be effective as a health promotion scientist and researcher or, for that matter, any occupation, requires an intrinsic interest in the subject matter. The first criterion in selecting a research topic is to select one that is of great interest to you. The second criterion is to select a topic that is salient to the field, something the field is wrestling with in terms of understanding how best to address the issue. The third criterion is to select a topic that has public health implications for society. This criterion suggests that the research be *applied* (in other words, research that has a practical, real-world application). Indeed, in the discipline of health promotion, our mission is *not* one of *basic* science (that is, research that may not have immediate or direct application to real-world issues).

A few ground rules may also help to weed out potential research topics. The first rule is don't select a research topic only because it is fashionable. Fashion in health promotion research, as in clothes, changes quickly. Choose something that you are passionate about studying, that needs additional research (which excludes almost nothing), and, if your study is done well, will have important implications for health promotion research and practice.

◆ ◆ ◆

In a Nutshell

Choose something that you are passionate about studying, that needs additional research (which excludes almost nothing), and, if your study is done well, will have important implications for health promotion research and practice.

◆ ◆ ◆

We will illustrate these concepts with an example from our own research. We have a strong interest and commitment to designing interventions to promote adolescents' adoption of condom use during sexual intercourse as a way to reduce their risk of becoming infected with STDs, including HIV. This interest allows us to identify potential research ideas and fuels our desire to test these ideas. Thus, criterion one (an idea driven by passion) for selecting a research topic is met. Currently, there are few HPPs that have demonstrated efficacy in enhancing adolescents' use of condoms during sexual intercourse. Thus, our second criterion (value to the discipline) is met. And, finally, there is an urgent need for the development of effective HPPs to promote safer sex behavior, as adolescents constitute a population at growing risk of HIV infection. Thus, our third criterion (value to society) has been met.

After meeting the prerequisite criteria for selecting a researchable topic, the next step is developing the research proposal. The research proposal itself has a number of sections. We'll use the Public Health Service (PHS) 398 forms as a template for heuristic purposes. As noted earlier, other proposal formats may be required, so pay careful attention to the requirements by reading the Request for Proposal (RFP), the Request for Application (RFA), or the Program Announcement (PA). Generally, the most liberal allotment for proposing a research plan is twenty-five single-spaced pages of text.

One formidable task that requires extreme attention is the preparation of an abstract (called the "Summary of the Proposed Research"). The goal of this space-limited paragraph is to provide a succinct yet comprehensive summary of the aims, significance, and proposed methodology. This will appear on a form page (see http://grants.nih.gov/grants/forms.htm for the PHS 398 forms; refer to form page 2) and does not count in the twenty-five-page limit. This paragraph will become your "first impression" to the Scientific Review Group (SRG), scientific peers who will evaluate the merits of your proposal. Thus, it is essential that the abstract be clear, articulate, and polished. This should be written only after the entire research plan has been developed, reviewed, modified, and finalized. If funded, this abstract will appear in the CRISP data file. (For a government-maintained listing of research projects, see www.http://crisp.cit.nih.gov/.)

Using the PHS 398 forms, the specific aims in a proposal are explicitly stated in Section A and labeled "Specific Aims." Typically, this section is approximately one page in length. An illustration of how to craft a specific aims section follows.

A.1 Specific Aims

1. To evaluate the efficacy of an HIV intervention relative to standard-of-care counseling in reducing HIV-associated sexual behaviors and incident STDs over a twelve-month follow-up period.
2. To evaluate the efficacy of an HIV intervention relative to standard-of-care counseling in enhancing theoretically important mediators of safer sex behavior over a twelve-month follow-up period.

The specific aims are the key research statements because they define clearly the research purpose and regulate the scope of the proposal. The aims must be parsimonious and unified. They should reflect succinctly the goals of the intended research ("less is more").

◆ ◆ ◆

In a Nutshell

The specific aims are the key research statements because they define clearly the research purpose and regulate the scope of the proposal.

◆ ◆ ◆

Corresponding hypotheses are also needed to fulfill the aims. The hypotheses must be in the form of testable statements. In this illustration, we composed the following hypotheses:

A.2 Primary Hypothesis

H1: A smaller proportion of adolescents in the HIV intervention condition compared to those receiving the standard-of-care counseling condition will engage in HIV-associated sexual behaviors and test positive for incident STDs over the twelve-month follow-up period.

H2: Adolescents in the HIV intervention condition, relative to those receiving the standard-of-care counseling condition, will demonstrate higher scores on psychosocial mediators of safer sex, including HIV prevention knowledge, self-efficacy to use condoms, communication with sex partners.

MINCUS AND DINCUS'S GRANT IS REVIEWED.

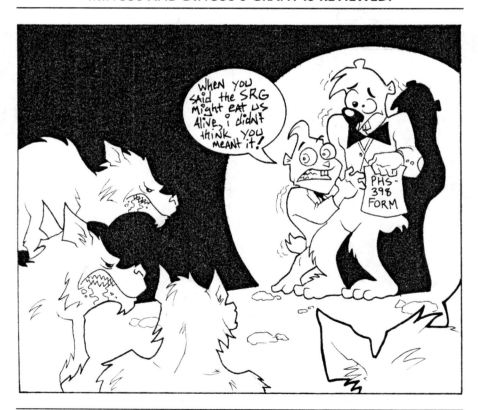

Copyright 2005 by Justin Wagner; reprinted with permission.

As shown, each specific aim has a corresponding research hypothesis, and each hypothesis is testable and directional. A hypothesis may be proposed as either a *null hypothesis* (that is, there are no differences between groups) or as a *motivator* or *alternative hypothesis*. Some people may also refer to the motivator or alternative hypothesis as a *research hypothesis*. Regardless of which one of these three terms is used, the meaning is identical (in other words, differences exist between groups). We are proposing a new intervention to enhance HIV-preventive behaviors and reduce adverse biological consequences of risky sexual behavior. Thus, in this instance, the motivator hypothesis is more meaningful than the null hypothesis because it reflects the investigators' desire to improve health conditions, practices, and programs. In proposing an intervention to enhance health behavior (or attitudes, beliefs, and so on), it is more relevant to offer a motivator hypothesis that states the direction of the HPP effects (for example, the HPP will yield positive effects). With the specific aims (Section A) clearly framed and written, the next step is Section B, "Background and Significance."

Background and Significance

The background and significance (B&S) section permits examination and framing of the existing empirical research relevant to the study. It is an opportunity to carefully consider data from diverse sources. A word of caution, however, is in order. Although the research literature may be replete with numerous studies, the B&S should be a targeted review. It is not a term paper, a master's thesis, or a dissertation. In fact, we suggest allocating only about three pages to this section. The goal of the B&S is to develop a rationale for the proposed study, for its conceptualization, and for its importance. Do not become mired in the review of the literature.

In constructing the B&S, it is important to understand the research literature—its strengths and weaknesses—so that an argument for the proposed study can be made. Indeed, if a satisfactory argument for the proposed study cannot be formulated, then the logical question arises: Why do the study? As you review the research literature, begin to make distinctions between studies. Some of these studies are well done and others are not. Some are observational and others are interventions. Not all studies are equally well designed, implemented, or analyzed. You, as a health promotion scientist, bring your unique skills to bear in analyzing the existing data. Thus, start to cull through the literature, identifying studies that may directly address your specific aims, some that may tangentially address your specific aims, and some that are unrelated to your aims but may have relevance to your intervention strategy or HPP techniques by virtue of having been used in other health promotion studies.

The B&S section for the illustration is constructed as follows, with subheadings reflecting specific sections of the B&S. Notice that topics progress from the broader to a more narrow focus.

B.1 Adolescents are at-risk for HIV infection.

B.2 Female adolescents are especially vulnerable to HIV/STD infection.

B.3 African American female adolescents are at significant risk of HIV infection.

B.4 Targeting adolescents at highest risk for HIV is a public health priority.

B.5 HIV interventions for adolescent females are needed.

B.6 Methodological limitations in assessing HIV intervention efficacy.

B.7 The importance of gender-tailored HIV interventions.

B.8 Psychosocial, gender, and relational correlates of HIV-preventive and risk behavior among adolescents and young adult women.

B.9 Peer approaches are a promising strategy for enhancing the efficacy of HIV interventions.

B.10 Significance of the proposed study for advancing the field of HIV prevention for adolescents.

This B&S section provides a brief review of the literature on adolescents and HIV, emphasizes the increased relative risk for females, and then African American adolescents. Indeed, subheadings B.1 to B.5 are crafted to make an inescapable point—this population is in urgent need of additional study to develop effective risk-reduction interventions. The B&S should firmly establish that the population is at risk, and thus there is a clear, cogent, and compelling need to address this health risk behavior among this population.

◆ ◆ ◆

In a Nutshell

The B&S should firmly establish that the population is at risk, and thus there is a clear, cogent, and compelling need to address this health risk behavior among this population.

◆ ◆ ◆

With the need to study the proposed population established, subheadings B.6 through B.9 are directly related to the proposed HPP and applicable methodological issues. These sections of the B&S provide a platform on which to build our HPP. First, however, we need to demonstrate that we are familiar with these different behavior change strategies, and that they have relevance to our proposed HPP. This is where many investigators falter. They can summarize the research literature with respect to identifying the problem (subheadings B.1 through B.5), but fail to provide an adequate discussion of the underlying theories, principles, strategies, and techniques that they will propose in their research methods. We cannot emphasize enough the importance of clearly demonstrating a thorough understanding of the underlying theories, principles, strategies, and techniques and how they are relevant to your proposed research. SRG members are often overburdened with having to read and critique many proposals in a relatively short amount of time. SRG members are not psychics or mind readers, and they may not be intimately familiar with all facets of your proposed research. When in doubt, write it out! In this instance, it is better to err on the side of redundancy than to make an error of omission by not including relevant information that is critical to building an argument to support funding your proposed study.

◆ ◆ ◆

In a Nutshell

SRG members are not psychics or mind readers, and they may not be intimately familiar with all facets of your proposed research. When in doubt, write it out!

◆ ◆ ◆

Finally, the B&S requires closure. Hopefully, you have carved a path through the morass of research literature. Now you are ready for a conclusion. How you conclude the B&S is critical. The conclusion may be what the members of the SRG remember most prominently about the B&S. We provide one more subheading that emphasizes the significance of the research to public health (B.10 Significance of the proposed study for advancing the field of HIV prevention for adolescents). Envision the information provided under each subheading as representing a piece to a puzzle. The SRG has read a number of pages, and its members are trying to put the pieces together and understand the "big picture." Thus, the last piece in the puzzle (that is, the significance to public health) is by far the most important.

What should be included in this last section? The objective is to enumerate and describe how the proposed study can significantly contribute to the field. Be brief, but be comprehensive. Also, here is an opportunity to express your passion and excitement. Research should not be a dispassionate enterprise. Quite the contrary, research is brimming with passion. Thus, you should include statements about how this study creates an exciting opportunity to interact with others from diverse scientific disciplines in a multidisciplinary approach; to develop new and innovative HP intervention strategies; and to apply HP strategies observed to be effective in other fields of health promotion research to your proposed study, population, and venue. Finally, add one statement that reiterates the clear, cogent, and compelling clinical and public health significance of your proposed study (for instance, "The proposed study of African American adolescent females will assess the efficacy of an intervention program designed to promote safer sex behaviors among a population at increasingly greater risk of STD and HIV infection").

◆ ◆ ◆

In a Nutshell

Research should not be a dispassionate enterprise. Quite the contrary, research is brimming with passion.

◆ ◆ ◆

Preliminary Studies

The next section of the PHS 398 is Section C: "Preliminary Studies" (PS). Typically, the PS section is approximately two to three pages in length and is designed to showcase previous relevant research or pilot studies conducted by the research team. This section should be tailored to the specific funding mechanism for which the proposal is written. For example, an R01 would require an extensive PS section and pilot data, whereas an R03 (a smaller developmental award) typically does not require pilot data. The team of investigators should be carefully chosen to provide a full complement of strengths to address the specific aims of the proposed research, and to develop, implement, and evaluate the research. This section is the opportunity to highlight the research team's expertise in research methods, survey design, development, implementation, and evaluation of primary prevention interventions, particularly with the proposed study population, and the use of newly developed tests or techniques. An appendix that contains relevant publications from the research team is also permitted. Describe some of the team's most relevant research; however, it is not necessary to enumerate every project or activity of the team. Although including every research experience by the team provides a cumulative index of the team's expansive array of skills and experiences, it often detracts from the focus of the skills needed to conduct the proposed study. Be judicious in selecting the research you plan to highlight. In the PS section, quality is much more important than quantity of information.

◆ ◆ ◆

In a Nutshell

This section is the opportunity to highlight the research team's expertise in research methods, survey design, development, implementation, and evaluation of primary prevention interventions, particularly with the proposed study population, and the use of newly developed tests or techniques.

◆ ◆ ◆

Most important, and this cannot be overstated, for large-scale research proposals, preliminary or *pilot research* (in other words, research that uses a small sample to inform the larger-scale research effort) is critical to convincing the SRG that the study proposed is feasible and has the potential to yield important findings that will advance the field of inquiry and benefit the population. The SRG does not expect a full-scale study; however, it does expect that you have initiated a pilot study to assess feasibility of recruiting the sample, evaluating the relevance and comprehension of the survey measures, implementing the HPP, and assessing participants' feedback about its developmental, cultural, or gender-relevance, as appropriate. Be sure to present the findings from the pilot study to justify the funding of the larger-scale proposed research. Assume that all the SRG members are from Missouri, "The Show Me State." So, show them the data! Data are critical to demonstrate that the proposed study has public health importance and significance.

Finally, the PS section requires closure. Up to this point in the section, you should have described the relevant skills, techniques, and expertise of the research team members that will enhance the probability for designing, implementing, and evaluating the proposed study. Now you need to close this section of the proposal. Again, how you "end" this section can influence strongly what the SRG remembers most about your team's skills and experience. We prefer to use a subheading titled "Significance of the Preliminary Studies for the Proposed Project." Narrative under this heading contains statements about how this study will create an "exciting opportunity" to harness the diverse array of skills and experiences of team members to conduct the proposed study.

Research Design and Methods (Overview, Site, and Eligibility)

The next section of the proposal is D: "Research Design and Methods." While all the elements of a research proposal are important, Section D is the most critical. This is where the proposed methodology and data analysis is described. This section should consume the vast majority of the twenty-five pages that are allowed when using the PHS 398 forms. There is no standard format for conceptualizing Section D. However, we provide a template that you can modify to suit your particular needs.

Step 1: Overview of the Research Design. The overview should contain the following elements: (1) the overarching aim; (2) the type of study (qualitative, cross-sectional, longitudinal, or intervention); (3) the primary outcome; (4) the sample selection; (5) the number of study participants; (6) a brief enumeration of the study's assessments procedures; (7) randomization procedures, if an intervention; (8) the theory underlying the study; (9) a brief description of the HPP, if an intervention; (10) the length of the follow-up period; and (11) data analysis.

Even with the elements articulated, it is not often intuitively comprehensible to decipher what exactly constitutes an overview. Thus, to be concrete we have provided an example of an overview.

Overview of the Research Design

The proposed study is an exciting opportunity to harness the experience and multi-disciplinary expertise of the research team to develop, implement, and evaluate the efficacy of a gender-sensitive and culturally relevant HIV intervention tailored toward high-risk African American female adolescents being treated for STDs, a vulnerable population in urgent need of intervention.

This study is a Phase III randomized, controlled trial designed to evaluate the efficacy of an HIV intervention relative to receiving the standard-of-care counseling that accompanies the treatment of STDs at the County Health Department. A random sample of 960 African American females, fifteen to nineteen years of age, will be recruited at the County Health Department STD Program following receipt of treatment and standard of care preventive counseling for STDs. At baseline, eligible adolescents will complete an audio-computer-assisted self-interview (A-CASI) and provide a urine specimen that will be analyzed using newly developed nucleic acid amplification assays to detect three prevalent STDs (chlamydia, gonorrhea, and trichomoniasis). The A-CASI interview, derived from Social Cognitive Theory and the Theory of Gender and Power, assesses sociodemographics, HIV-associated risk behaviors, cultural- and gender-relevant factors associated with risk and preventive practices, and other theoretically relevant mediators of HIV-risk and preventive behavior. After forty adolescents complete their baseline assessments, they will be recontacted and asked to return to the STD Program. When they return to the County Health Department they will be randomized to either the HIV intervention or the control condition. We expect approximately thirty-two adolescents to return for random assignment to study conditions. Adolescents randomized to the control condition will view a brief video about the importance of proper nutrition. Those randomized to the HIV intervention will participate in a group-format HIV intervention implemented over three consecutive Saturdays (four hours each day). The HIV intervention will be designed to be culturally sensitive and gender-relevant, and will be implemented by County Health Department health educators and facilitated by peer educators.

The intervention will emphasize the enhancement of (a) gender and ethnic pride; (b) HIV prevention knowledge; (c) self-efficacy for condom use skills, negotiation skills, and refusal skills; (d) norms supportive of abstaining from sex and using condoms if engaging in sexual behavior; and (e) building healthy relationships. All adolescents will be asked to return at six and twelve months postintervention to complete an A-CASI-administered psychosocial interview that is similar to the baseline interview and provide urine specimens for STD assay. An intent-to-treat analysis, controlling for baseline assessments, will determine the efficacy of the HIV intervention, relative to standard-of-care STD counseling only, in reducing HIV-associated sexual behaviors and incident STDs over a twelve-month follow-up period. Secondary analyses will evaluate the impact of the intervention condition, relative to the control condition, on hypothesized mediators of HIV-preventive behavior.

Although a succinct overview of the study provides a foundation on which to build Section D, it is usually useful to present a schematic representation of the proposed research design. A well-designed visual or figure is worth a thousand words, as it provides a snapshot of the entire project that the SRG can keep in mind as you begin to enumerate and describe, more fully, each element in the section. In Figure 15.1 we present an example of a figure outlining the research design.

◆ ◆ ◆

In a Nutshell

A well-designed visual or figure is worth a thousand words, as it provides a snapshot of the entire project that the SRG can keep in mind as you begin to enumerate and describe, more fully, each element in the section.

◆ ◆ ◆

Step 2: Description of the Study Site and Population. The next element in this section is often a description of the study site and population. This is an opportunity to demonstrate your familiarity with both the proposed study site and the

FIGURE 15.1. EXAMPLE OF A FIGURE OUTLINING THE RESEARCH DESIGN.

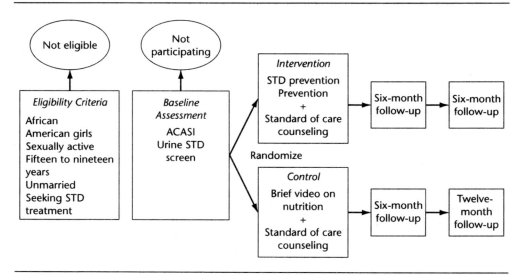

population in which you propose to conduct your study. Be succinct, but provide ample information about the site and population that is directly relevant to the proposed study. Here it is important to provide letters from site administrators that describe their support and enthusiasm for the proposed study, their willingness to commit site resources, and their willingness to provide access to the study population. Such letters are included as an appendix to the proposal. Box 15.1 provides a sample letter of support. Once the population and site(s) are adequately described, it is useful to articulate the eligibility criteria for participation in the study.

Step 3: Eligibility Criteria for Participation. In this section precisely articulate the criteria for participation in the proposed study. This typically includes the criteria such as age, race or ethnicity, gender, marital status, and presence or absence of a specific disease or risk behavior. The inclusion criteria should be tailored to correspond to the aims of the study. In addition to specifying the inclusion criteria, it is often useful to explicitly specify the exclusion criteria. An example follows:

To be eligible participants must be (a) African American females; (b) fifteen to nineteen years of age, inclusive at the time of enrollment into the project; (c) receiving STD treatment and counseling at the County Health Department STD Program; (d) unmarried; and (e) willing to provide written informed consent. Adolescents who refuse to provide written informed consent or have medical conditions that preclude participation in group-based educational programs (such as severe learning disorder) will be excluded.

Box 15.1. Sample Letter of Support

Baltimore

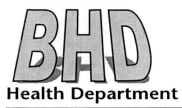

Health Department

475 South State Street, Baltimore MD 12745
555 444-8773

September 21, 2006

Gregory H. Hennington, Ph.D.
Maryland College of Public Health
1547 Baxter Road, NE
Room 542
Baltimore, MD 30322

RE: A Cancer Prevention Program for Young Women

Dear Dr. Hennington:

It was great to meet with you recently and learn about your proposal to test the feasibility of a three-session intervention designed for young women residing in Baltimore. Your idea to also test the efficacy of using support groups to promote behavior change is excellent. I fully support your proposal and will be glad to work with you to provide support for the project once you have secured funding. As you know, young women compose a large part of our clientele in our health depart-ment. Thus, we are naturally eager to assist in a research project designed to prevent them from developing both cervical and breast cancer. Clearly prevention efforts such as the one you have proposed are important to this population.

I understand that part of the project will involve hiring a health educator. I will gladly assist in the selection of this person. Good luck with your proposal for funding and please keep me posted about a possible start date for this project.

Sincerely,

Russell J. Hornby
Director
Baltimore Health Department

Research Design and Methods (Three Phases of the Research Plan)

At this juncture, let's review for a moment what we've accomplished in Section D. We have (1) provided a succinct overview of the proposed study, including a graphic representation of the proposed research design; (2) described the study site and population; and (3) specified the eligibility (inclusion and exclusion) criteria. Our next step is to begin describing the research plan.

There are countless ways in which you could present the research plan. We will show you one way to organize and present the research plan that we think provides a logical approach that the SRG can easily understand. We prefer to present the research plan in three sequential phases. Each phase represents a unique set of research activities and tasks that need to be completed to successfully develop, implement, and evaluate the proposed study. In this way we provide a logical and chronological sequence of research tasks and activities. The idea is for the research proposal to be an integrated whole, with each section of the proposal building on and informing subsequent sections. The more integrated the proposal, the easier it is to understand its flow and logic.

◆ ◆ ◆

In a Nutshell

The idea is for the research proposal to be an integrated whole, with each section of the proposal building on and informing subsequent sections. The more integrated the proposal, the easier it is to understand its flow and logic.

◆ ◆ ◆

We can categorize the research plan into three phases. Phase I describes program development, Phase II describes program implementation, and Phase III describes program evaluation. In the following sections, we review the elements commonly identified in each phase of the research plan. We describe a research plan designed to develop, implement, and evaluate an HPP. Of course, this plan is readily modifiable for observation studies (that is, for cross-sectional or longitudinal studies), as some of elements could be removed.

Phase I: Program Development

The primary Phase I activities include (1) hiring staff, (2) conducting focus groups, (3) describing the underlying theoretical framework guiding the study, (4) creating an advisory board, (5) developing the theoretically based HPP, (6) training the health educators to implement the HPP, (7) pilot testing the HPP, (8) specifying the data-collection procedures, (9) selecting measures for inclusion on the assessment instrument, (10) pilot testing the data-collection instrument, and (11) training staff to administer the data-collection instrument. In this section, we provide a brief description of each of the components included in Phase I.

Hiring Staff. In this section specify the names or position titles of staff to be hired. To facilitate the SRG's understanding of whether your staffing plan is appropriate to the research tasks and activities, it would be useful to list the project-year in which staff members are brought in (added to the project payroll). This demonstrates a degree of sophistication with respect to allocating staff time to complete project-related tasks. Unfortunately, this skill is not taught in many undergraduate or graduate courses. Experience and having conducted a feasibility study will be instrumental in guiding the assignment of staff time.

Conducting Formative Research. In many studies, *front loading* (building research activities in the beginning of the project) includes formative research to assist in tailoring the HPP. This is a sound research methodology. It's appropriate to specify the time period during which you propose to conduct formative research, for example, "During months 02 to 04 we will conduct a series of eight focus groups with adolescents recruited from the STD Program." Specify the purpose of the formative research, such as "Focus groups will be conducted to examine gender and culturally relevant causal factors potentially missing in our theoretical models that may influence African American female adolescents' sexual behavior." Next, it is useful to cite any prior experience by team members in conducting formative research; in this case, focus groups as well as those who will be designated to conduct the focus groups and analyze the resultant data. As a rule, if you propose a research activity, there should be someone specified in the research proposal that has the requisite skills and experience to conduct that activity.

◆ ◆ ◆

In a Nutshell

As a rule, if you propose a research activity, there should be someone specified in the research proposal that has the requisite skills and experience to conduct that activity.

◆ ◆ ◆

Describing the Underlying Theoretical Framework. As in the previous sections, specify the time frame when this activity or task is to be accomplished and describe the project staff dedicated to accomplishing the activity or task. Next, define the theoretical models that underlie the HPP. Briefly summarize model components and their relevance to the proposed HPP. A word of caution is called for. If more than one model or theory is specified and their conceptual components enumerated and articulated, it is important to state that you, after considerable thought, have decided that the multiple theories or models complement each other. Be sure that you fully describe how these models do so. (See DiClemente, Crosby, and Kegler, 2002, and Glanz, Lewis, and Rimer, 2003, for more information about complementary theories and models.) The obvious question from the SRG's perspective is, Why are multiple models or theories needed to guide the study? At this point, here is where it is appropriate to cite your prior research with these theories or models and their relevance and utility for explaining the phenomenon under study.

Creating a Community Advisory Board. Much of health promotion research is conducted within community settings. Thus, it is advantageous to propose a community advisory board (CAB) as part of the study. Specify the number and composition of the CAB members and how they will be identified, recruited, and compensated. Also, note the meeting schedule of the CAB and its scope of activities. One activity may be to review any project materials, such as the research survey, to ensure that they are culturally competent, comprehensive, and readable. Another activity is to ensure that the proposed HPP is culturally competent, addresses key concerns as identified by members of the target community, and is acceptable to community standards. Again, it is valuable to enclose letters of support from prospective CAB members. These letters can be attached to the proposal in an appendix.

Developing the HPP. Here is an opportunity to shine! You have read the empirical literature, you have conducted qualitative research and proposed additional research in this proposal, you have conducted a feasibility study, and you have pilot tested the HPP. Now it's time to demonstrate the culmination of this process. Begin this section by specifying the time frame in which the HPP will be developed (for example, during months 03 through 09) and the personnel who will develop the HPP. (For example, "Drs. DiClemente, Salazar, and Crosby will develop the STD prevention intervention in conjunction with the project health educators and peer educators with input from the CAB.")

Once you have described the "when" and "who," it is time to describe the HPP itself. A word of advice is to be sure to tightly integrate the HPP with the underlying models or theories. Models and theories are there to guide the development and implementation of the HPP; use them accordingly. It is critical to demonstrate a clear and obvious linkage between the underlying models or theories and your HPP activities. As an illustration, we refer to our aforementioned STD prevention study.

Social Cognitive Theory (SCT) will guide the design of the STD prevention intervention. According to SCT, behavior is the result of interactions among personal factors, environmental factors, and behavior. Personal factors include an individual's confidence in performing a certain behavior (self-efficacy), one's expectations about the outcomes associated with performing that specific behavior (outcome expectancies), and the individual's goals related to the behavior. Environmental factors include normative influences (peer norms) and the support that an individual may receive from others.

The aim of the proposed study is to enhance adolescents' confidence in their ability to self-regulate their sexual behavior. Thus, the STD prevention intervention will teach adolescents about safe and unsafe sexual practices as well as the outcomes associated with each. Given that the teens in the proposed study were treated for an STD, the intervention will teach youths about the link between having an STD and the increased risk of HIV infection. The STD prevention intervention will also teach teens skills such as (1) goal setting; (2) engaging in safer sexual behaviors (such as using condoms correctly and consistently, abstaining from sex, limiting their number of sexual partners); and (3) communicating effectively with one's sexual partner (that is, differentiating between passive, assertive, and aggressive communication styles and communicating the need to have one's partner tested for STDs). The STD prevention intervention will also be designed to create a normative atmosphere supportive of safer sex practices and self-protective communication styles. By supplying much-needed information and skills, we hope to enhance adolescents' self-efficacy to refuse risky sex and their ability to insist on condom use during sexual intercourse.

Again, the goal of this specific section is to make the connection between the underlying theory and the HPP activities transparent to the SRG. Intervention mapping, or enumerating each activity of the proposed HPP, and linking it to one of the model or theory constructs will be useful to assess how well you have used the model or theory in building your HPP.

Training the Health Educators to Administer the HPP. An important element often overlooked in research proposals by new and established investigators alike is specifying "*who*" will implement the HPP and "*how*" they will be trained. Now that you've carefully crafted your HPP, describe the personnel who will implement it. Describe their professional training (for example, M.P.H. in behavioral sciences or health education), their sociodemographic characteristics, if relevant to the effective implementation of the HPP (for example, African American health educators assisted by African American peer educators), and their background experiences (that is, prior experience in implementing an HPP with adolescents).

Once the personnel have been briefly described, it is useful to describe the training they will receive prior to implementing the HPP. This can be a brief paragraph that enumerates the training procedures used to train staff to proficiency. These could include any of the following: viewing videos, role-playing the HPP, role reversal in which the health educator may be asked to play the part of a study participant, group discussions, didactic instruction, and so on. It is useful to evaluate implementation personnel prior to their interacting with study participants. Also, have a plan available for corrective training and termination should an implementation staff member be unable or unwilling to conduct the HPP as designed. Noting that quality assurance procedures will be used to monitor implementation fidelity may be beneficial. Identifying the possibility of drift in interventions is important, as this requires remedial training of project staff.

Pilot Testing the HPP. Be sure to include language in your proposal that assures the SRG that the proposed HPP will be pilot tested. When the HPP is completed, the staff trained, and modification made to both the HPP and training protocols, a pilot test of the entire protocol is vital. In a pilot test, it is valuable to select participants from the target population who meet the eligibility criteria. The HPP will be assessed for feasibility and participant satisfaction; problems identified can be rectified, and the curriculum will be modified as necessary. Similarly, any difficulties encountered in implementing the HPP can be identified and rectified prior to actually starting the trial. A word of advice regarding this is to build in adequate time to conduct the pilot study and make modifications to the staff training protocol and HPP curriculum, and you should also specify the time frame in which the pilot study and modifications will be conducted.

Specifying the Data-Collection Procedures. This section is devoted to articulating the data-collection procedures used in the proposed study. If there are multiple procedures, it is critical to enumerate and adequately describe each procedure. For example, we used three data-collection procedures: (1) an A-CASI, (2) a urine specimen, and (3) a retrospective review of adolescents' clinic records. Describe the *first* data element with respect to time to completion. ("The A-CASI interview is approximately sixty minutes in length.") Describe where the data-collection procedure will be conducted. ("The A-CASI system will be implemented in a private room at the STD Program.") Finally, describe what type of data this procedure will yield. ("The A-CASI is designed to assess potential moderators, psychosocial beliefs, and sexual behaviors at baseline and six- and twelve-month followup.") Basically, describe each data-collection procedure in sufficient detail. Then proceed to describe the remaining data elements in a similar and systematic fashion.

Selecting Measures for Inclusion in the Assessment Instrument. A critical aspect of any study is selecting the measures (for example, scales, indexes, single-item measures) used to assess the constructs articulated in the proposal (see Chapter Nine). Furthermore, selection of constructs for assessment should be guided by a number of sources, including

- The underlying theoretical models guiding the proposed study
- A thorough review of the research literature examining potential moderators, mediators, and outcomes among the target population
- The research team's prior experience
- Input from the CAB
- Prior formative or qualitative research
- The results of the pilot study

Often, one or more of the just-enumerated factors is not available. However, the extent to which each source can contribute to the selection of constructs further strengthens the assessment component of the proposed study. Once the constructs are enumerated, select the measures to assess these constructs. Then, whenever feasible, these measures should have demonstrated reliability and validity with the target population (see Chapters Nine and Ten for a more detailed discussion of reliability and validity).

Pilot Testing the Data-Collection Instrument. As noted previously with respect to the HPP and the staff training, a pilot test can be very useful. Likewise, pilot testing the data-collection instrument(s) allows the research team to assess their utility; comprehension; and cultural, developmental, and gender relevance for the target population. This section should be brief. It should state that during a specified time period (for example, during months 08 through 10) the assessment instrument(s) will be pilot tested with a small sample selected from the target population. The pilot sample should be selected so that the individuals meet the purposed eligibility criteria. The data manager can calculate measures of internal consistency (that is, Cronbach's alpha) for all scales to determine their utility for this population. Items not well correlated with the entire scale can be deleted to improve the scale's psychometric properties. If entire scales are found to be unreliable, they should be replaced by a new measure that will undergo similar assessment procedures.

Training Staff to Administer the Data-Collection Instrument(s). Training is critical to avoid any ambiguity with respect to the study's protocol. Given the amount of time, energy, and emphasis placed on the results obtained from HPPs, training should be an integral component of any research plan. Depending on the data-collection instruments, it is useful to articulate the protocols that will be followed as well as the qualifications of the personnel involved in data collection (in other words, a trained research associate with experience in collecting similar data from the target population). Specify any training protocols that will ensure standard-ized data collection. This is increasingly important if there are multiple data collectors and the data will be collected using personal interviews, which are more susceptible to experimenter bias.

Phase II: Program Implementation

Phase II activities include

- Recruiting the study sample
- Screening and sampling procedures
- Administering the baseline assessment
- Randomizing participants to the study conditions
- Selecting and implementing the control condition
- Implementing the HPP
- Conducting quality assurance process evaluations
- Specifying follow-up procedures
- Defining strategies for enhancing retention

Recruiting the Study Sample. In this section you should propose (1) the projected sample size, (2) the time period during which it will be accrued, (3) the rate of accrual, and (4) from what population the sample will be recruited. For example, in our research the following statement was used: "We propose to enroll a sample of 960 youths over thirty months (32 adolescents per month) during months 13 through 42. Potential participants will be identified from the population of adolescents treated for STDs at the health department STD clinic."

Now that you've specified the sample, it is useful to project the participation rate. Estimating the participation rate is based on previous research, preferably by your team, or by a review of the relevant literature. For example, we noted that, "based on our previous research with African American female adolescents and young women, we projected approximately 80 percent of willing adolescents to actually return for assignment to study conditions."

A variety of recruitment strategies can be used to attract people to participate in HPP studies. Using recruitment procedures that have proven effective in other studies with the target population is invaluable. Again, experience with the target population will be useful in evaluating the type of strategies that are most effective.

To assist you we suggest that the following strategies be employed singly or in combination to enhance recruitment:

- Hire and train a recruitment-retention coordinator
- Provide a monetary allowance for completing the baseline assessment (the use of monetary incentives may significantly enhance participation in behavioral intervention trials) (DiClemente and Wingood, 1998)
- Describe the follow-up incentives to maintain interest
- Ensure confidentiality of the data and identifying information (for instance, all data will be maintained in a locked cabinet that is limited to access by key staff, only code numbers will be used on data forms and these will be kept separate from identifying information and code numbers)

Screening and Sampling Procedures. A brief section is often useful for describing the screening and sampling procedures. Again, *who* is conducting the screening? *Where* is it being conducted? *How* will it be conducted? This is important information for the SRG. Likewise, describe the sampling procedures. For example, in our research we used the following text to describe the sampling procedure: "The recruitment-retention coordinator will use a random numbers table to identify the sample of adolescents. This process will continue until the quota of forty adolescents has been recruited each month. The recruitment-retention coordinator will also collect sociodemographic information from adolescents who choose not to participate as well as their rationale for not participating in the study for later comparison with those adolescents who elect to participate." (See Chapter Five for more detail about this procedure.) If feasible, and not in violation of IRB regulations, collecting sociodemographic data from those potential participants who decline to be part of the study can provide a useful gauge of the representativeness of the final sample recruited. As in other aspects of the study, training the personnel responsible for screening and sampling is critical.

Administering the Baseline Assessment. In this section, describe the procedure for administering the baseline assessment. Again, it is vitally important to be specific in this description. The SRG is interested in knowing *who* will invite participants to complete the baseline assessment and *where* the assessment will be conducted.

Randomizing Participants to the Study Conditions. A central concern in any HPP that uses a randomized trial design (see Chapter Six) is the randomization protocol. In general, it is useful to specify *who* will determine the randomization sequence, *who* will conduct randomization, and *how* it will be implemented. Fortunately, there are a number of publications that address this important issue.

One procedure is to assign participants to the study conditions using concealment of allocation techniques (Schulz, 1995; Schulz and Grimes, 2002). These procedures have been designed to minimize bias in subject assignment to conditions in randomized trials. We have successfully used concealment of allocation procedures in our ongoing HPP interventions.

Selecting and Implementing the Control Condition. Selecting and implementing the control condition are also vital concerns when the HPP involves a between-groups design. Thus, it is useful to explain the rationale for selecting a particular control condition. A number of factors may need to be carefully weighed in selecting this control condition. First, the possibility of including a *placebo-attention condition* (structurally similar in terms of frequency, duration, and intensity, although the content should be irrelevant to the study outcomes) in the research design should be considered. This condition could reduce the likelihood that effects of the HPP could be attributed to nonspecific features (for example, group interaction and special attention should be considered). Second, consider if it is ethically feasible to include a "do nothing" control condition. For example, in testing an HPP to reduce HIV-associated risk behaviors among adolescents living in South Africa (a highly endemic area for HIV) can we ethically withhold any education related to HIV prevention? Thus, careful articulation of the rationale for selecting the control condition is imperative.

If a placebo-attention control condition is selected, implementation of the control condition, like the HPP, requires specification of *who, what, when,* and *where.* Describe the qualifications or relevant sociodemographic characteristics of the personnel responsible for implementing the control condition. Describe the control condition content. Describe when the control condition will be implemented. Finally, describe where the control condition will be implemented.

Implementing the HPP. There are two key elements that need careful clarification: (1) the personnel and logistics of implementing the HPP and (2) the content of the HPP.

First, it is important to specify *who, what, when, where,* and *how* of the HPP condition. For example, in our STD prevention intervention we noted that, "Participants randomized to the HIV intervention will receive three four-hour weekly group sessions, on consecutive Saturdays, implemented by two African American female health educators who will be assisted by two peer educators. The health educators will organize session materials, review session objectives at the beginning of every session, provide factual knowledge regarding HIV and associated risk behaviors, conduct didactic teachings, review homework, and provide reinforcement and social support. The peer educators will model social competency skills (assertive communication, refusal skills), coordinate group exercises, and provide reinforcement and social support. The health educators and peer educators will implement the HIV intervention following the guidelines in a structured implementation manual."

Describing the content of the HPP requires specifying each of the intervention elements. In a multisession HPP, specify the sessions in the sequence in which they are offered. While twenty-five pages may seem like a lot of space, you will find that being succinct is critical in preparing a coherent and comprehensive description of the HPP. A table that specifies the HPP activity and the mediator targeted by that activity can sometimes be useful as a summary mechanism.

Conducting Quality Assurance Process Evaluations.   One threat to the internal validity of any HPP study is variability in delivering either the intervention or the control condition. Often health educators and program facilitators have their own style of presenting information and providing skill-based education. Even though a protocol has been developed to promote standardization of HPP delivery, there is the potential for health educators to drift (that is, to adopt a somewhat different mode of delivery). This is particularly likely when the HPP is implemented over a protracted time period. To minimize the threat of differential implementation of the intervention, it is useful to develop a detailed, structured manual that includes each session activity, the goal and objectives for the session, the person responsible for implementing the activity (the health educator or the peer educator), and the time allocated to each activity. Facilitators should be required to follow these standardized implementation procedures. At the end of the session, the facilitators will complete a session log indicating whether each activity was covered, whether the appropriate amount of time was dedicated to each activity, and any problems that may have arisen for each activity. In addition, the principal investigator or project director should schedule weekly meetings with facilitators who will review any problems and concerns arising within the sessions. All HPP sessions should, when feasible, be audiotaped (permission must first be obtained from participants) and used to evaluate the consistency of presentation and adherence to the standardized implementation protocol, to address problems within the sessions, and to suggest strategies for dealing with problems or concerns that may arise. Also useful are standardized evaluation forms that participants complete anonymously. Completed forms can be used to rate HPP fidelity. We have used these procedures in our prior research and have found them to be highly informative and helpful in monitoring implementation fidelity.

Specifying Follow-Up Procedures. The aim of this section is to clearly delineate the follow-up assessment procedures. The procedures should be well articulated, specifying *who* will conduct the follow-up assessments, *when,* and *where.* If participants are compensated for completing follow-up assessments, specify the type and amount of compensation, and when it is provided to the participant. Also of importance, specify who will contact participants, when, and if transportation will be provided to assist in accessing the data-collection venue.

Defining Strategies for Enhancing Retention. A major concern in any longitudinal study is the maintenance of the study cohort. While there are a number of tracking procedures that have proven effective, a pilot study or previous research with the target population is invaluable in determining the optimal set of tracking procedures to be used in the proposed study. (See Chapters Five and Six for a more thorough discussion of procedures used to follow a cohort.)

Phase III: Program Evaluation (Assessing Whether the HPP Was Effective)

Phase III activities include (1) conducting the last data-management and verification checks, (2) implementing the data analytic plan, (3) describing the power analysis, and (4) outlining the project timeline. Clearly conveying to the SRG that you have thoughtfully planned each of these activities is important. Also, be sure that the planned analyses exactly match the stated aims and hypotheses shown in Section A. In developing the data analytic plan it is essential to have extensive input and guidance from a biostatistician. In the following sections, we provide general guidance to writing this part of the research plan.

Conducting the Last Data-Management and Verification Checks. Data reduction, cleaning, and entry and verification of participants' responses for analysis will be performed under the direction of the data analyst, usually a statistician with expertise in the relevant statistical techniques for analyzing the data. Generally, the data-entry procedure is programmed to flag impossible values, thus providing an instant range check. Usually there are two basic data files to maintain the study operation: a sampling file, which contains information on all participants in the study, and a merged file, which contains all data. Every effort should be made to demonstrate that the study will not be plagued by missing data. If feasible, proposed use of the A-CASI system provides one additional level of quality control by reducing missing data through onscreen reminders.

Implementing the Data Analytic Plan. The primary analysis evaluates the effectiveness of the HPP: (1) in improving relevant mediators of health-promoting behavior (in other words, knowledge and relevant beliefs and attitudes), and (2) in reducing high-risk behavior. While the randomized design does not ensure that the same outcome profile (that is, distribution of behavioral risk indicators and mediators) is expected in the HPP and control group, it does avoid systematic bias as well as enhancing the likelihood of comparability between conditions on unmeasured factors. However, certain individual characteristics may be important predictors of outcome or may influence the effectiveness of the intervention. Simple analytical techniques can be used in preliminary analyses to describe the profile of participants at entry and follow-up. To evaluate the effect of the HPP together with the effect of covariates and to evaluate the interaction, a variety of statistical techniques are available, repeated measures linear (for continuous outcomes) and logistic models (for categorical outcomes) in particular.

While defining specific statistical approaches is not within the scope of this chapter, the reader should consult Chapters Twelve and Thirteen as well as a biostatistician. However, we do suggest that any intervention can benefit by conducting a general description of the study group and simple comparisons of intervention and control groups. First, propose simple descriptive statistics (mean, median, percent), scatterplots, and histograms that can be used to evaluate the distribution of participants according to study measures, such as

- Sociodemographic variables including age, education, and income
- Summary scores derived from psychosocial mediators (such as depression, self-efficacy, perceived social norms, and so on)
- Outcomes of interest

Summary statistics for all of the measures should also be proposed. Simple correlation analyses can be conducted to evaluate the association between pairs of variables. Nonparametric statistics (for example, Spearman's rank correlation coefficient, Wilcoxon's rank-sum test) are appropriate to evaluate the significance of the associations. At this juncture, the assistance of a biostatistician who will be integrally involved in the study, preferably from its inception, will be indispensable to writing a successful proposal.

Describing the Power Analysis. One other aspect integrally related to the determination of the study sample is the power analysis. (See Chapter Twelve for a more detailed description of the power analysis.) Usually, to determine a proposed study's required sample size, the investigator examines an analysis for the primary hypothesis. Using other studies or previous research by the investigative team, the principal investigator posits an estimated effect size. A thorough rationale for the estimated effect size should be provided. For example, in our STD prevention study, we estimated an incidence of 25 percent for one or more of the STDs assessed during the twelve-month follow-up in the control group. To estimate our effect size, we relied on the most recent intervention research that incorporated STDs as a measure of program efficacy. We estimated a conservative effect size of 30 percent difference for STD re-infection rates between the STD prevention condition and the control condition. We used a one-tail test, setting alpha at $P = .05$, with power of 0.80 to calculate the sample size necessary under these conditions. Always take into account attrition. Thus, if the sample size needed is eight hundred, for instance, and you assume 20 percent attrition, then be sure to recruit one thousand participants (this includes the projected 20 percent loss to follow-up), which will yield an effective sample size of eight hundred participants.

◆ ◆ ◆

In a Nutshell

Using other studies or previous research by the investigative team, the principal investigator posits an estimated effect size. A thorough rationale for the estimated effect size should be provided.

◆ ◆ ◆

Outlining the Project Timeline. The project timeline is a final and important component of any proposal. The timeline is your estimation of the start and termination of specific research activities. Again, in the absence of experience, it is difficult to construct an accurate timeline. However, pilot research and previous experience can be invaluable in developing a "realistic" timeline. Figure 15.2 provides a template using a Gnatt chart format that provides a visual overview of research activities over the five-year duration of the project.

Summary

This chapter has been devoted to providing a "blueprint" for crafting a research proposal. We have described a number of elements that are critical to a successful proposal as well as to a valid study. We are quick to remind you, however,

FIGURE 15.2. TEMPLATE FOR A FIVE-YEAR PROJECT TIMELINE.

Activities	Project Month												
	1	5	10	15	20	25	30	35	40	45	50	55	60
Awarded funds	X												
Hire and train staff		XXXX											
Conduct focus groups			XXXX										
Develop HIV intervention			XXXX										
Pilot HIV intervention				XXX									
Develop the interview			XXXXXX										
Pilot the interview			XXXX										
Transfer and pilot the ACASI			XXXX										
Recruit for baseline assessments					XXXXXXXXXXXXXXXXXXXXXXXXX								
Begin four-month follow-up assessments						XXXXXXXXXXXXXXXXXXXXXXXX							
Begin eight-month follow-up assessments							XXXXXXXXXXXXXXXXXXXXXXXX						
Begin twelve-month follow-up assessments								XXXXXXXXXXXXXXXXXXXXXXXXX					
Data analysis and manuscript preparation												XXXXX	

that proposal writing is an incremental, iterative, and calibrated learning process. The suggestions presented in this chapter should be an asset to you once you begin this learning process. As you become engrossed in the process of proposal writing, we suggest that you consult a brief list of "tips" that we provide to you in Box 15.2.

We encourage readers to complement this chapter with more detailed texts. Foremost, we encourage readers to carefully consider the time, labor, and monetary needs necessary for designing, implementing, and evaluating an HPP. Given the importance of identifying effective HPPs, it is clearly worth the considerable expenditure of energy and resources to design the most rigorous study feasible. Keep in mind that writing effective grant proposals is an ongoing and iterative process. Ultimately, a prerequisite to success is dedicating ample time and effort.

Box 15.2. Tips for Successful Proposal Writing

H Have all instructions for assembling the application been carefully followed?

O On time (the deadline is not flexible!)

M Make sure your budget corresponds to the personnel allocation for each project year

E Exchange ideas with investigators of funded studies that may be similar to yours

R Realize that a successful proposal is 99 percent perspiration and only 1 percent inspiration—there is no substitute for unwavering determination!

U Understand the importance of carefully choosing the research team (this could be the beginning of a long and productive relationship)

N Never, ever, give up!

Furthermore, it is often useful to involve other colleagues in the proposal process. Selecting colleagues with the requisite skills needed to develop, implement, and evaluate the proposed study is one of the most important decisions you will make. Finally, keep in mind that perseverance and fortitude will pay off in the long run.

References

DiClemente, R. J., and Wingood, G. M. (1998). Monetary incentives: A useful strategy for enhancing enrollment and promoting participation in HIV/STD risk-reduction interventions. *Sexually Transmitted Infections, 74,* 239–240.

DiClemente, R. J., Crosby, R. A., and Kegler, M. (2002). *Emerging theories in health promotion practice and research.* San Francisco: Jossey Bass.

Glanz, K., Lewis, F. M., and Rimer, B. K. (2003). *Health behavior and health education: Theory, research, and practice.* San Francisco: Jossey Bass.

Schulz, K. F. (1995). Subverting randomization in controlled trials. *Journal of the American Medical Association, 274,* 1456–1458.

Schulz, K. F., and Grimes, D. A. (2002). Blinding in randomized trials: Hiding who got what. *Lancet, 359,* 696–700.

NAME INDEX

SUBJECT INDEX

A

Absolute measure, 357
Absolute zero point, 232, 322
Abstract writing: for manuscripts, 375–376, *377*, 391; for research proposals, 402–403
Abuse, history of, by researchers, 42–43, 58
Access: to participation in research, inclusion policies regarding, 46–47; to the target population, gaining, 108–110, 188, 273, 305. *See also* Sampling frame accessibility
Accident, meaning of, 31
Accurate recall, facilitating, 119–120
Action points, *16*
Active recruitment, 112
Activities, 204, *205*, *206*, 207, 209, 211
Adaptation, 95
Adjusted odds ratio, 338
Administrative buy-in, 108, 412
Adolescents and children: privacy rights of, 61; special protections for, 57, 58–60

Advanced investigations, *76*
Affordability, determining, 212
African American communities, distrust within, regarding research and researchers, 43
Aims, specific, proposal of, 401–405
Allocation procedures, concealment of, 136–137, 168–169, 350. *See also* Random assignment (randomization)
Alpha: defining, 325, 340; range of, 236
Alternative hypothesis: defined, 361; proposing an, 405
Alternative research method, 170–172
American Journal of Preventive Medicine, studies from, 144–146, 341–342
American Journal of Public Health, study from, 19–20
American Psychological Association (APA), 389, 390, 399
Analyses, cost, 212–216
Analysis of covariance (ANCOVA), 364–365, 366

Analysis of data. *See* Data analysis
Analysis of variance (ANOVA), 365–366
Anonymous mail contact, importance of, 123
Anonymous studies, waiving informed consent for, 56
Anthropology: cognitive, 179; cultural, 176
APA style, 389–390
Apgar Scale, 233
Archival data, 177
Archives of Pediatrics and Adolescent Medicine, study from, 340–341
Aristotelian perspective, 26
Arms: defined, 92; number of, to be employed, determining, 93
Artificial null findings, potential of, 140
Assent and permission, 59–60
Assessment: administering, time points for, 142–143; follow-up, 115; key issues in, 116–120; of the predictor before assessment of the outcome, 239; scheduling, of the control groups, 139–140; selecting measures for